STANDING ON PRINCIPLES

STANDING ON PRINCIPLES

COLLECTED ESSAYS

TOM L. BEAUCHAMP

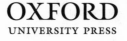

UNIVERSITY PRESS

2010

OXFORD

UNIVERSITY PRESS

Oxford University Press, Inc., publishes works that further
Oxford University's objective of excellence
in research, scholarship, and education.

Oxford   New York
Auckland   Cape Town   Dar es Salaam   Hong Kong   Karachi
Kuala Lumpur   Madrid   Melbourne   Mexico City   Nairobi
New Delhi   Shanghai   Taipei   Toronto

With offices in
Argentina   Austria   Brazil   Chile   Czech Republic   France   Greece
Guatemala   Hungary   Italy   Japan   Poland   Portugal   Singapore
South Korea   Switzerland   Thailand   Turkey   Ukraine   Vietnam

Library of Congress Cataloging-in-Publication Data
Beauchamp, Tom L.
Standing on principles : collected essays / Tom L. Beauchamp.
p. ; cm.
Contains articles published previously in various sources.
Includes bibliographical references and index.
ISBN 978-0-19-973718-5
1. Bioethics.   2. Human experimentation in medicine—Moral and ethical aspects.   I. Title.
[DNLM: 1. Bioethics—Collected Works.
2. Human Experimentation—Collected Works. WB 60 B371s 2010]
QH332.B425 2010
174'.957—dc22
2009033282

1   3   5   7   9   8   6   4   2

Printed in the United States of America
on acid-free paper

7292715

To
Ruth R. Faden
Partner for life and a magnificent human being in every way of being human.

CONTENTS

ACKNOWLEDGMENTS

Many parts of this book are connected to my work with James Childress. Our collaboration has been a two-way conversation, and he has been an abiding help in stimulating my thought on several of the essays in this volume. In 1978, Jim and I decided on the persons to whom we would dedicate the volume. On my side, I dedicated the volume to Ruth Faden and Donald Seldin, with whom I was in frequent conversation at the time about the embryonic but developing field of bioethics. I chose well. Now, more than 30 years later, they remain the deepest influences on my work on the subjects in this volume. Their personal dedication to me and their professional facilitation of my work have been remarkable. Wayne Davis, my department chair, deserves a similar acknowledgment for his support over the last 20 years. Perhaps no one is a perfect chair, but Wayne seems so, and he is a model of the honest philosopher.

Philosophers should learn from their critics, and I have had some dedicated critics over the years on several of the subjects addressed in this volume. I acknowledge in particular the many contributions made by John Arras, Bernard Gert, Danner Clouser, Albert Jonsen, Ronald Lindsay, Edmund Pellegrino, and David DeGrazia. All have offered trenchant criticisms. Other valued criticism has come from Oliver Rauprich, Rebecca Kukla, Carson Strong, Peter Herissone-Kelly, Avi Craimer, Frank Miller, and Robert Veatch.

Essay 1, "The Origins and Evolution of the *Belmont Report*," and Essay 2, "Codes, Declarations, and Other Ethical Guidance for Human Subjects Research: The *Belmont Report*," are centered on the years I worked for the National Commission for the Protection of Human Subjects (1975–1978), some of the most rewarding years of my life. I owe thanks to the many people who supported me in writing for the Commission, especially the writing of *Belmont*. I owe special acknowledgments to Patricia King, Michael Yesley, Donald Seldin, Albert Jonsen, Stephen Toulmin, Robert Levine, Barbara Mishkin, and Kenneth Ryan—and, for later criticisms, Ernest Marshall. They all caused me to rethink my ideas many times over. I am also grateful to Jay Katz, Samuel Gorovitz, LeRoy Walters, Tris Engelhardt, Charles McCarthy, and John Robertson for conversations and help in research during these years. For excellent editorial advice while writing Essay 2, I recognize the contribution made by Zeke Emanuel, Christine Grady, Robert A. Crouch, Reidar Lie, Frank Miller, and David Wendler, as editors of the book in which the piece appeared. Frank is owed special thanks for his efficient pursuit of my piece.

Essay 3, "The Four-Principles Approach to Health Care Ethics," and Essay 9, "Principles and Other Emerging Paradigms in Bioethics," are centered on principlism. The first of the two essays was written because Raanan Gillon persuaded me to compose it and then helped me make it as good as it could be. Raanan has been supportive throughout my career, and I thank him for contributions that reach far beyond this essay. I also owe Ed Pellegrino an acknowledgment for his many critiques of the four-principles approach, including a critique when I wrote this essay. My thinking on these issues has been pushed forward by some stimulating criticisms, published and unpublished, by Bernard Gert, Danner Clouser, Charles Culver, John Arras, David Smith, Alasdair Campbell, John Harris, and Dan Callahan. On the constructive side, I have enormously benefited from the work of my colleague Henry Richardson on the subject of specification. Henry has also been a supportive critic.

Essay 4, on "Informed Consent: Its History and Meaning," appeared because Bob Veatch persuaded me to write it and offered sound editorial advice during its drafting. Ruth Faden stimulated me to my best ideas on informed consent, and much of what I say here derives from our 1986 book, *A History and Theory of Informed Consent*. When writing that book we received wonderful support and criticism from Bettina Schöne-Seifert and Nancy King; and we were inspired at the time by the published work of, and personal consultation with, Jay Katz, Allen Buchanan, Robert Levine, Alan Meisel, and Sissela Bok.

Essay 5, "Who Deserves Autonomy and Whose Autonomy Deserves Respect?," came into being because I was persuaded by James Stacey Taylor to rethink and deepen my previous publications on autonomy. On the matters of autonomy treated in this essay, many people have contributed to my thinking. Almost certainly, the deepest influences have come from work with Ruth Faden and through discussions with Joel Feinberg, who was working on his theory of autonomy as I was first developing mine. I still today regard Feinberg as the soundest writer on many of the subjects I address. In what seems a lifetime ago, I had several discussions with Gerald Dworkin that helped me get my thoughts straight on various issues about autonomy.

Essay 6, "The Concept of Paternalism in Biomedical Ethics," is the final phase, I hope, in my long history of probing the subject of paternalism. Jim Childress and I have struggled together through the muddy conceptual issues in this area. Although we have never come to complete agreement, Jim has convinced me to moderate my skeptical views about soft paternalism. Jim and Ruth Faden have been instrumental in helping me get my thoughts straight. In the early years of my thinking about the key problems (dating to 1975), I was influenced by Joel Feinberg, with whom I had stimulating conversations on the subject. My work stands in the shadow of Feinberg's seminal writing on the subject.

Essay 7, "When Hastened Death Is neither Killing nor Letting Die, brings together much of my thinking about physician-hastened dying. Tim Quill and Peg Battin were my editors and advisors when I wrote this essay. The compactness and directness of the argument in this essay owe much to them. I've learned a great deal about what to say and not say about these issues from conversations with, and the publications of, Dan Brock and James Rachels. I have had several public debates with Ed Pellegrino on the topic. Ed has many times helped me understand views that I don't hold; he has a wonderful ability to make them clear and plausible. In the early years in which my views on these subjects were developing, I acknowledge how much I enjoyed examining ideas through conversations with Arnold Davidson. Every philosopher should have as much fun as Arnold and I had in those years.

Essay 8, "The Exploitation of the Economically Disadvantaged in Pharmaceutical Research," was originally written for a conference. I thank the organizer of the conference, Denis Arnold. At the conference, I received useful criticism from Dan Callahan, Norman Daniels, and Dan Wikler. My work on pharmaceutical research in all its dimensions has been greatly facilitated by many years of discussing these issues with Robert Levine. In working on the subject of global justice and the economically disadvantaged, I have had stimulating interactions with Ruth Faden, Madison Powers, and Thomas Pogge.

Essay 10, "A Defense of the Common Morality," and Essay 11, "From Morality to Common Morality," are devoted to the subject of common morality. As anyone can see by reading the second of the two essays, I owe an immense amount to Bernard Gert, not only for his criticisms of me, but for the constructive side of his moral theory. It is a pleasure to be able to acknowledge the influence of his bold criticisms and his constructive theories. My essay was written for and delivered at Dartmouth College on the occasion of Gert's retirement and 50th year of teaching at Dartmouth. I was helped in formulating my topic by Jim Moor, Bernie's colleague at Dartmouth. Dan Brock, Ron Green, and Don Marquis gave me stimulating criticisms during the visit to Dartmouth that helped me redraft. More generally on the subjects of common morality and principlism, much in my work has been either motivated by or improved by the work of other critics, especially David DeGrazia, Carson Strong, and Ronald Lindsay.

Essay 12, "On Eliminating the Distinction Between Applied Ethics and Ethical Theory," and Essay 13, "Does Ethical Theory Have a Future in Bioethics?," are two of my forays into the waters of ethical theory and its limitations. The first, Essay 12, was written long ago; it was invited by the two editors of the *Monist* in those years, Eugene Freeman and John Hospers. Not much had been published on this subject at the time, but I did greatly benefit by Gert's early work on the subject. I owe the idea behind Essay 13, and criticism of it, to Jeff Kahn and Anna Mastroianni, the two editors of the journal issue in which this essay appeared.

Essay 14, "The Failure of Theories of Personhood," was first delivered as an address in Hong Kong, where I had the good fortune to receive excellent criticism from Gerhold Becker, John Harris, and Michael Quante. Later I received equally helpful criticisms from Robert Veatch and Henry Richardson when presenting the paper at Georgetown. Throughout the period of my writing this essay, I had many discussions about the issues with Raymond Frey.

Essay 15, "Looking Back and Judging Our Predecessors," was published in the form of an exchange between Allen Buchanan and me. Allen and I largely agreed on every major issue, but I was given a distinct advantage when writing my essay: Allen sent his draft first, and I was able to learn a good bit from him. I owe much in my presentation to the structure he laid out in his essay, and both of us owe much to the work of the Advisory Committee on Human Radiation Experiments (ACHRE), *Final Report of the Advisory Committee on Human Radiation Experiments* (New York: Oxford University Press, 1996), on whose conclusions Allen and I were commenting. In getting straight on the history surrounding the radiation experiments, I learned a great deal from Ruth Faden, Jonathan Moreno, and Susan Lederer.

In the Introduction to this volume, I have supplied the names of publishers and full bibliographical and copyright information pertaining to all original sources of these *Collected Essays*.

INTRODUCTION

This volume collects essays and treatises on several subjects that I have written over the course of 25 years. All are on philosophical and moral issues in the field of biomedical ethics. The topics range from the historical origins of modern research ethics to substantive issues in bioethics about moral principles and methodology. Despite the diversity of topics, a specific unity holds the three parts of this collection together. The unifying theme is the transparent connection of these essays to many of the topics and chapters in *Principles of Biomedical Ethics* (hereafter *Principles*), which I coauthored with James Childress. All readers familiar with the basic structure of that book will see that these *Collected Essays* augment, develop, and defend some of its central positions and arguments. A few essays take off in new directions, but all have a connection to themes in *Principles*. I have tried to select only essays that expand and deepen, while not duplicating, material in *Principles*.

This introduction explains the publishing history and content of these essays, as well as ways in which they augment and develop the so-called "principlist" theory that Childress and I developed together. The year, source, and place of publication and an abstract of each essay are supplied.

The book is divided into three parts. The first part is entitled "The *Belmont Report* and the Rise of Principles." The two essays in this part explain the emerging importance of frameworks of principles in bioethics in the mid-1970s. The primary sources at the time of the rise of these frameworks were *Principles* and the *Belmont Report*. The latter is a government report that I drafted for the National Commission for the Protection of Human Subjects of Biomedical and Behavioral Research. The history of the writing of both of these works and their crossover influence are explained and analyzed in Part I.

The second part is entitled "Principlism and Practice." This section treats several issues about moral principles and their practical use in bioethics as well as the nature of "principlism." This word was coined by Danner Clouser and Bernard Gert principally to refer to the theory Childress and I developed. The first essay in this second section adopts the language of "The Four-Principles Approach," an expression originally coined by Raanan Gillon to refer to the theory in *Principles*. The material in Part II develops some themes Childress and

I address in Chapters 4 through 7 of *Principles* (using 6th edition chapter numbers).

The third part concentrates on questions of theory and method in ethics—long my major teaching and publishing interest in bioethics. This part treats the idea that the four-principles approach provides a theoretical framework or paradigm for bioethics together with some ideas about theory and method that include discussion of the nature and role of the common morality. This part also probes whether ethical theory has a strong role to play in the future of bioethics and whether so-called "applied ethics" should be sharply distinguished from general ethical theory. Two other essays investigate whether the concept of person has a significant role to play in bioethics and how judgments can be made of the actions and character of persons who lived in past decades and centuries when they embraced significantly different moral standards. The material in the third part develops answers to various problems that Childress and I address in Chapters 1, 2, 3, 9, and 10 of *Principles*.

During the preparation of this volume I have lightly edited almost all of these essays for purposes of clarity and style. I have added content to three of the essays. This supplementary content has in every case been drawn from other parts of my published work. In no case have I altered the basic structure or argument found in the original publication. I have altered a title only in the case of the fourth essay: "Informed Consent: Its History and Meaning"; it was originally published under the less specific title "Informed Consent."

I also explain below precisely what I have done to alter the few essays in which material has been added in these *Collected Essays*.

PART I. THE *BELMONT REPORT* AND THE RISE OF PRINCIPLES

Essay 1. "The Origins and Evolution of the *Belmont Report*"

Publication Data. This essay was published in *Belmont Revisited: Ethical Principles for Research with Human Subjects.* Copyright © 2005 by Georgetown University Press. From *Belmont Revisited: Ethical Principles for Research with Human Subjects,* James Childress, Eric Meslin, and Harold Shapiro, Editors, pp. 12–25. Reprinted with permission. www.press.georgetown.edu. This essay, as here slightly revised, also draws on a small body of material in an essay I wrote in *The Story of Bioethics,* also published by Georgetown University Press. Reprinted with permission.

Abstract. This 2005 article recounts my work in delineating a framework of principles of research ethics when I was in the position of consultant philosopher at the National Commission for the Protection of Human Subjects of Biomedical and Behavioral Research (U.S. Congress and NIH, 1974–78). The article starts with the historical context in which principles rose to prominence in biomedical ethics.

I concentrate here on research ethics. The project of creating a framework of basic principles for all federally funded research had been mandated by a public law enacted by the U.S. Congress. I was at work on the volume with Childress when I accepted an assignment with the National Commission to write its *Belmont Report*. I explain both the history of my drafting of this *Report*, how it was revised in the course of deliberations at the National Commission, and the connection of this drafting to my concurrent work with Childress. I discuss how the National Commission viewed these principles as embedded in preexisting public morality and how it regarded its set of principles as a universally valid resource for the formulation of public and institutional policies of research ethics. I outline how the views in *Belmont* express the basic structure for research ethics as it developed in the last quarter of the twentieth century and remains today.

Essay 2. "Codes, Declarations, and Other Ethical Guidance for Human Subjects Research: The *Belmont Report*"

Publication Data. This essay was published in *The Oxford Textbook of Clinical Research Ethics*, ed. Ezekiel Emanuel, Christine Grady, Robert Crouch, Reidar Lie, Franklin Miller, and David Wendler (New York: Oxford University Press, 2008), 149–155. By permission of Oxford University Press (New York).

Abstract. This essay was commissioned by a group of scholars in bioethics in the Department of Bioethics at the National Institutes of Health. It picks up the discussion of the *Belmont Report* roughly where I ended the discussion in the first essay. This second essay further examines the history of the *Report* together with an explanation of the National Commission's larger body of publications, which comprised 17 volumes. It discusses the moral content of the principles that were adopted and the idea that the principles form a basic moral framework for research ethics.

The essay contains a critical evaluation of the philosophical roots of the principles and includes a section that examines philosophical questions about and weaknesses in the principles (as they are expressed in the *Belmont Report*), including some weaknesses that persist still today in research ethics. The essay concludes with a section on the influence and ongoing significance of the *Belmont Report*, which still stands as an internationally influential government-commission statement of moral requirements in research ethics. It is possibly more widely known than any document in research ethics other than the Declaration of Helsinki, which at present seems to be in a stage of declining influence. *Belmont* was eventually adopted by all relevant agencies of the U.S. government as a statement of the obligations scientific investigators must discharge in conducting human research. I explain how *Belmont* has been one of the few documents to have influenced almost every sphere of activity in bioethics: moral theory and general standards of professional ethics, government regulatory activity, bioethics consultation, and even medical practice.

PART II. PRINCIPLISM AND PRACTICE

Essay 3. "The Four Principles Approach to Health Care Ethics"

Publication Data. This essay was published in *Principles of Health Care Ethics*, 2nd ed., Richard Ashcroft, Angus Dawson, Heather Draper, and John Macmillan, eds. (London: John Wylie, 2007), 3–10. By permission of Wiley-Blackwell, 9600 Garsington Road, Oxford OX4 2DQ.

Abstract. This essay was first published in the early 1990s with the goal of explaining and critically examining the four principles or "principlist" account of biomedical ethics to an international audience. The first edition of the *Principles of Health Care Ethics* was the creation of British physician and medical ethics scholar Raanan Gillon. This anthology was devoted primarily to critical appraisal of the *Principles* book that Childress and I published. My essay on "The Four-Principles Approach" was the opening essay in both the first and the second editions. (The essay is published here as it was revised and updated for the second edition.) The essay is a basic and reasonably comprehensive explanation of the four-principles approach, clarifying various of its claims and attempting to straighten out assorted misunderstandings of the *Principles* book. The following topics are discussed: the origins of principled frameworks in bioethics, the nature of the framework that Childress and I use, the centrality of the common morality in our work, the prima facie character of principles and rules, the specification of principles and rules, and the role of the method of coherence in moral justification.

Essay 4. "Informed Consent: Its History and Meaning"

Publication Data. This essay was published in *Medical Ethics*, ed. Robert M. Veatch (Boston and London: Jones and Bartlett Publishers, Inc., 1st edition 1989; 2nd edition, 1997), 186–205. Copyright © 1997 Jones and Bartlett Publishers, Sudbury, MA. www.jbpub.com. Reprinted with permission. Some supplementary historical material has been added that derives from the book I coauthored with Ruth Faden entitled *A History and Theory of Informed Consent* (New York: Oxford University Press, 1986). By permission of Oxford University Press.

Abstract. This essay is a comprehensive treatment of the history, nature, and moral importance of informed consent. It begins by treating the near absence of requirements of informed consent in the history of medicine. I trace how informed consent obligations and requirements gradually emerged from legal cases, regulatory interventions, government-appointed commissions, and intra-professional events in the last half of the twentieth century. Following this history, I present an analysis of the concept of informed consent, including an analytical treatment of its basic elements and conceptual conditions. This analysis might seem to provide a solid foundation for a definition of "informed consent," but I argue that this term needs a deeper analysis. It must be understood in terms of two common, entrenched, and irreducibly different meanings of "informed consent." I establish the two senses as (1) autonomous choice and (2) institutional consent. I note that assessment of the quality of the consent is important for understanding both senses of "informed consent" and for understanding requirements of obtaining consent. I argue that the quality of consent should be judged by several different considerations, including the level of understanding of disclosed infor-mation and whether undue influence is present in making a request for consent. Finally, I examine various justifications for waiving or at least not requiring informed consent. Some are found to be valid reasons for not obtaining consent, and others are found to be unjustified.

Essay 5. "Who Deserves Autonomy and Whose Autonomy Deserves Respect?"

Publication Data. This essay was published in *Personal Autonomy: New Essays in Personal Autonomy and Its Role in Contemporary Moral Philosophy*, ed. James Taylor (Cambridge: Cambridge University Press, 2005), 310–329. Copyright © 2005 Cambridge University Press. Reprinted with the permission of Cambridge University Press. A few paragraphs of supplementary material have been added from my "Consent and Autonomy," in Frank Miller and Roger Wertheimer, eds., *The Ethics of Consent* (New York: Oxford University Press, 2010). By permission of Oxford University Press (New York).

Abstract. I distinguish between "autonomy," "respect for autonomy," and "rights of autonomy." Whereas "respect for autonomy" and "rights of autonomy" are moral notions, "autonomy" and "autonomous person" are not obviously moral notions. To some philosophers they seem metaphysical rather than moral. However, this distinction between the metaphysical and the moral has fostered precarious claims in moral philosophy such as these: (1) analysis of autonomy is a conceptual and metaphysical project, not a moral one; (2) a theory of autonomy should not be built on moral notions, but rather on a theory of mind, self, or person; (3) the concept of autonomy is intimately connected to the concept of person, which alone anchors the concept of moral status. I assess each of these claims with the objective of determining who qualifies as autonomous and which level (or degree) of autonomy deserves respect.

I argue that moral notions—in particular, respect for autonomy—should affect how we construct theories of autonomous action and the autonomous person on grounds that a theory of autonomy should be kept consistent with the substantive assumptions about autonomy implicit in the principle of respect for autonomy. However, theories of autonomy should only be *constrained* by the principle of respect for autonomy, not wholly *determined* by it. I offer an abbreviated theory of conceptually necessary conditions of autonomy. My conditions differ substantially from prominent accounts in the literature, such as Harry Frankfurt's theory, which I criticize in section 4 of this paper. My discussion of the claim that the concept of autonomy is intimately connected to the concept of person leads directly to the content of essay 14 in these *Collected Essays*.

Essay 6. "The Concept of Paternalism in Biomedical Ethics"

Publication Data. This essay was published in the *Jahrbuch für Wissenschaft und Ethik* (2009). Berlin: Walter de Gruyter GmbH & Co. KG; Mies-van-der-Rohe-Str. 1; 80807 München, Germany. Permission by Rights & Licenses Department.

Abstract. This essay pulls together in one place the several strands of my thought over 35 years on the problem of paternalism (principally medical paternalism). In the literature of biomedical ethics, paternalism has been both defended and attacked in several areas of clinical medicine, public health, health policy, and government agency policies (e.g., the policies of the Food and Drug Administration). I argue that it is unclear in much of this literature what paternalism is and which types of paternalism, if any, are justified. The position closest to a consensus position in the literature is that so-called strong (or hard) paternalism is not justified, but I argue that strong paternalism can be justified and that it is the only interesting and controversial form of paternalism. I try to show that questions of the justification and the definition of paternalism are closely connected, and that there is a definition that is grounded in fidelity to the principle of respect for autonomy. I then discuss several of the most prominent practical problems about paternalism in biomedical ethics. In each case I focus on how obligations of respect for autonomy and beneficence need to be balanced when making a judgment about whether a paternalistic intervention is justified.

Essay 7. "When Hastened Death Is Neither Killing nor Letting Die"

Publication Data. This essay was published in Timothy E. Quill and Margaret P. Battin, eds., *Physician-Assisted Dying: The Case for Palliative Care and Patient*

Choice, pp. 118–129. Copyright © 2004. The Johns Hopkins University Press. Reprinted with the permission of the Johns Hopkins University Press.

Abstract. This essay covers a broad range of issues in what is today commonly categorized as "physician-assisted suicide." I start with a brief discussion of the recent history of the issues, from the Quinlan case to the present. I then discuss issues about rights of autonomous choice, including whether the capacity for autonomy is likely to be reduced in circumstances of making a choice to hasten death and whether so-called "coercive situations" sometimes deprive a person of autonomous choice. I consider the justification of physician involvement in hastening death and whether the physician's intention makes a morally relevant difference. I also analyze conceptual features of the language generally used to discuss these subjects, including "suicide," "hastened death," "killing," and "letting die." These concepts can make a critical moral difference to how we think about whether an intentionally hastened death constitutes either a suicide, a killing, or a letting die.

The meaning of these terms also can determine whether "suicide," as used both in medicine and beyond, entails disapproval and whether it is proper to use the language of "causing death," which suggests liability, when characterizing the physician's action of hastening death. Also assessed are whether "the right to die" is a meaningful notion and, if so, how it differs from the right to refuse treatment, the right to avoid suffering, and the right to death with dignity.

Essay 8. "The Exploitation of the Economically Disadvantaged in Pharmaceutical Research"

Publication Data. This essay was published in Denis Arnold, ed., *Ethics and the Business of Biomedicine* (Cambridge: Cambridge University Press, 2009). Copyright © 2009 Cambridge University Press. Reprinted with the permission of Cambridge University Press.

Abstract. I evaluate some searing criticisms of the power and influence of the pharmaceutical industry that have appeared in various published sources. The industry stands accused of a sea of injustices and corruptions, including aggressive and deceptive marketing schemes, exploitative uses of research subjects, a corrupting influence on universities, suppression of and amateurism in handling scientific data, and conflicts of interest that bias research investigators. Each charge of injustice derives from concern about some form of unfair *influence* exerted by pharmaceutical companies. The array of alleged forms of influence is vast, and I here telescope to one area: the recruitment and enrollment in clinical research of vulnerable human subjects, in particular the economically disadvantaged. I focus on the charge that subjects in clinical trials are unjustly exploited by manipulative and unfair payment schemes.

I treat three problems. The first is whether the economically disadvantaged constitute a vulnerable group. I argue that classification as a "group" is a misleading characterization that may cause paternalistic overprotection. The second problem is whether the vulnerable poor are exploited by payments that constitute either an undue influence or an undue industry profit. I argue that such assessments should be made situationally, not categorically. The third problem is whether the poor are likely to give compromised or nonvoluntary consents. I argue that this third problem, like the second, is subtle and complicated, but practically manageable, and I add that pharmaceutical research involving the poor and vulnerable can, with proper precaution, be carried out in an ethically responsible manner. Whether the research *is* so conducted is another matter, an empirical problem beyond the scope of my argument.

PART III. THEORY AND METHOD

Essay 9. "Principles and Other Emerging Paradigms in Bioethics"

Publication Data. Tom L. Beauchamp, as published in 69 *Indiana Law Journal*: 1–17 (1994). Copyright © 1994 by the Trustees of Indiana University. Reprinted with permission. For the present volume I have added a few paragraphs to this essay.

Abstract. This article is centered on several accounts of biomedical ethics that allegedly challenge the principles account that Childress and I defend. Leading critics of our principles (Bernard Gert, Danner Clouser, Albert Jonsen, Stephen Toulmin, Carson Strong, John Arras, Edmund Pellegrino, and others) have, since the late 1980s, defended some types of theory or method proposed as alternatives to or substitutes for principlism. These types include casuistry, virtue theory, and impartial rule theory. These accounts were first emerging to prominence in bioethics at the time this article was written. I welcome these developments in this essay, because they improve the range, precision, and quality of thought in the field. I also acknowledge the contribution those who embrace these paradigms have made to the improvement of my own thought. However, I argue that impartial rule theory, casuistry, and virtue ethics should not be presented as rivals to principlism, because they neither replace the principles in principlism nor are inconsistent with those principles. I argue that all leading "alternatives" are compatible with, and not alternatives to, an approach based on principles. Finally, I point to some limitations of the principle-based approach, in light of these paradigms, and reflect on how those limitations should be handled.

Essay 10. "A Defense of the Common Morality"

Publication Data. This essay was published in *Kennedy Institute of Ethics Journal* 13:3 (2003): 259–274. Copyright © 2003. The Johns Hopkins University Press. Reprinted with the permission of the Johns Hopkins University Press.

Abstract. Phenomena of moral conflict and disagreement have led writers in ethics to two antithetical conclusions: Either moral distinctions hold universally or they hold only relative to a particular and contingent moral framework. If the latter, they cannot claim universal validity. In this essay I defend a universalistic account of the most general norms of morality in the course of responding to some critics of the common morality theory that Childress and I defend in *Principles.* In particular, I respond to criticisms by David DeGrazia and Leigh Turner, both of whom take "common morality" to refer to a broader and quite different body of norms than I do.

I maintain that one can consistently deny universality to some justified moral norms while claiming universality for others. I argue that universality is located in the common morality and that nonuniversality is to be expected in other parts of the moral life, which I call "particular moralities." The existence of universal moral standards is defended in terms of (1) a theory of the objectives of morality, (2) an account of the norms that achieve those objectives, and (3) an account of normative justification (both pragmatic and coherentist). This defense in terms of (1) through (3) sets the stage for the next essay in the volume (#11, as abstracted immediately below).

Essay 11. "From Morality to Common Morality"

Publication Data. This essay is forthcoming in a volume to be entitled, roughly, *Bernard Gert and Applied Philosophy.* It is being edited at Dartmouth College as the present volume goes to press. Published by permission of Jim Moor and Bernard Gert. ©

Abstract. For some 19 years, Bernard Gert has criticized my views about moral philosophy and the principles of biomedical ethics. In this article I focus on the major issue addressed in his moral theory: the justification of morality—that is, the justification of the common morality. I concentrate on a body of claims that he and I both defend about the common morality, and I emphasize our similarities rather than our differences. I orient the discussion around his account and develop my own account in the process.

My objectives in this paper are threefold: first, to argue that the common morality is a reasonable basis for both moral theory and practical ethics;

second, to identify and defend three forms of justification of the common morality; and third, to show precisely where Gert and I agree and disagree. The main question I address is, "Which types of justification of the common morality are needed, and for which types of claims about the common morality are they suitable?" I present three distinct strategies of justification: (1) normative theoretical justification, resting on ethical theory; (2) normative conceptual justification, resting on conceptual analysis, and (3) empirical justification, resting on empirical research. Each of these three types justifies a different conclusion about the common morality. I do not produce a justification of any one of the three strategies, although I outline the form such justifications would take. That is, my limited aim is to identify three available types of justification and to identify the conclusions each type can be expected to reach. In particular, I distinguish justification of the norms of the common morality (Gert's principal project) from the justification of claims that the common morality exists (which, as yet, is of little or no interest to Gert, though is of interest to me).

The first half of the paper is devoted to finding points of agreement in our theories. In the second half, I am critical of Gert's lack of attendance to a few important issues, especially his neglect of empirical claims, including ones that he himself seems to rely on. On the whole, this essay presents my account of the methods of justification of common morality, and therefore is not limited to a criticism of Gert's views.

Essay 12. "On Eliminating the Distinction Between Applied Ethics and Ethical Theory"

Publication Data. This essay was published in *The Monist* 67 (October 1984): 514–531. Copyright © *The Monist: An International Quarterly Journal of General Philosophical Inquiry.* Open Court Publishing Co., Chicago, Illinois. Reprinted by permission.

Abstract. I motivate this 1984 paper by noting that so-called "applied ethics"—a recently coined term—has become a major growth area in the curricular offerings in North American philosophy, but that its actual standing in philosophy is insecure. Many philosophers regard the literature in applied ethics as lightweight and perhaps philosophically barren. However, I argue that understanding and teaching the best literature in applied ethics can be as difficult as mastering material in more abstract regions of ethical theory, but I also argue that no significant differences distinguish ethical theory and applied ethics as philosophical activities or methods. I do not maintain that there are no differences in content. I argue only that good applied philosophers do what philosophers have always done: They analyze concepts; submit to critical scrutiny various strategies that are used to justify beliefs, policies, and actions; examine hidden presuppositions; and offer both moral criticism and constructive theories.

Early in the paper I argue for eliminating the distinction between applied ethics and ethical theory. I turn, in later sections, to methodological considerations, paying particular attention to the "case method" and the way analytical argument surrounds it in law, business, and medicine. I argue that philosophers can profit in both a scholarly and a pedagogical way from certain uses of the case method. At various points in the paper I examine some of the work and the claims of Norman Daniels, Bernard Gert, and Dan Clouser.

Essay 13. "Does Ethical Theory Have a Future in Bioethics?"

Publication Data. This essay was published in the *Journal of Law, Medicine & Ethics* 32 (2004): 209–217. © 2004 by the American Society of Law, Medicine & Ethics.

Abstract. This article assesses whether ethical theory is likely to continue in upcoming years to play the prominent role it has in the previous 25 years of published literature and curriculum development in bioethics. What transpired during these years suggests that the field enjoys a successful and stable marriage to philosophical ethical theory. However, the marriage became shaky as bioethics became a more interdisciplinary and practical field. A practical price is paid for theoretical generality in philosophy, and it is not clear that contemporary bioethics is willing to pay that price. It is also often unclear whether and, if so, how theory is to be brought to bear on dilemmatic problems, public policy, moral controversies, and moral conflict. I envision that the next 25 years could be very different because of this now troubled marriage. The most philosophical parts of bioethics seem headed toward a retreat to philosophy departments and philosophy journals, while bioethics continues on its current course toward becoming a more interdisciplinary and practical field.

One piece of evidence of philosophy's declining influence is that many individuals in law, theological ethics, political theory, the social and behavioral sciences, and the health professions now carefully address mainstream issues of bioethics without finding ethical theory essential or even particularly useful or insightful. Another is that philosophers have yet to offer detailed statements of a method for moving from philosophical theories to the practical commitments of the theories. Although many moral philosophers are at present actively involved in problems of biomedical ethics such as clinical and corporate consulting, policy formulation, and committee review, it is an open question what their role *as moral philosophers* should be and whether they can successfully bring ethical theories and methods to bear on problems of practice.

My concerns in this essay are with the types of theory and method that have been under discussion in bioethics in the last quarter-century. Three interconnected areas have been prominent: (1) normative moral theories (from utilitarian and Kantian theories to principlism, casuistry, virtue ethics, feminist ethics, particularism, etc.); (2) moral and conceptual analyses of basic moral notions (informed consent, the killing/letting-die distinction, etc.); and (3) methodology (how bioethics proceeds—e.g., by use of cases, narratives, specified principles, theory application, reflective equilibrium, legal methods, etc.). I leave it an open question whether (2) or (3) can be successfully addressed without addressing (1), an unresolved problem in philosophical ethics. However, I question philosophy's success in all three areas, laying emphasis on its weaknesses in connecting theory to practice.

In assessing the contemporary literature and how it needs to change, I confine attention to three substantive areas of the intersection between bioethics and ethical theory: cultural relativity and moral universality, moral justification, and conceptual analysis. In each case I argue that philosophers need to develop theories and methods more closely attuned to practice. The work of several philosophers, including Ruth Macklin, Norman Daniels, and Gerald Dworkin, is examined. In their writings there is a methodological gap between philosophical theory (and method) and practical conclusions. The future of philosophical ethics in interdisciplinary bioethics may turn on whether such gaps can be closed. If not, bioethics may justifiably conclude that philosophy is of little practical value for the field.

Essay 14. "The Failure of Theories of Personhood"

Publication Data. This essay was published in *Kennedy Institute of Ethics Journal* 9:4 (1999): 309–324. Copyright © 1999. The Johns Hopkins University Press. Reprinted with the permission of the Johns Hopkins University Press.

Abstract. This article focuses on the pervasive belief in popular culture, philosophy, religion, law, and science (e.g., in research ethics) that some special property of persons, such as self-consciousness, rationality, language use, or dignity, confers a unique moral status. I discuss the distinction between moral persons and metaphysical persons and also the connection or lack of connection between the theory of autonomy and the theory of persons. I argue that no set of cognitive properties alone confers moral standing and that metaphysical personhood is not sufficient for either moral personhood or moral standing. Cognitive theories fail to capture the depth of commitments embedded in using the language of "person," and it is more assumed than demonstrated in cognitive theories that nonhuman animals lack a relevant form of self-consciousness or its functional equivalent. Although nonhuman animals are not plausible candidates for moral persons, humans, too, fail to qualify as moral persons if they lack one or more of the conditions of moral personhood. If moral personhood were the sole basis of moral rights, then these humans would lack rights for the same reasons that nonhuman animals are often held to lack rights.

I also argue that the vagueness and the inherently contestable nature of the concept of person are not likely to be dissipated by philosophical theories of the nature of persons and that we would be better off if we eliminated the language of "person" from moral theory altogether and replaced it with more specific concepts.

Essay 15. "Looking Back and Judging Our Predecessors"

Publication Data. This essay was published in *Kennedy Institute of Ethics Journal* 6:3 (1996): 251–270. Copyright © 1996. The Johns Hopkins University Press. Reprinted with the permission of the Johns Hopkins University Press.

Abstract. This essay is on the problem of retrospective moral judgment. It considers how moral theory and related methods of assessment should be used to address the following question: "Can persons and institutions be held responsible for actions taken decades ago, when moral standards, practices, and policies were strikingly different, or even nonexistent?" The question is whether the principles and rules that we currently embrace are unfairly retrofitted when we use them to make judgments about the medical ethics of our predecessors. This seemingly straightforward question requires making several distinctions and using different forms of argument to untangle the issue(s). For example, issues of wrongdoing need to be disengaged from questions of culpability and exculpation. Also, even if institutions can be found guilty of wrongdoing, it does not follow that particular individuals in those institutions can be found to be either wrongdoers or culpable.

To illustrate the problems of theory and method present in these questions, I consider two morally and politically important examples of how these questions have arisen in biomedical ethics. Both come from research ethics, and the two are intimately connected. The first source is a set of moral problems addressed in the *Report of the Advisory Committee on Human Radiation Experiments* that was appointed by President William Clinton to investigate questionable experiments funded by the U.S. government after World War II. The second is the work of an Ad Hoc faculty committee at the University of California, San Francisco ("Report of the UCSF Ad Hoc Fact Finding Committee on World War II Human Radiation Experiments") that investigated the ethics of the actions of its own administration and faculty in its involvement in the human radiation experiments.

The Advisory Committee identified six basic ethical principles as relevant to its work and then appropriately argued that persons and institutions can be held responsible for actions taken even if the standards, practices, and policies at the time on the use of research subjects were strikingly different than those we call upon today. I argue that in reaching its conclusions, the Advisory Committee did not altogether adhere to the language and commitments of its own ethical framework. In its *Final Report*, the Advisory Committee emphasizes judgments of *wrongdoing*, to the relative neglect of *culpability*; I argue that the Advisory Committee properly treats mitigating conditions that are exculpatory, but does not provide a thoroughgoing assessment of either culpability or exculpation. It also fails to judge the culpability of particular individuals, though it was positioned to do so.

I am thus critical of the Advisory Committee's findings, but I am especially critical of the more serious deficiencies in the Ad Hoc Committee's deliberations and conclusions. The latter group reaches no significant judgments of either wrongdoing or culpability, but almost certainly should have. A balanced investigation would have more critically assessed (1) physician wrongdoing, (2) the culpability of specific agents, and (3) institutional responsibility.

Part I

THE *BELMONT REPORT* AND THE RISE OF
PRINCIPLES

THE ORIGINS AND EVOLUTION OF THE
BELMONT REPORT

When, on December 22, 1976, I agreed to join the staff of the National Commission for the Protection of Human Subjects of Biomedical and Behavioral Research, my first and only major assignment was to write the "Belmont Paper," as it was then called. At the time, I had already drafted substantial parts of *Principles of Biomedical Ethics* with James Childress.[1] Subsequent to my appointment, the two manuscripts were drafted simultaneously, often side by side, the one inevitably influencing the other.

I here explain how the "Belmont Paper" evolved into the *Belmont Report*.[2] I will also correct some common but mistaken speculation about the emergence of frameworks of principles in research ethics and the connections between *Belmont* and *Principles*.

THE BEGINNINGS OF *BELMONT*

The idea for the "Belmont Paper" originally grew from a vision of shared moral principles governing research that emerged during a break-out session at a four-day retreat held February 13–16, 1976, at the Smithsonian Institution's Belmont Conference Center in Maryland.[3] Albert Jonsen has reported on the contributions at this meeting of Stephen Toulmin, Karen Lebacqz, Joe Brady, and others.[4] However, this meeting predates my work on the *Belmont Report*, and I leave it to Jonsen and the others in attendance to relate the story of the retreat.

A few months after this conference at Belmont, I received two phone calls: the first from Toulmin, who was the staff philosopher at the National Commission, and the second from Michael Yesley, staff director. They asked me to write a paper for the National Commission on the nature and scope of the notion of justice. Yesley told me that the commissioners sought help in understanding theories of justice and their applications to the moral problems of human subject research. I wrote this paper and assumed that my work for the National Commission was concluded.[5]

However, shortly after I completed the paper, Toulmin returned to full-time teaching at the University of Chicago, and Yesley inquired whether I was available to replace him on the staff. This appointment met some resistance. Two commissioners who later became my close friends—Brady and Donald Seldin—were initially skeptical of the appointment. Nonetheless, Yesley prevailed, likely with the help of Chairperson Kenneth Ryan and my colleague Patricia King, and I joined the National Commission staff.

On my first morning in the office, Yesley told me that he was assigning me the task of writing the "Belmont Paper."[6] I asked Yesley what the task was. He pointed out that the National Commission had been charged by Congress to investigate the ethics of research and to explore basic ethical principles.[7] Members of the staff were at work on various topics in research ethics, he reported, but no one was working on basic principles. He said that an opening round of discussions of the principles had been held at the Belmont retreat. The National Commission had delineated a rough schema of three basic ethical principles: respect for persons, beneficence, and justice. I asked Yesley what these moral notions meant to the commissioners, to which he responded that he had no well-formed idea and that it was my job to figure out what the commissioners meant—or, more likely, to figure out what they should have meant.

So, I found myself with the job of giving shape and substance to something called the "Belmont Paper," though at that point I had never heard of Belmont or the paper. It struck me as an odd title for a publication. Moreover, this document had never been mentioned during my interview for the job or at any other time until Yesley gave me the assignment. My immediate sense was that I was the new kid on the block and had been given the dregs of National Commission work. I had thought, when I decided to join the National Commission staff, that I would be working on the ethics of psychosurgery and research involving children, which were heated and perplexing controversies at the time. I was chagrined to learn that I was to write something on which no one else was working and that had its origins in a retreat that I had not attended. Moreover, the mandate to do the work had its roots in a federal law that I had not seen until that morning.

Yesley proceeded to explain that no one had yet worked seriously on the sections of the report on principles because no one knew what to do with them. This moment of honesty was not heartening, but I was not discouraged either, because Childress and I were at that time well into the writing of our book on the role of basic principles in biomedical ethics. It intrigued me that the two of us had worked relatively little on research ethics, which was the sole focus of the National Commission. I saw in my early conversations with Yesley that these two projects, *Principles* and *Belmont*, had many points of intersecting interest and could be mutually beneficial. And so it would be.

Yesley also gave me some hope by saying that a crude draft of the "Belmont Paper" already existed, though a twinkle in his eye warned me not to expect too much. That same morning I read the "Belmont draft."[8] Scarce could a new recruit have been more dismayed. So little was said about the principles that to call it a "draft" of principles would be like calling a dictionary entry a scholarly treatise. Some sections were useful, especially a few handsome pages that had been written largely by Robert Levine on the subject of "The Boundaries Between Biomedical and Behavioral Research and Accepted and Routine Practice" (later revised under the subtitle "Boundaries Between Practice and Research" and made the first section of the *Belmont Report*). Apart from Levine's contribution, however, this draft of *Belmont* had almost nothing to say about the principles that were slated to be its heart.

In the next few weeks, virtually everything in this draft pertaining to principles would be thrown away either because it contained too little on principles or because it had too much on peripheral issues. At the time, these peripheral issues constituted almost the entire document, with the exception of the section written by Levine, which was neither peripheral nor on principles. The major topics addressed were the National Commission's mandate, appropriate review mechanisms, compensation for injury, national and international regulations and codes, research design, and other items that did not belong in the *Belmont Report*. These topics, being peripheral, were therefore eliminated. Except for Levine's section on boundaries, everything in this draft landed on the cutting-room floor.[9]

Once the "Belmont draft" was left with nothing in the section on principles, Yesley suggested that I might find the needed content from the massive compendium on research titled *Experimentation with Human Beings*, edited by Jay Katz with the assistance of Alexander Capron and Eleanor Swift Glass.[10] Drawn from sociology, psychology, medicine, and law, this book was at the time the most thorough collection of materials on research ethics and law. Yesley informed me that I should endeavor to learn all the information presented in this book, but after days of poring over this wonderful resource, I found that it offered virtually nothing on *principles* suitable for an analytical discussion of research ethics. The various codes and statements by professional associations found in this book had occasional connections with my task and with the National Commission's objectives, but only distant ones.[11]

THE HISTORICAL ORIGINS OF THE PRINCIPLES
OF THE *BELMONT REPORT*

Fortunately, Childress and I had gathered a useful collection of materials on principles and theories, largely in the writings of philosophers. I had been influenced in my thinking about principles by the writings of W. D. Ross and William Frankena. My training led me to turn to these and other philosophical treatments, which had already proved helpful in my work on *Principles*.

However, it would be misleading to suggest that the principles featured in the *Belmont Report* derived from the writings of philosophers. Their grounding is ultimately in what I would eventually call, following Alan Donagan, "the common morality." The *Belmont Report* makes reference to "our cultural tradition" as the basis of its principles, and it is clear that these principles derive from the common morality rather than a particular philosophical work or tradition. However, what *Belmont* means by our "tradition" is unclear, and I believe the import of the *Belmont* principles cannot be tied to a particular tradition, but rather to a conviction that there is a universally valid point of view. I believe, and I think that the commissioners believed, that these principles are norms shared by all morally informed and committed persons.

The commissioners almost certainly believed that these principles are already embedded in public morality and are presupposed in the formulation of public and institutional policies. The principles do not deviate from what every morally sensitive person knows to be right, based on his or her own moral training and experience. That is, every morally sensitive person believes that a moral way of life requires that we respect persons and take into account their well-being in our actions. *Belmont's* principles are so woven into the fabric of morality that no responsible research investigator could conduct research without reference to them.[12]

THE RELATIONSHIP BETWEEN THE *BELMONT* PRINCIPLES AND THE
PRINCIPLES IN *PRINCIPLES OF BIOMEDICAL ETHICS*

Many have supposed that the *Belmont Report* provided the starting point and the abstract framework for *Principles of Biomedical Ethics*.[13] They have wrongly assumed that *Belmont* preceded and grounded *Principles*.[14] The two works were written simultaneously, the one influencing the other.[15] There was reciprocity in the drafting, and influence ran bilaterally. I was often simultaneously drafting material on the same principle or topic both for the National Commission and for my colleague Childress, while he was at the same time writing material for me to inspect. I would routinely write parts of the *Belmont Report* during the day at the National Commission headquarters on Westbard Avenue in Bethesda, then go to my office at Georgetown University in the evening and draft parts of chapters for Childress to review. Despite their entirely independent origins, these projects grew up and matured together.

Once I grasped the moral vision the National Commission initiated at Belmont, I could see that Childress and I had major substantive disagreements with the National Commission. The names of the principles articulated in the *Belmont Report* bear notable similarities to some of the names Childress and I were using and continued to use, but the two schemas of principles are far from constituting a uniform name, number, or conception. Indeed, the two frameworks are inconsistent.

I regarded the National Commission as confused in the way it analyzed the principle of respect for persons. It seemed to blend a principle of respect for autonomy and a principle of beneficence that required protection of, and avoidance of the causation of harm to, incompetent persons. Childress and I both thought at the time that we should make our analysis turn on sharp distinctions between the principle of beneficence, the principle of nonmaleficence, and the principle of respect for autonomy, though the National Commission did not make such sharp distinctions. This matter was connected to an additional problem: The National Commission may have had a fundamentally utilitarian vision of social beneficence without adequate internal controls in its framework to protect subjects against abuse when there is the promise of major benefit for other sick or disabled persons.

The differences between the philosophy in *Principles* and the National Commission's views in *Belmont* have occasionally been the subject of published commentary.[16] Some commentators correctly see that we developed substantially different moral visions and that neither approach was erected on the foundations of the other. By early 1977, I had come to the view that the National Commission, especially in the person of its chair, Kenneth Ryan, was sufficiently rigid in its vision of the principles that there was no way to substantively alter the conception, although I thought that all three principles were either defective or underanalyzed. From this point forward, I attempted to analyze principles for the National Commission exclusively as the commissioners envisioned them. *Principles of Biomedical Ethics* became the sole work expressing my deepest philosophical convictions about principles.

THE DRAFTING AND REDRAFTING OF *BELMONT*

While Yesley gave me free rein in the drafting and redrafting of *Belmont*, the drafts were always subject to revisions and improvements made by the commissioners and staff members.[17] All members of the staff did their best to formulate ideas that were responsive to changes suggested by the commissioners. Commissioner Seldin encouraged me with as much vigor as he could muster, which was and remains today considerable, to make my drafts as philosophical as possible. Seldin wanted some Mill here, some Kant there, and the signature of philosophical argument sprinkled throughout the document. I tried this style, but other commissioners wanted a streamlined document and minimalist statement relatively free of the trappings of philosophy. Seldin, Yesley, and I ultimately relented,[18] and bolder philosophical defenses of the principles were gradually stripped from the body of *Belmont.*

Public deliberations in National Commission meetings were a staple source of ideas, but a few commissioners spoke privately to me or to Yesley about desired changes, and a few commissioners proposed changes to Assistant Staff Director Barbara Mishkin, who then passed them on to me. Most of these suggestions were accepted, and a serious attempt was made to implement them. In this respect, the writing of this document was a joint product of commissioner–staff interactions. However, most of the revisions made by the commissioners, other than through their comments in public deliberations, concerned small matters, and the commissioners were rarely involved in tendering written changes or detailed suggestions.

An exception to this generalization is found in a meeting on *Belmont* involving a few members of the staff and a few commissioners that occurred during September 1977 in the belvedere (or rooftop study) of Jonsen's home in San Francisco. The small group in attendance attempted to revise the "Belmont Paper" for presentation at the next meetings during which the commissioners were scheduled to debate it. As Jonsen reports in *The Birth of Bioethics* and elsewhere, the purpose of this meeting was to revisit previous drafts and deliberations of the commissioners.[19]

The history of drafting and redrafting that I have outlined may suggest that the document grew in size over time, but the reverse is true. The document grew quickly in the early drafting and then was contracted over time. I wrote much more for the National Commission about respect for persons, beneficence, and justice than eventually found its way into the *Belmont Report.* When various materials I had written were eliminated from *Belmont,* I would scoop up the reject piles and fashion them for *Principles of Biomedical Ethics.* Several late-written chunks of this book, in its parts on research ethics, were fashioned from the more philosophical but abjured parts of what I wrote for the National Commission that never found their way into the final draft of *Belmont.*

EXPLICIT AND IMPLICIT IDEAS ABOUT AN APPLIED RESEARCH ETHICS

Michael Yesley deserves credit for one key organizing conception in this report. He and I were in almost daily discussion about the "Belmont Paper." We spent many hours discussing the best way to develop the principles to express what the commissioners wanted to say, and even how to sneak in certain lines of thought that the commissioners might not notice. One late afternoon we were discussing the overall enterprise. We discussed each principle, whether the principles were truly independent, and how the principles related to the topics in research ethics under consideration by the National Commission. Yesley said, as a way of summarizing our reflections, "What these principles come to is really quite simple for our purposes: Respect for persons applies to informed consent, beneficence applies to risk-benefit assessment, and justice applies to the selection of subjects." Yesley had articulated the following abstract schema:

Principle of	*Applies to*	*Guidelines for*
Respect for persons		Informed consent
Beneficence		Risk–benefit assessment
Justice		Selection of subjects

This schema may seem trifling today, and it was already nascent in preexisting drafts of the report and in the National Commission's deliberations. But no one at the time had articulated these ideas in precisely this way, and Yesley's summary was immensely helpful in peering through countless hours of discussion to see the underlying structure and commitment at work in the principles destined to be the backbone of *Belmont*. Yesley had captured what would soon become the major portion of the table of contents of the *Belmont Report*, as well as the rationale of its organization. I then attempted to draft the document so that the basic principles could be applied to develop guidelines in specific areas and could also serve as justification for guidelines.

In light of this schema, a general strategy emerged for handling problems of research ethics, namely, that each principle made moral demands in a specific domain of responsibility for research. For example, the principle of respect for persons demands informed and voluntary consent. Under this conception, the purpose of consent provisions is not protection from risk, as many earlier federal policies seemed to imply, but the protection of autonomy and personal dignity, including the personal dignity of incompetent persons incapable of acting autonomously, for whose involvement a duly authorized third party must consent.

I wrote the sections on principles in the *Belmont Report* based on this model of each principle applying to a zone of moral concern. In this drafting, the focus of the document shifted to include not only abstract principles and their analysis, but also a moral view that is considerably more concrete and meaningful for those engaged in the practice of research. Explication of the value being advanced was heavily influenced by the context of biomedicine, and rather less influenced by contexts of the social and behavioral sciences. *Belmont*, in this way, moved toward an applied, professional morality of research ethics.

Although *Belmont* takes this modest step in the direction of an applied research ethics, there was never any ambition or attempt to make this document specific and practical. This objective was to be accomplished by the other volumes the National Commission issued. *Belmont* was meant to be, and should be remembered as, a moral framework for research ethics. Commissioners and staff were always aware that this framework is too indeterminate *by itself* to decide practice or policy or to resolve moral conflicts. The process of making the general principles in *Belmont* sufficiently concrete is a progressive process of reducing the indeterminateness and abstractness of the general principles to give them increased action-guiding capacity.[20] *Belmont* looks to educational institutions, professional associations, government agencies, institutional review boards, and the like to provide the particulars of research ethics.

PRINCIPLISM, CASUISTRY, OR BOTH?

Another misunderstanding of both *Principles* and *Belmont* has emerged in recent treatments of casuistry. Some commentators have misinterpreted the National Commission's work by overreading it as fundamentally a casuistry, and other commentators have misinterpreted *Principles of Biomedical Ethics* by underreading it as competitive with, and possibly undermined by, casuistry. However, a better interpretation is available: The National Commission demonstrably used casuistical reasoning in its deliberations, but its commitment to basic principles was never challenged throughout its years of deliberation. Similarly, Childress and I have from our first edition used casuistical reasoning in the treatment of cases, and we do not believe that there is any inconsistency between this form of reasoning and a commitment to principles. In the histories of both the National Commission and *Principles of Biomedical Ethics*, it is difficult to understand how the two commitments could be seen as other than complementary.

The final editing of the *Belmont Report* was done by three people in a small classroom at the NIH.[21] Al Jonsen, Stephen Toulmin, and I were given this assignment by the National Commission. Some who have followed the later writings of Jonsen and Toulmin on casuistry may be surprised to learn that throughout the National Commission's deliberations, as well as in this final drafting, Jonsen and Toulmin contributed to the clarification of the *principles* in the report. There was never an objection by either that a strategy of using principles should be other than central to the National Commission's statement of its ethical framework. Jonsen has often repeated his support for these principles.

However, Jonsen has also said that commissioners stated their views as principlists, but deliberated as casuists. He is suggesting that the National Commission's deliberations constituted a casuistry of reasoning about historical and contemporary cases,[22] despite the commissioners' commitment to and frequent reference to the *Belmont* principles. Jonsen and Toulmin once explicated this understanding of the National Commission's work in terms of the individual commissioners coming to agreement not on matters of moral theory and universal principles, but rather on how to make judgments about specific kinds of cases. Agreement, they argue, could never have been derived from the principles.[23]

This interpretation gives insight into the National Commission, but it needs careful qualification to avoid misunderstanding. Casuistical reasoning more so than moral theory or universal abstraction often did function to forge agreement during National Commission deliberations. The commissioners appealed to particular cases and families of cases, and consensus was reached through agreement on cases and generalization from cases when agreement on an underlying theoretical rationale would have been impossible.[24] Commissioners would never have been able to agree on a single ethical theory, nor did they even attempt to buttress the *Belmont* principles with a theory. Jonsen and Toulmin's treatment of the National Commission is, in this regard, entirely reasonable, and a similar line of argument can be taken to explicate the methods of reasoning at work in other bioethics commissions.[25]

Nonetheless, this methodological appraisal is consistent with a firm commitment to moral principles; the commissioners, including Jonsen, were emphatic in their support of and appeals to the general moral principles delineated in the *Belmont Report*.[26] The transcripts of the National Commission's deliberations show a constant movement from principle to case and from case to principle. Principles supported arguments about how to handle a case, and precedent cases supported the importance of commitment to principles. Cases or examples favorable to one point of view were brought forward, and counterexamples then advanced. Principles were invoked to justify the choice and use of both examples and counterexamples. On many occasions an argument was offered that a case judgment was irrelevant or immoral in light of the commitments of a principle.[27] The National Commission's deliberations and conclusions are best understood in terms of reasoning in which principles are interpreted and specified by the force of examples and counterexamples that emerge from experience with cases.

It is doubtful that Jonsen ever intended to deny this understanding of principles and their roles, despite the widely held view that casuistry dispenses with principles. Jonsen has said that "casuistic analysis does not deny the relevance of principle and theory,"[28] and, in an insightful statement in his later work, he has written that:

> when maxims such as "Do no harm," or "Informed consent is obligatory," are invoked, they represent, as it were, cut-down versions of the major principles relevant to the topic, such as beneficence and autonomy, cut down to fit the nature of the topic and the kinds of circumstances that pertain to it.[29]

Jonsen goes on to point out that casuistry is "complementary to principles" and that "casuistry is not an alternative to principles: No sound casuistry can dispense with principles."[30]

Casuists and those who support frameworks of principles like those in *Belmont* and *Principles of Biomedical Ethics* should be able to agree that when they reflect on cases and policies, they rarely have in hand either principles that were formulated without reference to experience with cases or paradigm cases lacking a prior commitment to general norms. Only a false dilemma makes us choose between the National Commission as principlist or casuist. It was both.

Notes

1. A contract for the book was issued by Oxford University Press on August 19, 1976. The manuscript was completed in late 1977; galleys arrived in October 1978, bearing the 1979 copyright date.

2. See also Appendices I and II to the *Belmont Report*. The *Belmont Report* was completed in late 1977 and published on September 30, 1978: *The Belmont Report: Ethical Guidelines for the Protection of Human Subjects of Research* (Washington, DC: DHEW Publication OS 78-0012). It first appeared in the Federal Register on April 18, 1979.

The National Commission for the Protection of Human Subjects of Biomedical and Behavioral Research was established July 12, 1974, under the National Research Act, Public Law 93-348, Title II. The first meeting was held December 3–4, 1974. The 43rd and final meeting was on September 8, 1978.

3. See the archives of the National Commission, 15th meeting, February 13–16, 1976, vol. 15A—a volume prepared for the Belmont meeting. This meeting book contains a "staff summary" on the subject of "ethical principles" as well as expert papers prepared by Kurt Baier, Alasdair MacIntyre, James Childress, H. Tristram Engelhardt, Alvan Feinstein, and LeRoy Walters. The papers by Engelhardt and Walters most closely approximate the moral considerations ultimately treated in the "Belmont Paper," but neither quite matches the National Commission's three principles. Walters, however, comes very close to a formulation of the concerns in practical ethics to which the National Commission applies its principles. All meeting books are housed in the archives of the Kennedy Institute of Ethics Library, Georgetown University.

4. "On the Origins and Future of the *Belmont Report*," in *Belmont Revisited: Ethical Principles for Research*, ed. James F. Childress, Eric M. Meslin, and Harold T. Shapiro (Washington, DC: Georgetown University Press, 2005), 3–11.

5. The paper was published as "Distributive Justice and Morally Relevant Differences," in *Appendix I to the Belmont Report*, 6.1–6.20. This paper was distributed at the 22nd meeting of the National Commission, held in September 1976, seven months after the retreat at the Belmont Conference House.

6. My first day in attendance at a National Commission meeting was the Saturday meeting of the National Commission on January 8, 1977.

7. The National Research Act, P.L. 93-348, July 12, 1974. Congress charged the National Commission with recommending regulations to the Department of Health, Education, and Welfare (DHEW) to protect the rights of research subjects and developing ethical principles to govern the conduct of research. In this respect, the *Belmont Report* was at the core of the tasks the National Commission had been assigned by Congress. DHEW's conversion of its grants administration *policies* governing the conduct of research involving human subjects into formal *regulations* applicable to the entire department was relevant to the creation of the National Commission. In the U.S. Senate, Senator Edward Kennedy, with Jacob Javits's support, was calling for a permanent, *regulatory* commission independent of the National Institutes of Health (NIH) to protect the welfare and rights of human subjects. Paul Rogers in the House supported the NIH in advocating that the commission be *advisory* only. Kennedy agreed to yield to Rogers if DHEW published satisfactory regulations. This compromise was accepted. Regulations were published on May 30, 1974; then, on July 12, 1974, P.L. 93-348 was modified to authorize the National Commission as an advisory body. Charles McCarthy helped me understand this history. For a useful framing of the more general regulatory history, see Joseph V. Brady and Albert R. Jonsen (two commissioners), "The Evolution of Regulatory Influences on Research with Human Subjects," in *Human Subjects Research*, ed. Robert Greenwald, Mary Kay Ryan, and James E. Mulvihill, (New York: Plenum Press, 1982), 3–18.

8. This draft had a history beginning with the 16th meeting (March 12–14, 1976), which contained a draft dated March 1, 1976, and titled "Identification of Basic Ethical Principles." This document summarized the relevant historical background and set forth the three "underlying ethical principles" that came to form the National Commission's framework. Each principle was discussed in a single paragraph. This document was slightly recast in a draft of June 3, 1976 (prepared for the ninth meeting, June 11–13, 1976), in which the discussion of principles was shortened to little more than one page devoted to all three principles. Surprisingly, in the summary statement (p. 9), "respect for persons" is presented as the principle of "autonomy." No further draft was presented to the National Commission until ten months later, at the 29th meeting (April 8–9, 1977). I began work on the document in January 1977.

Transcripts of the National Commission's meetings are also available in the archives of the Kennedy Institute of Ethics at Georgetown University. See National Commission for the Protection of Human Subjects of Biomedical and Behavioral Research. Archived Materials 1974–78, General Category: "Transcript of the Meeting Proceedings" (for discussion of the "Belmont Paper" at the following meetings: February 11–13, 1977; July 8–9, 1977; April 14–15, 1978; and June 9–10, 1978).

9. Cf. the radical differences between the draft available at the 19th meeting (June 1–13, 1976) and the draft at the 29th meeting (April 8–9, 1977). The drafts show that the critical period that gave shape to the *Belmont* principles was the period between January and April 1977. Less dramatic improvements were made between April 1977 and eventual publication more than a year later.

10. Jay Katz, with the assistance of Alexander Capron and Eleanor Glass, eds., *Experimentation with Human Beings* (New York: Russell Sage Foundation, 1972).

11. The first and only footnote in the *Belmont Report* is a reference to this background reading. Typical materials that I examined during this period include *United States v. Karl Brandt, Trials of War Criminals Before the Nuremberg Military Tribunals Under Control Council Law* No. 10, 1948–49, Military Tribunal I (Washington, DC: U.S. Government Printing Office, 1948–1949), vols. 1 and 2, reproduced in part in Katz, *Experimentation with Human Beings,* 292–306; American Medical Association, House of Delegates, Judicial Council, "Supplementary Report of the Judicial Council," *Journal of the American Medical Association* 132 (1946): 90; World Health Organization, 18th World Medical Assembly, Helsinki, Finland, "Declaration of Helsinki: Recommendations Guiding Medical Doctors in Biomedical Research Involving Human Subjects," *New England Journal of Medicine* 271 (1964): 473, reprinted in Katz, *Experimentation with Human Beings,* 312–313. Less helpful than I had hoped was Henry Beecher, "Some Guiding Principles for Clinical Investigation," *Journal of the American Medical Association* 195 (1966): 1135–1136. For behavioral research, I started with Stuart E. Golann, "Ethical Standards for Psychology: Development and Revisions, 1938-1968," *Annals of the New York Academy of Sciences* 169 (1970): 398–405, and American Psychological Association, Inc., *Ethical Principles in the Conduct of Research with Human Participants* (Washington, DC: APA, 1973).

12. For a clearer presentation of this viewpoint in a later document by a government-initiated commission, see several chapters in Advisory Committee on Human Radiation Experiments (ACHRE), *Final Report of the Advisory Committee on Human Radiation Experiments* (New York: Oxford University Press, 1996).

13. See, e.g., Eric Meslin et al., "Principlism and the Ethical Appraisal of Clinical Trials," *Bioethics* 9 (1995): 399–403; Bernard Gert, Charles M. Culver, and K. Danner Clouser, *Bioethics: A Return to Fundamentals* (New York: Oxford University Press, 1997), 72–74; and Jonathan D. Moreno, *Deciding Together: Bioethics and Consensus* (New York: Oxford University Press, 1995), 76–78. Meslin et al. say that "Beauchamp and Childress's *Principles of Biomedical Ethics* . . . is the most rigorous presentation of the principles initially described in the *Belmont Report*" (p. 403). Gert et al. see *Principles* as having "emerged from the work of the National Commission" (p. 71). Moreno presumes that Beauchamp and Childress "brought the three [*Belmont*] principles into bioethical analysis more generally." The thesis that the idea of an abstract framework of principles for bioethics originated with the National Commission has been sufficiently prevalent that authors and lecturers have occasionally cited the principles as Childress and I have named and articulated them and then felt comfortable in attributing these same principles to the National Commission.

14. The draft of *Belmont* that appeared in typescript for the National Commission meeting of December 2, 1977 (37th meeting) shows several similarities to various passages in the first edition *of Principles of Biomedical Ethics.* Childress and I had completed our manuscript by this date, but *Belmont* would be taken through five more drafts presented to the commissioners, the last being presented at the final (43rd) meeting (September 8, 1978).

15. Prior to my involvement with the National Commission, and prior to the *Belmont* retreat, Childress and I had lectured and written about principles of biomedical ethics. In early 1976, coincidentally at about the same time of the *Belmont* retreat, Childress and I

wrote a programmatic idea for the book, based on our lectures, which we submitted to Oxford University Press. We had already developed a general conception of what later came to be called by some commentators "midlevel principles."

For more on the nature, history, and defensibility of a commitment to such midlevel principles in bioethics, see Gert, Culver, and Clouser, *Bioethics: A Return to Fundamentals,* 72ff; Tom Beauchamp and David DeGrazia, "Principlism," in *Bioethics: A Philosophical Overview,* vol. 1 of *Handbook of the Philosophy of Medicine,* ed. George Khusfh (Dordrecht, Netherlands: Kluwer, 2002); James Childress, "Ethical Theories, Principles, and Casuistry in Bioethics: An Interpretation and Defense of Principlism," in *Religious Methods and Resources in Bioethics,* ed. Paul F. Camenisch (Boston: Kluwer, 1994), 181–201; Beauchamp, "The Four Principles Approach to Medical Ethics," in *Principles of Health Care Ethics,* ed. R. Gillon, (London: John Wiley & Sons, 1994), 3–12; Beauchamp, "The Role of Principles in Practical Ethics," in *Philosophical Perspectives on Bioethics,* ed. L. W. Sumner and J. Boyle (Toronto: University of Toronto Press, 1996); and Earl Winkler, "Moral Philosophy and Bioethics: Contextualism versus the Paradigm Theory," in *Philosophical Perspectives on Bioethics,* ed. L. W. Sumner and J. Boyle (Toronto: University of Toronto Press, 1996).

16. Particularly insightful is Ernest Marshall, "Does the Moral Philosophy of the *Belmont Report* Rest on a Mistake?" *IRB: A Review of Human Subjects Research* 8 (1986): 5–6. See also John Fletcher, "Abortion Politics, Science, and Research Ethics: Take Down the Wall of Separation," *Journal of Contemporary Health Law and Policy* 8 (1992): 95–121, esp. sect. 4, "Resources in Research Ethics: Adequacy of the *Belmont* Report."

17. Albert Jonsen, a commissioner, reports in *The Birth of Bioethics* (New York: Oxford University Press, 1998) that I was "working with [Stephen] Toulmin on subsequent drafts" of the *Belmont Report* in 1977. Although I sat next to Stephen in National Commission meetings and conversed with him about many subjects during meetings of the National Commission throughout 1977, we never jointly drafted, worked on, or discussed *Belmont* until it was in near-final form and already approved by the commissioners. Stephen had been assigned to a project on recombinant DNA and did not participate in *Belmont* drafts after I came to the National Commission.

18. Yesley was my constant critic, more so than anyone else. Seldin was my constant counsel, forever exhorting me to make the document more philosophically credible. Patricia King taught me more about the National Commission and its commissioners than anyone else. It was she who helped me understand why a really philosophical document was not the most desirable result.

19. Jonsen reports in *The Birth of Bioethics* (p. 103) that "the date is uncertain" of this meeting at his home (and see his "On the Origins and Future of the *Belmont Report,*" p. 5). In fact, the date is the afternoon of September 21 through September 23, 1977 (which includes the travel period). Jonsen correctly remarks that one purpose of this meeting was to revisit "the February 1977 deliberations" of the commissioners, but he incorrectly reports that the meeting was called "to revise the June 1976 draft." Except for a section on boundaries written by Robert Levine, the June 1976 draft had been so heavily recast that *Belmont* was by September a completely different document. Seven months of continual redrafting of *Belmont* had occurred, from February to September 1977, prior to the meeting

at his home. The National Commission did not discuss the draft reports at its meetings during those seven months. (The last discussion occurred in February). However, "staff drafts" of the "Belmont Paper" were distributed at two meetings during this period, namely, the 29th meeting (April 8–9, 1977) and the 30th meeting (May 13–14, 1977). All drafts are now housed in the archives of the Kennedy Institute of Ethics Library.

20. See Henry S. Richardson, "Specifying Norms as a Way to Resolve Concrete Ethical Problems," *Philosophy and Public Affairs* 19 (1990): 279–310; Richardson, "Specifying, Balancing, and Interpreting Bioethical Principles," *Journal of Medicine and Philosophy* 25 (2000): 285–307, an updated version of which appears in *Belmont Revisited: Ethical Principles for Research*, ed. Childress, Meslin, and Shapiro, 205–227. See also Tom Beauchamp and James Childress, *Principles of Biomedical Ethics*, 5th ed. (New York: Oxford University Press, 2001), 15–19; David DeGrazia, "Moving Forward in Bioethical Theory: Theories, Cases, and Specified Principlism," *Journal of Medicine and Philosophy* 17 (1992): 511–539; DeGrazia and Beauchamp, "Philosophical Foundations and Philosophical Methods," in *Method in Medical Ethics*, ed. Jeremy Sugarman and Daniel P. Sulmasy (Washington, DC: Georgetown University Press, 2001), esp. 31–46.

21. I have diary notes that our editing meetings occurred May 31–June 1, 1978, just prior to the National Commission's 42nd and penultimate meeting, on June 9–10, 1978. Thus, the wording at the 42nd meeting was the final wording unless a commissioner raised an objection at that meeting or the next.

22. As used here, *casuistry* implies that some forms of moral reasoning and judgment neither appeal to nor rely upon principles and rules, but rather involve appeals to the grounding of moral judgment in narratives, paradigm cases, analogies, models, classification schemes, and even immediate intuition and discerning insight. Each change in the circumstances changes the case. The casuistic method begins with cases whose moral features and conclusions have already been decided and then compares the salient features in the paradigm cases with the features of cases that require a decision. See Albert Jonsen and Stephen Toulmin, *Abuse of Casuistry* (Berkeley: University of California Press, 1988), 251–254, 296–299; Jonsen, "On the Origins and Future of the *Belmont Report*," in *Belmont Revisited*, 3–11; Jonsen, "Casuistry as Methodology in Clinical Ethics," *Theoretical Medicine* 12 (1991): 299–302; John Arras, "Principles and Particularity: The Role of Cases in Bioethics," *Indiana Law Journal* 69 (1994): 983–1014. See also Toulmin, "The Tyranny of Principles," *Hastings Center Report* 11 (1981): 31–39.

23. Jonsen and Toulmin, *Abuse of Casuistry*, 16–19.

24. A few years ago, I reviewed all the National Commission transcripts pertaining to *Belmont*, primarily to study the National Commission's method of treating issues in research ethics. I found that Jonsen and Toulmin had occasionally mentioned casuistry, but they clearly understood the National Commission's casuistry as consistent with its invocation of moral principles. For additional discussion, see Stephen Toulmin, "The National Commission on Human Experimentation: Procedures and Outcomes," in *Scientific Controversies: Case Studies in the Resolution and Closure of Disputes in Science and Technology*, ed. H. T. Engelhardt Jr. and A. Caplan (New York: Cambridge University Press, 1987), 599–613, and Jonsen, "Casuistry as Methodology in Clinical Ethics."

25. See, e.g., Alexander Capron, "Looking Back at the President's Commission," *Hastings Center Report* 13, no. 5 (1983): 8–9.

26. See Jonsen's own summation to this effect in "Casuistry," *Methods of Bioethics*, ed. Sugarman and Sulmasy, 112–113, and his Introduction to a reprinting of the *Belmont Report* in *Source Book in Bioethics*, ed. Albert Jonsen, Robert M. Veatch, and LeRoy Walters (Washington, DC: Georgetown University Press, 1998).

27. Albert Jonsen, "Case Analysis in Clinical Ethics," *Journal of Clinical Ethics* 1 (1990): 65.

28. Jonsen, "Case Analysis in Clinical Ethics": 65.

29. Jonsen, "Casuistry: An Alternative or Complement to Principles?" *Kennedy Institute of Ethics Journal* 5 (1995): 237–251.

30. Jonsen, "Casuistry: An Alternative or Complement to Principles?" 244–249. See also Jonsen, "The Weight and Weighing of Ethical Principles," in *The Ethics of Research Involving Human Subjects: Facing the 21st Century,* ed. Harold Y. Vanderpool (Frederick, MD: University Publishing Group, 1996), 59–82.

2

CODES, DECLARATIONS, AND OTHER ETHICAL GUIDANCE FOR HUMAN SUBJECTS RESEARCH: THE *BELMONT REPORT*

The *Belmont Report* is a short document on moral principles that was published in 1978 by the National Commission for the Protection of Human Subjects of Biomedical and Behavioral Research (hereafter the National Commission). Since that time it has provided a basic framework for analyzing ethical issues that arise during medical research in the United States as well as in other countries.

HISTORY

The National Commission was established in 1974 by the U.S. Congress with a charge to identify ethical principles and develop guidelines to govern the conduct of research involving humans. It was hoped the guidelines would ensure that the basic ethical principles would become embedded in the U.S. research oversight system, so that meaningful protection was afforded to research participants. Another mandated goal was to distinguish the boundaries between the accepted and routine practice of medicine on the one hand, and biomedical and behavioral research on the other.

The National Commission held its first meeting on December 3–4, 1974, and its 43rd and final meeting on September 8, 1978.[1] It completed a draft of the *Belmont Report* in late 1977, and issued it in final published form on September 30, 1978. The report was then republished in the *Federal Register* on April 18, 1979—a date now commonly cited as the original date of publication.

The National Commission also published 16 other reports and appendix volumes, most focused on ethical issues in research involving vulnerable populations. Its more than 100 recommendations for reform went directly to the Secretary of the Department of Health, Education and Welfare (DHEW)—later remodeled and made the Department of Health and Human Services (DHHS). Many of the National Commission's recommendations were eventually codified as federal regulations.[2] The *Belmont Report* itself was not written in the style of federal regulations and was never so codified. It was the National Commission's statement of a general, principled moral framework. The foundation of this "analytical framework," as it is called in the report, was a collection of moral principles appropriate for research that first emerged during discussions at a retreat the National Commission held on February 13–16, 1976, at the Smithsonian Institution's Belmont Conference Center in Elkridge, Maryland. There had been no draft or planning for this framework prior to the retreat. This conference center's name was then appropriated, and the report was published under the full title of *The Belmont Report: Ethical Principles and Guidelines for the Protection of Human Subjects of Research.*

The National Commission came into existence in the aftermath of public outrage and congressional uncertainty over the Tuskegee syphilis experiments and other questionable uses of humans in research. The socioeconomic deprivation of the African American men who were enrolled in the Tuskegee experiments made them vulnerable to overt and unjustifiable forms of manipulation at the hands of health professionals, as had been widely reported in news media and widely circulated in the report of an advisory panel to the DHEW in 1973.[3] Other reports of the abuse of fetuses, prisoners, children, and "the institutionalized mentally infirm" appeared in the news media.

The law that created the National Commission specified that no more than 5 of the Commission's 11 members could be research investigators (see Table 1). This stipulation testified to congressional determination at the time that research activities of the biomedical and behavioral sciences be brought under the critical eye, and possibly the control, of persons outside of the sciences. At that time, the research system generally placed responsibility for the protection of humans in research on the shoulders of individual investigators. That is, federal policies relied on the discretion and good judgment of investigators to determine the conditions under which research should be conducted. Federal involvement and review committees were then in the formative stages. They were destined to undergo rapid change toward protectionism under the guidance of the National Commission.

Carol Levine offers the following sobering and accurate statement of the context in which the National Commission deliberated:

The Belmont Report ... reflected the history of the 30 years immediately preceding it. This emphasis is understandable, given the signal event in the modern history of clinical-research ethics [Nazi experimentation]. American public opinion was shaped by the revelations of unethical experiments such as the Willowbrook hepatitis B studies,... the Jewish Chronic Disease Hospital studies,... and, especially, the Tuskegee Syphilis Study.... Our

TABLE 2.1   Members of the National Commission for the Protection of Human Subjects of Biomedical and Behavioral Research

- Kenneth John Ryan, M.D., Chairman, Chief of Staff, Boston Hospital for Women
- Joseph V. Brady, Ph.D., Professor of Behavioral Biology, Johns Hopkins University
- Robert E. Cooke, M.D., President, Medical College of Pennsylvania
- Dorothy I. Height, President, National Council of Negro Women, Inc.
- Albert R. Jonsen, Ph.D., Associate Professor of Bioethics, University of California at San Francisco
- Patricia King, J.D., Associate Professor of Law, Georgetown University Law Center
- Karen Lebacqz, Ph.D., Associate Professor of Christian Ethics, Pacific School of Religion
- David W. Louisell, J.D., Professor of Law, University of California at Berkeley
- Donald W. Seldin, M.D., Professor and Chairman, Department of Internal Medicine, Southwestern Medical School, University of Texas
- Eliot Stellar, Ph.D., Provost of the University and Professor of Physiological Psychology, University of Pennsylvania
- Robert H. Turtle, LL.B., Attorney, VomBaur, Coburn, Simmons and Turtle, Washington, D.C.

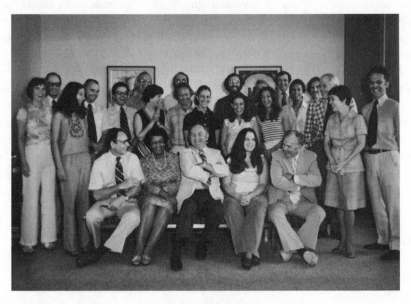

FIGURE 2.1   Commissioners and Staff of the National Commission for the Protection of Human Subjects of Biomedical and Behavioral Research, 1977.

basic approach to the ethical conduct of research and approval of investigational drugs was born in scandal and reared in protectionism. Perceived as vulnerable, either because of their membership in groups lacking social power or because of personal characteristics suggesting a lack of autonomy, individuals were the primary focus of this concern.[4]

CONTENT AND CORE STRENGTHS

The *Belmont Report* is best known for its framework of basic moral principles, which are still today referred to as the *"Belmont* principles." The National Commission identified three general principles as underlying the conduct of research: respect for persons, beneficence, and justice. The key organizing conception underlying the National Commission's presentation of these principles and their use was the following: Respect for persons applies to informed consent; beneficence applies to risk–benefit assessment; and justice applies to the selection of research participants. The following abstract schema represents this conception:

Principle of	*Applies to*
Respect for persons	Informed consent
Beneficence	Risk–benefit assessment
Justice	Selection of research subjects

In this way, each moral principle makes moral demands in a specific domain of responsibility for research. This conception of the connection between abstract moral principles and applied bioethics has been enduring. Many engaged in research ethics carry this general conception with them today.

The principle of respect for persons demands that the choices of autonomous persons not be overridden or otherwise disrespected and that persons who are not adequately autonomous be protected by the consent of an authorized third party who is likely to appreciate their circumstances and will look after their best interests. This principle in effect requires valid permission before investigators can proceed with research. To achieve this goal, the principle insists on the individual's informed consent, analyzed in terms of the conditions of information disclosure, comprehension, and voluntariness. The National Commission proposed "the reasonable volunteer" as an appropriate standard for judging the adequacy and clarity of information disclosure. Investigators are held responsible for ascertaining that research participants have comprehended the information they have been given about the proposed research. The purpose of consent provisions is not protection from risk, as earlier federal policies seemed to imply, but protection of autonomy and personal dignity, including the personal dignity of incompetent persons incapable of acting autonomously. The report went on to suggest that third parties should be encouraged to follow the research as it proceeds and should be aware of the right to withdraw an incompetent person from his or her research participation throughout the process.

The principle of beneficence is an abstract norm that includes rules such as "Do no harm," "Balance benefits against risks," and "Maximize possible benefits and minimize possible harms." This principle is satisfied in the research context by refraining from intentionally causing injury and by ensuring that risks are reasonable in relation to probable benefits. The National Commission required that there be an array of data pertaining to benefits and risks and of alternative ways of obtaining the benefits (if any) sought from involvement in research. It demanded that, if possible, systematic and nonarbitrary presentations of risks and benefits be made to research participants as part of the informed consent process and that the assessment of risks and safeguards be considered by an institutional review board (IRB) in weighing the justifiability of research protocols. The National Commission stated that participants ought not to be asked or allowed to consent to more risk than is warranted by anticipated benefits and that forms of risk incommensurate with participants' previous experience should not be imposed in the case of groups such as children, who might be overburdened and possibly disturbed or terrified. However, the report recognized that risks must be permitted during the course of many forms of research in order for investigators to be positioned to distinguish harmful from beneficial outcomes.

The principle of justice requires fairness in the distribution of both the burdens and the benefits of research. The National Commission insisted that this principle requires special levels of protection for vulnerable and disadvantaged parties. This principle demands that researchers first seek out and select persons best prepared to bear the burdens of research (e.g., healthy adults) and that they not offer research only to groups who have been repeatedly targeted (e. g., mentally retarded children). The National Commission noted that, historically, the burdens of research were placed heavily on the economically disadvantaged, the very sick, and the vulnerable, owing to their ready availability. This conclusion was based on published data, reports in the media, public testimony to the National Commission, and some onsite visits to places such as prisons. The overutilization of readily available, and often compromised, segments of the U.S. population was a matter of deep moral concern to the National Commission. The theme of justice and proper selection of research participants was the *Belmont Report's* way of saying that because medical research is a social enterprise for the public good, it must be accomplished in a broadly inclusive and participatory way. If participation in research is unwelcome and falls on a narrow spectrum of citizens because of their ready availability, then it is unwarranted. Likewise, the National Commission recommended that persons who are already burdened by some form of disability or institutionalization should not be asked to accept the burdens of research—unless, as occurs in some cases, other participants cannot be located or are otherwise inappropriate.

The *Belmont Report* includes not only these three abstract principles and their analysis but also a moral view that moves modestly in the direction of an applied research ethics. Just as there is a distinction between theoretical or general ethics and applied or practical ethics, so the National Commission thought of the *Belmont Report* as its statement of a brief theoretical framework. Because of its practical and policy objectives, the explanation of the principles had a notably applied character. Even so, the National Commission had no ambition to make the report itself specific and practical for institutions that conduct research. This objective was to be accomplished by the other 16 volumes on problems of research ethics and recommendations for public policy that the National Commission issued. The *Belmont Report* itself was intended to provide only a general framework of basic principles.

National Commission members and staff were keenly aware that this framework was too indeterminate by itself to decide practice or policy or to resolve moral conflicts. The process of molding the general principles in the *Belmont Report* so that they become sufficiently concrete is a process of reducing the indeterminateness and abstractness of the principles to give them increased action-guiding capacity. The report looks to educational institutions, professional associations, government agencies, and IRBs to provide the more specific rules and judgments required for research ethics.

The works of philosophers such as W. D. Ross and William Frankena were often consulted in the drafting of the *Belmont Report,* but the moral principles featured in the report should not be read as deriving from the writings of philosophers. The *Belmont Report* made reference to values "generally accepted in our cultural tradition" as the basis of its principles. These principles derived from National Commission members' understanding of social morality, and these commissioners may have been confusing social morality with universal morality. We will never know what the commissioners meant by our "tradition," but the import of the *Belmont* principles is not to be tied to the unique views of a particular tradition or nation. The National Commission apparently conceived of its principles as universally valid norms. That is, the principles were taken to be applicable to all contexts of human research, not merely to some local region, such as an institution or a nation. The presumption is that no responsible research investigator could conduct research without reference to these principles; these principles form the core of any policy worthy of the name "research ethics."

WEAKNESSES, DEFICIENCIES, AND UNCLARITIES

Despite the *Belmont Report's* wide acceptance, several issues have been or can be raised about the adequacy of the *Belmont* principles. Here are six possible problems.

1. The way the principles are delineated is arguably confused, especially the principle of respect for persons. This principle appears to confusingly blend two principles: a principle of respect for autonomy and a principle of protecting and avoiding harm to incompetent (nonautonomous) persons. The National Commission said that it was attempting to protect both autonomous persons and those with "diminished autonomy," that is, those who are incapable of self-determination. Both are persons, it said, and both are entitled to protection.

The question is whether protections for persons who are incapable of self-determination can be justified in any way other than by the principle of beneficence. If not, the criticism goes, then the National Commission has adopted an incoherent position in thinking that respect for persons and beneficence are independent principles. Robert Veatch seems to both criticize and defend the National Commission for this apparent confusion:

> The Belmont Report offers a three-principle theory that uses the Kantian term: "respect for persons." It subsumes autonomy under this broader notion, but in a strange way it also subsumes the welfare of the incompetent under respect for persons. This is hard to defend. Autonomy may be an element of a more fundamental notion of respect for persons, but it seems that the duty to serve the welfare of the incompetent is straightforwardly a part of the duty of beneficence. Nevertheless, if respect for persons includes autonomy, it could include other elements as well ... [I myself include] principles other than autonomy as part of respect for persons. If respect for persons includes only respect for autonomy, then nonautonomous persons are left stranded... Respecting persons must involve... Veracity... Fidelity to promises... [and] Avoidance of killing.[5]

Veatch is suggesting that although the National Commission erred in its explication of respect for persons, its general viewpoint could be reconstructed and rendered viable.

However, there remains the problem of whether there is any meaningful way to justify protections for persons who are incapable of self-determination except by appeal to a principle such as beneficence or justice. What is it to respect an incompetent person if it is not to act beneficently or justly in regard to the person? Accordingly, the appropriate principle to determine one's commitments would seem to be either beneficence or justice, or both. It is the *welfare* of the incompetent person that the National Commission seeks to protect, not the *personhood* of the incompetent person. If this view is correct, then the National Commission has adopted an incoherent position by thinking that respect for persons and beneficence, and perhaps justice, are independent principles.

However, there is apparently a hidden target implicitly at work in the National Commission's choice of the language of "persons." The principle of respect for persons seems to be functioning to give incompetent persons a *moral status* that is functionally equivalent to the moral status autonomous persons possess. That is, the principle is functioning for the National Commission as a way of saying that the absence of autonomy must not lead to the neglect, disadvantage, or lowered esteem of incompetent individuals and those in vulnerable populations, and that such persons have a right to appropriate third-party consent. In short, the National Commission was attempting to handle issues of the moral status of incompetent individuals through its interpretation of the principle of respect for persons.

2. The National Commission was very concerned that using utilitarian justifications of research had become too easy in the biomedical world. The Nazi experiments, Tuskegee, and the Jewish Chronic Disease Hospital cases all seemed to have been driven by a very utilitarian view of (social) beneficence that justified using humans on grounds of benefit to the broader public. However, the National Commission itself has been accused of having inadequate internal controls in its moral framework to protect research participants against abuse when there is the promise of major benefit for society. Two National Commission members, Robert Cooke and Robert Turtle, sternly criticized the National Commission's report on children on grounds that it had presented an unjustifiable utilitarian justification of research that placed children at undue risk.[6,7]

Whatever the merits of this criticism, the *Belmont Report* was written with the intent to rectify what was perceived as an imbalance favoring social utility in the justification of research. That is, a major purpose of the report was to properly balance the interests of research participants with those of science and society. Considerations of autonomy, justice, and risk control were set out to limit utilitarian overbalancing and investigator discretion. However, it is doubtful that the question of how best to control utilitarian balancing was ever resolved by the National Commission.

3. Paradoxically, the *Belmont Report,* and the National Commission more generally, can be criticized for being overly protective of research participants— and, consequently, as insufficiently utilitarian to meet the needs of certain classes of persons. The National Commission's emphasis was on the protection of persons from research injury. Research participation was conceived as a burden that individuals accepted in order to advance the public good and that should be distributed equitably. It is unclear why this assumption was so deep in the National Commission's work, but it can likely be explained by the atmosphere of scandal that had emerged at the time. The nature and acceptability of the public's interest in research and the goals of research were little-explored matters in the *Belmont Report*. The notion that research is not always viewed by partici- pants as burdensome was underexamined.

The AIDS epidemic altered this mindset, perhaps forever. Whereas the *Belmont Report* sought to protect research participants, AIDS activists sought not protec- tion from, but inclusion in, the research process. They wanted justice and respect for their autonomy, but not along the lines of justice and autonomy staked out in the *Belmont Report*. They wanted to be able to choose unapproved drugs; con- siderations of justice, they thought, should be used to allow them access to clinical trials. To them, the *Belmont* principles could be interpreted as protectionist to the point of excluding those who might benefit from research and from access to potentially beneficial drugs. In the end, this push for inclusion in research and broader access to the potential benefits of research altered the course of research ethics. Whether this development constitutes an expansion in the scope and use of the *Belmont* principles or a confrontation with these principles is debatable, but it certainly reconfigured research ethics.[4,8]

4. The *Belmont Report* has also been criticized for its abstractness and inability to resolve or otherwise treat practical moral problems. The report anticipated this criticism and cautioned that its principles "cannot always be applied so as to resolve beyond dispute particular ethical problems. The objective is [only] to provide an analytical framework that will guide the resolution of ethical problems arising from research involving human subjects." The National Commission thus warned readers that they should not expect to use *Belmont* principles as a checklist of federal regulations or as guidelines like recipes in cooking. Nonetheless, several critics have asked whether these principles are in any meaningful respect practical, or even useful. The concern is that norms as general as the *Belmont* principles underdetermine almost all moral judgments because they are abstract and contain too little content to determine concrete judgments.

Danner Clouser and Bernard Gert have objected to the *Belmont* principles and all related analytical frameworks, contending that principles function more like chapter headings in a book than as directive rules and theories. Therefore, receiving no directive guidance from the principle, anyone who is working on a problem in bioethics is left free to deal with that principle in his or her own way and may give it whatever meaning and significance he or she wishes. Consider justice. The *Belmont* principle of justice in the selection of research participants instructs a moral agent to be alert to various matters of justice, but does such a general principle actually guide conduct? Other moral considerations besides the principle(s) of justice, such as moral intuitions and ethical theories, may be needed to do the real work of ethical reflection.[9-11]

This criticism merits careful attention, but can any system of principles, rules, or general guidelines escape this problem? Clouser and Gert maintain that some general moral rules can provide deep and directive substance, but these authors have had difficulty in clarifying and justifying this claim. Their point is no doubt correct for unspecified principles, but all abstract principles and rules will need some sort of specification in context to become directive. The National Commission anticipated this problem. It did not advance the *Belmont* principles as sufficient for resolving problems, but only as a starting point. The National Commission noted that "other principles may be relevant" and that its principles should be able to "serve as a basic justification for" more "particular prescriptions and evaluations."

5. The *Belmont Report* has also been faulted for another, but closely related, reason: It gave no indication of how to prioritize or weigh its principles. Several commentators assert that the National Commission should have argued that one or more of its principles has priority—for example, that considerations of respect for persons and justice take priority over considerations of social benefit.[5,7,12] These critics support a model of basic moral principles and protections that cannot be violated under any circumstances, even if there is a clear and substantial benefit for society. Such restrictions—often said to be deontological in contrast to utilitarian—are analogous to constitutional rights that constrain conduct and prohibit balancing of interests in various political and social matters. Some who propose such an ordinal or priority ranking of principles argue that it is the morally correct view, but others are more concerned to show that the National Commission has not found a way out of situations in which its own principles come into conflict. Some critics also point out that a priority ranking of the sort they propose to mitigate conflict between beneficence and either autonomy or social justice would allow the National Commission to escape the accusation that its schema too readily invites utilitarian justifications of research protocols.

Other commentators have argued that the National Commission was correct in its assumption that the principles are more or less weighty depending on the particular circumstances in which they are to be applied. Accounts of this sort are often referred to as balancing theories. Such theories do not allow any principle in the basic analytical framework to have an ordered priority over any other principle. That is, there is neither a hierarchical ranking of principles nor an a priori weighting of principles. When principles conflict, the balance of right over wrong must be determined by assessing the weight of competing considerations as they emerge in the circumstance. What agents ought to do is determined by what they ought to do, all things considered. This appears to be the view presumed in the *Belmont Report*, and it seems also to be the view currently accepted in federal regulations for protocol review, waivers of consent, and the like.[13–15]

6. One former National Commission member, Albert Jonsen, and one staff member, Stephen Toulmin, have jointly questioned whether the National Commission actually used its framework of *Belmont* principles to support or defend its own bioethical conclusions. They have argued that the National Commission members wrote their documents as principlists, but actually worked as casuists. This thesis is not a criticism of the National Commission's substantive work, only a methodological comment on the use and limits of its principles. These authors hold that the National Commission's actual moral deliberations proceeded by the consideration of influential cases rather than by appeal to universal principles, and they think, more generally, that this paradigm of reasoning is the best method in bioethics. Jonsen and Toulmin present this understanding of the National Commission's work as follows:

> The one thing [individual Commissioners] could not agree on was why they agreed.... Instead of securely established universal principles,... giving them intellectual grounding for particular judgments about specific kinds of cases, it was the other way around.... The *locus of certitude* in the Commissioners' discussions... lay in a shared perception of what was specifically at stake in particular kinds of human situations.... That could never have been derived from the supposed theoretical certainty of the principles to which individual Commissioners appealed in their personal accounts.

The point is that National Commission members reasoned by appeal to particular cases and families of cases, and reached consensus through agreement on central cases and on generalization from sets of cases. Principles were therefore of lesser importance than readers might suppose when they read the *Belmont Report*. Although the *Belmont* principles are important guiding ideals, they are, in this estimate, overrated if revered for their practicality. Although Jonsen has supported the moral principles delineated in the *Belmont Report*, he has also maintained that in practical ethics, these principles must be interpreted and specified by the force of examples and counterexamples that emerge from experience with cases.[18] From this perspective, the National Commission used principles primarily as general guiding ideals.

ENDURING LEGACY AND INFLUENCE

The *Belmont Report* is one of the few documents to influence almost every sphere of activity in bioethics: moral theory and general standards of research ethics, government regulatory activity, bioethics consultation, and even medical practice. Its influence has arguably been as extensive in practice as in theory.

Many interested in the role of moral theory and principles in bioethics have honored the *Belmont Report* for its framework of principles, even if those principles have not been widely analyzed in this literature. As Dan Brock has observed, "The Belmont Report... had great impact on bioethics because it addressed the moral principles that underlay the various reports on particular aspects of research."[19] Brock is noting the influence of the idea that a body of principles can be used to frame and discuss a wide range of practical moral problems.

In federal regulatory oversight and law, the *Belmont Report* has at times assumed a near canonical role. The Advisory Committee on Human Radiation Experiments noted in 1995 that

> Many conditions coalesced [historically] into the framework for the regulation of the use of human subjects in federally funded research that is the basis for today's system. . . . [T]his framework is undergirded by the three Belmont principles. The federal regulations and the conceptual framework built on the Belmont principles became so widely adopted and cited that it might be argued that their establishment marked the end of serious shortcomings in federal research ethics policies.[20]

Similarly, an Institute of Medicine report, issued by its Committee on Assessing the System for Protecting Human Research Participants, stated in 2002 that "The ethical foundations of research protections in the United States can be found in the three tenets identified in the Belmont Report."[21] Moreover, the *Belmont* principles found their way into every document the National Commission published, and these became the backbone of federal law. From this perspective, as Christine Grady has observed, "probably the single most influential body in the United States involved with the protection of human research subjects was the National Commission."[22]

The legacy of *Belmont* may be most enduring in areas of practice. Federal regulations require that all institutions receiving federal funds for research

espouse a statement of principles for the protection of human research participants. Virtually all such institutions have subscribed to the *Belmont* principles as
the basis of their efforts to assess research protocols from an ethical point of view.
Professional associations, too, have widely recognized the authority and historical
significance of the *Belmont* principles.[23] Eric Cassell has even argued that the
Belmont principles have "permeated clinical medicine" as extensively as they have
medical research.[24] His claim is that the *Belmont* principles were a significant force
in a broad cultural shift in medicine toward a reworking of the relationship
between doctor and patient.

Whatever the influence and enduring legacy of *Belmont,* it is not clear
that scientists who are involved today in research with humans are any more
familiar with the *Belmont* principles than their predecessors of several decades
ago were familiar with documents such as the Nuremberg Code. When the
National Commission deliberated, it seemed to some observers that the general
system of protecting human research participants in the United States was in
need of serious repair, that research investigators were not educated about
research ethics, and that participants were not adequately protected. To some
observers, the system seems today caught in a similar state of disrepair. From
1997 to 2002, a large number of hearings, bills, and reports by official, prestigious
government bodies and government-mandated bodies in the United States
concluded that the system of IRB review and the practice of informed consent—the core of research ethics established by the National Commission—are
seriously defective.[8,21]

The National Commission and its *Belmont Report* may have succeeded both in
"resolving" some major problems of research ethics and in bringing "oversight" to
the research context, as historian David Rothman has claimed,[25] but this fix may
have been temporary and time-bound. Today, the *Belmont* principles may be
more revered than they are understood and practiced.

Notes

1. The National Commission for the Protection of Human Subjects of Biomedical and
Behavioral Research. *The Belmont Report: Ethical Principles and Guidelines for the Protection
of Human Subjects of Research.* Washington, DC: Department of Health, Education and
Welfare; DHEW Publication OS 78-0012 1978. Available at: http://www.hhs.gov/ohrp/
humansubjects/guidance/belmont.htm.

2. Department of Health and Human Services, National Institutes of Health, and Office
for Human Research Protections. The Common Rule, Title 45 (Public Welfare), Code of
Federal Regulations, Part 46 (Protection of Human Subjects). Available at: http://www.hhs.
gov/ohrp/humansubjects/guidance/45cfr46.htm.

3. Jones JH. *Bad Blood*, 2nd ed. New York: The Free Press; 1993.

4. Levine C. "Changing views of justice after Belmont: AIDS and the inclusion of 'vulnerable' subjects." In: Vanderpool HY, ed. *The Ethics of Research Involving Human Subjects: Facing the 21st Century*. Frederick, MD: University Publishing Group; 1996: 105–126.

5. Veatch RM. "Resolving conflicts among principles: Ranking, balancing, and specifying." *Kennedy Institute of Ethics Journal* 1995; 5: 199–218.

6. National Commission for the Protection of Human Subjects of Biomedical and Behavioral Research. Archived Materials 1974–78. Transcript of the Meeting Proceedings (for discussion of the Belmont Paper at the following meetings: February 11–13, 1977; July 8–9, 1977; April 14–15, 1978; and June 9–10, 1978), Kennedy Institute Library, Georgetown University, Washington, DC.

7. Marshall E. "Does the moral philosophy of the Belmont Report rest on a mistake?" *IRB: A Review of Human Subjects Research* 1986; 8(6): 5–6.

8. Moreno JD. "Goodbye to all that: The end of moderate protectionism in human subjects research." *Hastings Center Report* 2001; 31(3): 9–17.

9. Clouser KD, Gert B. "Morality vs. principlism." In: Gillon R, Lloyd A, eds. *Principles of Health Care Ethics*. London, England: John Wiley and Sons; 1994: 251–266.

10. Gert B, Culver CM, Clouser KD. *Bioethics: A Return to Fundamentals*. New York: Oxford University Press; 1997: 72–75.

11. Clouser KD, Gert B. "A critique of principlism." *Journal of Medicine and Philosophy* 1990; 15: 219–236.

12. Veatch RM. "From Nuremberg through the 1990s: The priority of autonomy." In: Van-derpool HY, ed. *The Ethics of Research Involving Human Subjects: Facing the 21st Century*. Frederick, MD: University Publishing Group; 1996: 45–58.

13. Ackerman TF. "Choosing between Nuremberg and the National Commission: The balancing of moral principles in clinical research." In Vanderpool HY, ed. *The Ethics of Research Involving Haman Subjects: Facing the 21st Century*. Frederick, MD: University Publishing Group; 1996, 83–104.

14. Beauchamp TL, Childress JF. *Principles of Biomedical Ethics*, 6th ed. New York: Oxford University Press; 2009: Chapters 1, 10.

15. Jonsen AR. "The weight and weighing of ethical principles." In: Vanderpool HY. *The Ethics of Research Involving Human Subjects: Facing the 21st Century*. Frederick, MD: University Publishing Group; 1996: 64–65.

16. Jonsen AR, Toulmin S. *The Abuse of Casuistry*. Berkeley, CA: University of California Press; 1988: 16–19.

17. Toulmin S. "The National Commission on human experimentation: Procedures and outcomes." In: Engelhardt HT Jr., Caplan A, eds. *Scientific Controversies: Case Studies in the Resolution and Closure of Disputes in Science and Technology*. New York: Cambridge University Press; 1987: 599–613.

18. Jonsen AR. "Casuistry." In: Sugarman J, Sulmasy DP, eds. *Methods of Bioethics*. Washington, DC: Georgetown University Press; 2001: 112–113.

19. Brock D. "Public policy and bioethics." In: Reich WT, ed. *Encyclopedia of Bioethics*, 2nd ed. New York: Macmillan Reference; 1995: 2181–2188.

20. Advisory Committee on Human Radiation Experiments. *Final Report of the Advisory Committee on Human Radiation Experiments.* New York: Oxford University Press; 1996.

21. Institute of Medicine, Committee on Assessing the System for Protecting Human Research Participants (Federman DE, Hanna KE, Rodriguez LL, eds.). *Responsible Research: A Systems Approach to Protecting Research Participants.* Washington, DC: National Academies Press; 2002.

22. Grady C. *The Search for an AIDS Vaccine: Ethical Issues in the Development and Testing of a Preventive HIV Vaccine.* Bloomington, IN: Indiana University Press; 1995: 42.

23. Pincus HA, Lieberman JA, Ferris S. *Ethics in Psychiatric Research.* Washington, DC: American Psychiatric Publishing, Inc.; 1999.

24. Cassell EJ. "The principles of the Belmont Report revisited: How have respect for persons, beneficence, and justice been applied to clinical medicine?" *Hastings Center Report* 2000; 30(4): 12–21.

25. Rothman DJ. "Research, human: Historical aspects." In: Reich WT, ed. *Encyclopedia of Bioethics*, 2nd ed. New York: Macmillan Reference; 1995: 2256.

Part II

PRINCIPLISM AND PRACTICE

3

THE FOUR PRINCIPLES APPROACH TO
HEALTH CARE ETHICS

My objective in this essay is to explain the so-called "four principles" approach and to explain the philosophical and practical roles these principles play. I start with a brief history and then turn to the four-principles framework, its practical uses, and philosophical problems of making the abstract framework specific.

THE ORIGINS OF PRINCIPLES IN HEALTH CARE ETHICS

Prior to the early 1970s, there was no firm ground in which a commitment to principles or even ethical theory could take root in biomedical ethics. This is not to say that physicians and researchers had no principled commitments to patients and research subjects. They did, but moral principles, practices, and virtues were rarely discussed. The health care ethics outlook in Europe and America was largely that of maximizing medical benefits and minimizing risks of harm and disease. The Hippocratic tradition had neglected many problems of truthfulness, privacy, justice, communal responsibility, the vulnerability of research subjects, and the like.[1] Views about ethics had been confined largely to the perspectives of those in the professions of medicine, public health, and nursing. No sustained work combined concerns in ethical theory and the health care fields.

Principles that could be understood with relative ease by the members of various disciplines figured prominently in the development of biomedical ethics during the 1970s and early 1980s. Principles were used to present frameworks of evaluative assumptions so that they could be used by, and readily understood by, people with many different forms of professional training. The distilled morality found in principles gave people a shared and serviceable group of general norms for analyzing many types of moral problems. In some respects, it could even be claimed that principles gave the embryonic field of bioethics a shared method for attacking its problems, and this gave some minimal coherence and uniformity to bioethics.

There were two primary sources of the early interest in principles in biomedical ethics. The first was the *Belmont Report* (and related documents) of the National Commission for the Protection of Human Subjects,[2] and the second was the book entitled *Principles of Biomedical Ethics*, which I coauthored with James F. Childress. I here confine discussion to the latter.

Childress and I began our search for the principles of biomedical ethics in 1975. In early 1976, we drafted the main ideas for the book, although only later would the title *Principles of Biomedical Ethics* be placed on it.[3] Our goal was to develop a set of principles suitable for biomedical ethics. One of our proposals was that health care's traditional preoccupation with a beneficence-based model of health care ethics be augmented by an autonomy model, while also incorporating a wider set of social concerns, particularly those focused on social justice. The principles are understood as standards of conduct on which many other moral claims and judgments depend. A principle, then, is an essential norm in a system of moral thought and one that is basic for moral reasoning. More specific rules for health care ethics can be formulated *by reference to* these four principles, but neither rules nor practical judgments can be straightforwardly *deduced* from the principles.

THE FRAMEWORK OF PRINCIPLES

The principles in our framework have always been grouped under four general categories: (1) respect for autonomy (a principle requiring respect for the decision-making capacities of autonomous persons), (2) nonmaleficence (a principle requiring not causing harm to others), (3) beneficence (a group of principles requiring that we prevent harm, provide benefits, and balance benefits against risks and costs), and (4) justice (a group of principles requiring appropriate distribution of benefits, risks, and costs fairly). I will concentrate on an explication of each of the principles and how they are to be understood collectively as a framework.

Respect for Autonomy

Respect for autonomy is rooted in liberal moral and political traditions of the importance of individual freedom and choice. In moral philosophy, personal autonomy refers to personal self-governance: personal rule of the self by adequate understanding while remaining free from controlling interferences by others and from personal limitations that prevent choice. *Autonomy* means freedom from external constraint and the presence of critical mental capacities such as understanding, intending, and voluntary decision making.[4] The autonomous individual acts freely in accordance with a self-chosen plan, analogous to the way an independent government manages its territories and sets its policies. A person of diminished autonomy, by contrast, is in some respect controlled by others or incapable of deliberating or acting on the basis of his or her desires and plans.

To respect an autonomous agent is to recognize with due appreciation that person's capacities and perspectives, including his or her right to hold certain views, to make certain choices, and to take certain actions based on personal values and beliefs. The moral demand that we respect the autonomy of persons can be expressed as a *principle* of respect for autonomy that states both a negative obligation and a positive obligation. As a negative obligation, autonomous actions should not be subjected to controlling constraints by others. As a positive obligation, this principle requires respectful treatment in informational exchanges and in other actions that foster autonomous decision making.

Many autonomous actions could not occur without others' material cooperation in making options available. Respect for autonomy obligates professionals in health care and research involving human subjects to disclose information, to probe for and ensure understanding and voluntariness, and to foster adequate decision making. True respect requires more than mere noninterference in others' personal affairs. It includes, at least in some contexts, building up or maintaining others' capacities for autonomous choice while helping to allay fears and other conditions that destroy or disrupt their autonomous actions. Respect, on this account, involves acknowledging the value and decision-making rights of persons and enabling them to act autonomously, whereas disrespect for autonomy involves attitudes and actions that ignore, insult, demean, or are inattentive to others' rights of autonomy.

Many issues in professional ethics concern failures to respect a person's autonomy, ranging from manipulative underdisclosure of pertinent information to nonrecognition of a refusal of medical interventions. For example, in the debate over whether autonomous, informed patients have the right to refuse medical interventions, the principle of respect for autonomy suggests that an autonomous decision to refuse interventions must be respected. Although it was not until the late 1970s that serious attention was given to the rights of patients to refuse, this is no reason for thinking that respect for autonomy as now understood is a newly added principle in our moral perspective. It simply means that the implications of this principle were not widely appreciated until recently.[5]

Controversial problems with the principle of respect for autonomy, as with all moral principles, arise when we must interpret its significance for particular contexts, determine precise limits on its application, and decide how to handle situations in which it conflicts with other moral principles. Many controversies involve questions about the conditions under which a person's right to autonomous expression demands actions by others, as well as questions about the restrictions society may rightfully place on choices by patients or subjects when these choices conflict with other values. If restriction of the patient's autonomy is in order, the justification will always rest on some competing moral principle such as beneficence or justice.

Nonmaleficence

Physicians have long avowed that they are obligated to avoid doing harm to their patients. Among the most quoted principles in the history of codes of health care ethics is the maxim *primum non nocere*: "Above all, do no harm." British physician Thomas Percival furnished the first developed modern account of health care ethics. He maintained that a principle of nonmaleficence fixes the physician's primary obligations and triumphs even over respect for the patient's autonomy in a circumstance of potential harm to patients:

> To a patient... who makes inquiries which, if faithfully answered, might prove fatal to him, it would be a gross and unfeeling wrong to reveal the truth. His right to it is suspended, and even annihilated; because... it would be deeply injurious to himself, to his family, and to the public. And he has the strongest claim, from the trust reposed in his physician, as well as from the common principles of humanity, to be guarded against whatever would be detrimental to him.[6]

Some basic rules in the common morality are requirements to avoid causing a harm. They include rules such as do not kill; do not cause pain; do not disable; do not deprive of pleasure; do not cheat; and do not break promises.[7] Similar but more specific prohibitions are found across the literature of biomedical ethics, each grounded in the principle that intentionally or negligently caused harm is a fundamental moral wrong.

Numerous problems of nonmaleficence are found in health care ethics today, some involving blatant abuses of persons and others involving subtle and unresolved questions. Blatant examples of failures to act nonmaleficently are found in the use of physicians to classify political dissidents as mentally ill, thereafter treating them with harmful drugs and incarcerating them with insane and violent persons.[8] More subtle examples are found in the use of medications for the treatment of aggressive and destructive patients. These common treatment modalities are helpful to many patients, but they can be harmful to others.

A provocative question about nonmaleficence and physician ethics has been raised by Paul S. Appelbaum in an investigation of "the problem of doing harm" through testimony in criminal contexts and civil litigation— for example, by omitting information in the context of a trial, after which a more severe punishment is delivered to the person than likely would have been delivered. Appelbaum presents the generic problem as one of nonmaleficence:

> If physicians are committed to doing good and avoiding harm, how can they participate in legal proceedings from which harm may result? If, on the other hand, physicians in court abandon medicine's traditional ethical principles, how do they justify that deviation? And if the obligations to do good and avoid harm no longer govern physicians in the legal setting, what alternative principles come into play?... Are physicians in general bound by the principles of beneficence and nonmaleficence?[9]

Beneficence

The physician who professes to "do no harm" is not usually interpreted as pledging never to cause harm, but rather to strive to create a positive balance of goods over inflicted harms. Those engaged in medical practice, research, and public health know that risks of harm presented by interventions must often be weighed against possible benefits for patients, subjects, and the public. Here we see the importance of beneficence as a principle beyond the scope of nonmaleficence.

In ordinary English, the term *beneficence* connotes acts of mercy, kindness, charity, love, and humanity. In its most general meaning, it includes all forms of action intended to benefit other persons. In health care ethics beneficence commonly refers to an action done to benefit others, whereas benevolence refers to the character trait or virtue of being disposed to act for the benefit of others. The principle of beneficence refers to a moral obligation to act for the benefit of others. No demand is more important in taking care of patients: The welfare of patients is medicine's context and justification. Beneficence has long been treated as a foundational value—and sometimes as *the* foundational value[10]—in health care ethics.

The principle of beneficence requires us to help others further their important and legitimate interests, often by preventing or removing possible harms. This principle includes rules such as "maximize possible benefits and minimize possible harms" and "balance benefits against risks." Many duties in medicine, nursing, public health, and research are expressed in terms of a positive obligation to come to the assistance of those in need of treatment or in danger of injury. The harms to be prevented, removed, or minimized are the pain, suffering, and disability of injury and disease. The range of benefits that might be considered relevant is broad. It could even include helping patients find appropriate forms of financial assistance and helping them gain access to health care or research protocols. Sometimes the benefit is for the patient, at other times for society.

Some writers in health care ethics suggest that certain duties not to injure others are more compelling than duties to benefit them. They point out that we do not consider it justifiable to kill a dying patient in order to use the patient's organs to save two others, even though benefits would be maximized, all things considered. The obligation not to injure a patient by abandonment has been said to be stronger than the obligation to prevent injury to a patient who has been abandoned by another (under the assumption that both are moral duties). Despite the attractiveness of these notions that there is a hierarchical ordering rule, Childress and I reject such hierarchies on grounds that obligations of beneficence do, under many circumstances, outweigh those of nonmaleficence. A harm inflicted by not avoiding causing it may be negligible or trivial, whereas the harm that beneficence requires we prevent may be substantial. For example, saving a person's life by a blood transfusion clearly justifies the inflicted harm of venipuncture on the blood donor. One of the motivations for separating nonmaleficence from beneficence is that these principles themselves come into conflict. Since the weights of the two principles can vary, there can be no mechanical decision rule asserting that one obligation must always outweigh the other.

Perhaps the major theoretical problem about beneficence is whether the principle generates general moral duties that are incumbent on everyone—not because of a professional role, but because morality itself makes a general demand of beneficence. Many analyses of beneficence in ethical theory (most notably utilitarianism[11]) seem to demand severe sacrifice and extreme generosity in the moral life—for example, giving a kidney for transplantation or donating bone marrow to a stranger. However, many moral philosophers have argued that such beneficent action is virtuous and a moral ideal, but not an obligation; therefore, there is no principle of beneficence of the sort proclaimed in the four-principles approach.

I agree that the line between what is required and what is not required by the principle is difficult to draw, and that drawing a precise line independent of context is impossible. I do not agree, however, with the radical view that there are no obligations of beneficence—both general and specific obligations. I return to this problem of weighing, judging, and specifying later in this essay in a discussion of the notion of prima facie duties.

Justice

Every civilized society is a cooperative venture structured by moral, legal, and cultural principles of justice that define the terms of cooperation. A person in any such society has been treated justly if treated according to what is fair, due, or owed. For example, if equal political rights are due to all citizens, then justice is done when those rights are accorded. The more restricted notion of *distributive justice* refers to fair, equitable, and appropriate distribution in society. Usually this term refers to the distribution of primary social goods, such as economic goods and fundamental political rights, but burdens are also within its scope. Paying for forms of national health insurance is a distributed burden; medical-welfare checks and grants to do research are distributed benefits.

There is no single principle of justice in the four-principles approach. Somewhat like principles under the heading of beneficence, there are several principles, each requiring specification in particular contexts. But common to almost all theories of justice—and accepted in the four-principles approach—is the minimal (formal) principle that like cases should be treated alike, or, to use the language of equality, equals ought to be treated equally and unequals unequally. This elementary principle, or formal principle of justice, states no particular respects in which people ought to be treated. It merely asserts that whatever respects are relevant, if persons are equal in those respects, they should be treated alike. Thus, the formal principle of justice does not tell us how to determine equality or proportion in these matters, and it lacks substance as a specific guide to conduct.

Many controversies about justice arise over what should be considered the relevant characteristics for equal treatment. Principles that specify these relevant characteristics are often said to be "material" because they identify relevant properties for distribution. Childress and I take account of the fact that philosophers have developed diverse theories of justice that provide sometimes conflicting material principles. We try to show that there are some merits in egalitarian theories, libertarian theories, and utilitarian theories; and we defend a mixed use of principles in these theories. We regard these three theories of justice as appropriately capturing some of our traditional convictions about justice, and we think that they can all be tapped as resources that will help to produce a coherent conception of justice.

However, many issues of justice in health care ethics are not easily framed in the context of traditional principles and abstract moral theories.[12] For example, some basic issues in health care ethics in the last three decades center on special levels of protection and aid for vulnerable and disadvantaged parties in health care systems. These issues cut across clinical ethics, public health ethics, and research ethics. The four-principles approach tries to deal with several of these issues, without producing a grand theory for resolving all issues of justice. For example, we address issues in research ethics about whether research is permissible with groups who have been repeatedly used as research subjects, though the advantages of research are calculated to benefit all in society. We argue that since medical research is a social enterprise for the public good, it must be accomplished in a broadly inclusive and participatory way, and we try to specify the commitments of such generalizations. In this way, we incorporate principles of justice but do not produce a general theory of justice.

THE CHOICE OF FOUR PRINCIPLES AND THE EVOLUTION OF THE THEORY

The choice of our four types of moral principle as the framework for moral decision making in bioethics derives in part from professional roles and traditions. As I noted earlier, the obligations and virtues of health professionals have for centuries, as found in codes and learned writings on ethics, been framed by professional commitments to provide medical care and to protect patients from disease, injury, and system failure. Our principles build on this tradition, but they also significantly depart from it by including parts of morality that traditionally have been neglected in health care ethics, attending especially to the traditional neglect of principles of respect for autonomy and justice. All four types of principles are needed to provide a comprehensive framework for biomedical ethics, but this general framework is abstract and spare until it has been further specified—that is, interpreted and adapted for particular circumstances.

Principles of Biomedical Ethics has evolved appreciably since the first edition in its understanding of abstractness and the demands of particular circumstances. This is not because the principles have changed, but because over the years Childress and I have altered some of our views about the grounding of the principles and about their practical significance. Two major changes deserve special attention. The first is our development of the idea that the four principles are already embedded in public morality—a universal common morality—and are presupposed in the formulation of public and institutional policies.

The second is our adoption of Henry Richardson's account of the specification of moral norms. These supplements to our theory and their significance will be discussed in the next two sections.

The Centrality of the Common Morality

The source of the four principles is what Childress and I call *the common morality* (a view only incorporated at the point of the third edition of *Principles*, following the language of Alan Donagan). The common morality is applicable to all persons in all places, and all human conduct is rightly judged by its standards. The following are examples of *standards of action* (here rules of obligation) in the common morality: (1) don't kill, (2) don't cause pain or suffering to others, (3) prevent evil or harm from occurring, (4) rescue persons in danger, (5) tell the truth, (6) nurture the young and dependent, (7) keep your promises, (8) don't steal, (9) don't punish the innocent, and (10) treat all persons with equal moral consideration.

Why have such norms become parts of a common morality, whereas other norms have not? To answer this question, I start with an assumption about the primary goal—that is, objective—of the social institution of morality. This objective is to promote human flourishing by counteracting conditions that cause the quality of people's lives to worsen. The goal is to prevent or limit problems of indifference, conflict, suffering, hostility, scarce resources, limited information, and the like. Centuries of experience have demonstrated that the human condition tends to deteriorate into misery, confusion, violence, and distrust unless norms of the sort just listed—the norms of the common morality—are observed. When complied with, these norms lessen human misery and preventable death. It is an overstatement to maintain that all of these norms are necessary for the survival of a society (as some philosophers and social scientists have maintained[13]), but it is not too much to claim that these norms are necessary to ameliorate or counteract the tendency for the quality of people's lives to worsen or for social relationships to disintegrate.[14]

These norms are what they are, and not some other set of norms, because they have proven over time that their observance is essential to realize the objectives of morality. What justifies them is that they achieve the objectives of morality, not the fact that they are universally shared across cultures. It is conceivable, of course, that the set of norms that is shared universally is not the same set of norms as the set pragmatically justified by their conformity to the objectives of morality. I agree that if another set of norms would better serve the objectives of morality, then that set of norms ought to displace the norms currently in place. However, there are no clear candidates as alternatives to these norms.

What Childress and I call "principles" are the most general and basic norms of the common morality. In *Principles of Biomedical Ethics,* we devote an entire chapter to each principle in the attempt to explain its nature, content, specification, and the like. The assumption behind the argument in each chapter is that our framework of four principles should incorporate and articulate the most general values of the common morality.

Our framework encompasses several types of moral norms, including not only principles but also rules, rights, and moral ideals. We treat principles as the most general and comprehensive norms, but we make only a loose distinction between rules and principles. Rules, we argue, are more precise and practical guides to action that depend on the more general principles for their justification. We defend several types of rules, all of which should be viewed as specifications of principles. These include substantive rules (e.g., truth telling, confidentiality, and privacy rules), authority rules (e.g., rules of surrogate authority and rules of professional authority), and procedural rules (e.g., rules for determining eligibility for organ transplantation and rules for reporting grievances to higher authorities).

The Prima Facie Character of Principles and Rules

These principles and rules (or other norms in the common morality) can in some circumstances be justifiably overridden by other moral norms with which they conflict. For example, we might justifiably not tell the truth in order to prevent someone from killing another person, and we might justifiably disclose confidential information about a person in order to protect the rights of another person. Principles, duties, and rights are not absolute (or unconditional) merely because they are universal. There are exceptions to all principles, each of which is merely presumptive in force.

Oxford philosopher W. D. Ross developed a theory that has been influential on *Principles* since the first edition. Ross's theory is intended to assist in resolving problems of conflict between principles. His views are based on an account of prima facie duties, which he contrasts with actual duties. A prima facie duty is one that is always to be acted upon unless it conflicts on a particular occasion with another duty. One's *actual* duty, by contrast, is determined by an examination of the respective weights of competing prima facie duties in particular situations. When principles contingently conflict, no supreme principle is available—in the four-principles approach—to determine an overriding obligation. Therefore, discretionary judgment becomes an inescapable part of moral thinking in our approach.

Here is an example. A physician has confidential information about a patient who is also an employee in the hospital where the physician practices. The employee is seeking advancement in a stress-filled position, but the physician has good reason to believe this advancement would be devastating for both the employee and the hospital. The physician has duties of confidentiality, nonmaleficence, and beneficence in these circumstances: Should the physician break confidence? Could the matter be handled by making thin disclosures only to the hospital administrator and not to the personnel office? Can such disclosures be made consistent with one's general commitments to confidentiality? Addressing these questions through a process of moral justification is required to establish one's actual duty in the face of these conflicts of prima facie duties. Once we acknowledge that all general principles have exceptions, we are free to view every moral conclusion that is supported by a principle and every principle itself as subject to modification or reformulation. Change of this sort is to be accomplished through *specification*, the means by which principles come to have their practical value.

The Specification of Norms and Moral Coherence

To say that principles have their origins in and find support in the common morality and in traditions of health care is not to say that their appearance in a developed system of biomedical ethics is identical to their appearance in the traditions from which they spring. Prima facie principles underdetermine moral judgments because there is too little content in abstract principles to determine concrete outcomes. Every norm and theory contains regions of indeterminacy that need reduction through further development of their commitments in the system, augmenting them with a more specific moral content. I turn, then, to these questions: How does the prima facie conception of principles work in practical bioethics? How are general principles to reach down to concrete policies? How does one fill the gap between abstract principles and concrete judgments?

The Method of Specification

The answer is that principles must be specified to suit the needs and demands of particular contexts, thus enabling principles to overcome their lack of content and to handle moral conflict. Specification is a process of reducing the indeterminateness of abstract norms and providing them with specific action-guiding content.[15] For example, without further specification, "do no harm" is too abstract to help in thinking through problems such as whether physicians may justifiably hasten the death of patients. The general norm has to be specified for this particular context.

Specification is not a process of either producing or defending general norms such as those in the common morality; it assumes that they are available. Specifying the norms with which one starts (whether those in the common morality or norms that were previously specified) is accomplished by *narrowing the scope* of the norms, not by explaining what the general norms *mean*. The scope is narrowed, as Henry Richardson puts it, by "spelling out where, when, why, how, by what means, to whom, or by whom the action is to be done or avoided."[16] For example, the norm that we are obligated to "respect the autonomy of persons" cannot, unless specified, handle complicated problems of what to disclose or demand in clinical medicine and research involving human subjects. A definition of "respect for autonomy" (as, say, "allowing competent persons to exercise their liberty rights") might clarify one's meaning in using the norm, but would not narrow the general norm or render it more specific.

Specification adds content to general norms. For example, one possible specification of "respect the autonomy of persons" is "respect the autonomy of competent patients when they become incompetent by following their advance directives." This specification will work well in some medical contexts, but will not be adequate in others, thus necessitating additional specification. Progressive specification can continue indefinitely, gradually reducing the conflicts that abstract principles themselves cannot resolve. However, to qualify all along the way as a specification, a transparent connection must always be maintained to the initial norm that gives moral authority to the resulting string of norms.

Now we come to a critical matter about particular moralities, by contrast to the common morality. There is always the possibility of developing more than one line of specification of a norm when confronting practical problems and moral disagreements. It is simply part of the moral life that different persons and groups will offer different (sometimes conflicting) specifications, potentially creating multiple particular moralities. On any problematic issue (such as abortion, animal research, aid in disaster relief, health inequities, and euthanasia), competing specifications are likely to be offered by reasonable and fair-minded parties, all of whom are committed to the common morality. We cannot hold persons to a higher standard than to make judgments conscientiously in light of the relevant basic and specified norms while attending to the available factual evidence. Conscientious and reasonable moral agents will understandably disagree with equally conscientious persons over moral weights and priorities in circumstances of a contingent conflict of norms.

Nothing in the model of specification suggests that we can always eliminate circumstances of intractable conflicting judgments. However, we should always try to do so by justifying the specification we put forward. This suggests that specification as a method needs to be connected to a model of justification that will support some specifications and not others. Only brief attention can be paid here to this difficult philosophical problem.

Justifying Specifications Using the Method of Coherence

A specification is justified, in the four-principles approach, if and only if it maximizes the coherence of the overall set of relevant, justified beliefs. These beliefs could include empirically justified beliefs, justified basic moral beliefs, and previously justified specifications. This is a version of so-called wide reflective equilibrium.[17] No matter how wide the pool of beliefs, there is no reason to expect that the process of rendering norms coherent by specification will come to an end or be perfected. Particular moralities are, from this perspective, continuous works in progress—a process rather than a finished product. There is no reason to think that morality can be rendered coherent in only one way through the process of specification. Many particular moralities present coherent ways to specify the common morality. Normatively, we can demand no more than that agents faithfully specify the norms of the common morality with an attentive eye to overall coherence.

The following are some of the criteria for a coherent (and therefore, according to this model, justified) set of ethical beliefs: consistency (the avoidance of contradiction), argumentative support (explicit support for a position with reasons), intuitive plausibility (the feature of a norm or judgment being secure in its own right), compatibility or coherence with reasonable nonmoral beliefs (in particular, coherence with available empirical evidence), comprehensiveness (the feature of covering the entire moral domain, or as much of it as possible), and simplicity (reducing the number of moral considerations to the minimum possible without sacrifice in terms of the other criteria).[18]

CONCLUSION

I have explained, and argued in defense of, what has often been called the four-principles approach to biomedical ethics and is now increasingly called *principlism*.[19] The four clusters of principles derive from both considered judgments in the common morality and enduring and valuable parts of traditions of health care. Health care ethics has often been said to be an "applied ethics," but this metaphor may be more misleading than helpful. It is rarely the case that we can directly apply a principle to resolve a tough problem. We will almost always be engaged in collecting evidence, reasoning, and specifying general principles. This is how problems should be treated and how progress can be made in health care ethics. From this perspective, the four principles form only a starting point—the point where the practical work begins.

Notes

1. Albert R. Jonsen, *The Birth of Bioethics* (New York: Oxford University Press, 1998), 3ff; Edmund D. Pellegrino and David C. Thomasma, *The Virtues in Medical Practice* (New York: Oxford University Press, 1993), 184–189.

2. National Commission for the Protection of Human Subjects of Biomedical and Behavioral Research, *The Belmont Report: Ethical Principles and Guidelines for the Protection of Human Subjects of Research* (Washington, DC: DHEW Publication OS 78-0012 1978); James F. Childress, Eric M. Meslin, Harold T. Shapiro, eds. *Belmont Revisited: Ethical Principles for Research with Human Subjects* (Washington, DC: Georgetown University Press, 2005).

3. Tom L. Beauchamp and James F. Childress, *Principles of Biomedical Ethics*, 1st edition (New York: Oxford University Press, 1979).

4. H. Tristram Engelhardt, Jr., *The Foundations of Bioethics* (New York: Oxford University Press, 1996), 2nd edition; Jay Katz, *The Silent World of Doctor and Patient* (New York: The Free Press, 1984); James F. Childress, "The Place of Autonomy in Bioethics," *Hastings Center Report* 20 (January/February 1990): 12–16; Rebecca Kukla, "Conscientious Autonomy: Displacing Decisions in Health Care," *Hastings Center Report* (March-April 2005): 34–44.

5. Ruth R. Faden and Tom L. Beauchamp, *A History and Theory of Informed Consent* (New York: Oxford, 1986).

6. Thomas Percival, *Medical Ethics; or a Code of Institutes and Precepts, Adapted to the Professional Conduct of Physicians and Surgeons* (Manchester: S. Russell, 1803), 165–166. Percival's work was the pattern for the American Medical Association's (AMA) first code of ethics in 1847.

7. Compare Bernard Gert, *Morality: Its Nature and Justification* (New York: Oxford, 2005).

8. See, for example, Sidney Bloch and Peter Reddaway, *Soviet Psychiatric Abuse: The Shadow over World Psychiatry* (Boulder, CO: Westview Press, 1984), esp. ch. 1.

9. Paul S. Appelbaum, "The Parable of the Forensic Physician: Ethics and the Problem of Doing Harm," *International Journal of Law and Psychiatry* 13 (1990): 249–259, esp. 250–251.

10. Edmund Pellegrino and David Thomasma, *For the Patient's Good: The Restoration of Beneficence in Health Care* (New York: Oxford University Press, 1988); Pellegrino, "The Four Principles and the Doctor-Patient Relationship: The Need for a Better Linkage," in Raanan Gillon, ed. *Principles of Health Care Ethics* (Chichester, England: John Wiley & Sons, 1994).

11. Peter Singer, "Living High and Letting Die," *Philosophy and Phenomenological Research* 59 (1999): 183–187. Peter Singer, *Practical Ethics*, 2nd edition (Cambridge: Cambridge University Press, 1993); Shelly Kagan, *The Limits of Morality* (Oxford:

Clarendon Press, 1989); Richard W. Miller, "Beneficence, Duty, and Distance," *Philosophy & Public Affairs* 32 (2004): 357–383.

12. For diverse accounts of justice in biomedical ethics, see Norman Daniels, *Just Health Care* (New York: Cambridge University Press, 1985); Daniels, *Just Health* (New York: Cambridge University Press, 2006); Madison Powers and Ruth Faden, *Social Justice: The Moral Foundations of Public Health and Health Policy* (New York: Oxford University Press, 2006); Allen Buchanan, "Health-Care Delivery and Resource Allocation," in *Medical Ethics,* ed. Robert Veatch, 2nd edition (Boston: Jones and Bartlett Publishers, 1997); Allen Buchanan, Dan Brock, Norman Daniels, and Daniel Wikler, *From Chance to Choice: Genetics and Justice* (New York: Cambridge University Press, 2000).

13. Sissela Bok, *Common Values* (Columbia, MO: University of Missouri Press, 1995), 13–23, 50–59.

14. G. J. Warnock, *The Object of Morality* (London: Methuen & Co., 1971), esp. 15–26; John Mackie, *Ethics: Inventing Right and Wrong* (London: Penguin, 1977), 107ff.

15. Henry S. Richardson, "Specifying Norms as a Way to Resolve Concrete Ethical Problems," *Philosophy and Public Affairs* 19 (Fall 1990): 279–310; Richardson, "Specifying, Balancing, and Interpreting Bioethical Principles," *Journal of Medicine and Philosophy* 25 (2000): 285–307; David DeGrazia, "Moving Forward in Bioethical Theory: Theories, Cases, and Specified Principlism," *Journal of Medicine and Philosophy* 17 (1992): 511–539; and DeGrazia and Tom L. Beauchamp, "Philosophical Foundations and Philosophical Methods," in *Methods of Bioethics,* ed. D. Sulmasy and J. Sugarman (Washington, DC: Georgetown University Press, 2001), esp. 33–36.

16. Richardson, "Specifying, Balancing, and Interpreting Bioethical Principles," 289.

17. Norman Daniels, "Wide Reflective Equilibrium and Theory Acceptance in Ethics," *Journal of Philosophy* 76 (1979): 256–282; Daniels, "Wide Reflective Equilibrium in Practice," in L.W. Sumner and J. Boyle, *Philosophical Perspectives on Bioethics* (Toronto: University of Toronto Press, 1996).

18. DeGrazia and Beauchamp, "Philosophical Foundations and Philosophical Methods"; and David DeGrazia, "Common Morality, Coherence, and the Principles of Biomedical Ethics," *Kennedy Institute of Ethics Journal* 13 (2003): 219–230.

19. See, for example, B. Gert, C. M. Culver, and K. D. Clouser, *Bioethics: A Return to Fundamentals* (New York: Oxford University Press, 1997), ch. 4; John H. Evans, "A Sociological Account of the Growth of Principlism," *Hastings Center Report* 30 (Sept.–Oct. 2000): 31–38; Earl Winkler, "Moral Philosophy and Bioethics: Contextualism versus the Paradigm Theory," in L. W. Sumner and J. Boyle, eds. *Philosophical Perspectives on Bioethics*; John D. Arras, "Principles and Particularity: The Role of Cases in Bioethics," *Indiana Law Journal* 69 (1994): 983–1014; and Carson Strong, "Specified Principlism," *Journal of Medicine and Philosophy* 25 (2000): 285–307.

4

INFORMED CONSENT: ITS HISTORY AND MEANING

The practice of obtaining informed consent has its history in medicine and biomedical research, where the disclosure of information and the withholding of information are aspects of the daily encounters between patient and physician, as well as subject and investigator. Although discussions of disclosure and justified nondisclosure have played a role in the history of medical ethics, the term *informed consent* emerged only in the 1950s, and discussions of the concept as it is used today began only around 1972. Concomitantly, a revolution was occurring in standards of appropriate patient–physician interaction. Medical ethics moved from a narrow focus on the physician's or researcher's obligation to disclose information to the quality of a patient's or subject's understanding of information and right to authorize or refuse a biomedical intervention.

HISTORICAL BACKGROUND

Many writers have proposed that managing medical information in encounters with patients is a basic moral responsibility of physicians. Pioneering ventures are found in classic documents in the history of medicine, such as the Hippocratic writings (fifth to fourth century, BC), Percival's *Medical Ethics* (1803), and the first *Code of Ethics* (1846–1847) of the American Medical Association, as well as in the historically significant didactic writings on medical ethics in the eighteenth and nineteenth centuries, sometimes referred to as the "learned" tradition, comprising discursive study of medical ethics through treatises and books.

These codes and writings present a disappointing history from the perspective of the right to give informed consent. The Hippocratic writings did not hint at obligations of veracity or disclosure, and throughout the ancient, medieval, and early modern periods, medical ethics developed predominantly within the profession of medicine. With few exceptions, no serious consideration was given to issues of either consent or self-determination by patients and research subjects. The central concern was how to make disclosures without harming patients by revealing their condition too abruptly and starkly. The emphasis on the principle "first, do no harm" promoted the idea that a health care professional is obligated not to make disclosures because to do so would be to risk a harmful outcome.

The Eighteenth Century

Benjamin Rush and John Gregory have sometimes been acknowledged for their enlightenment-inspired views about disclosure and public education in the eighteenth century. However, neither was advocating informed consent. They wanted patients to be sufficiently educated so that they could understand their physician's recommendations and therefore be motivated to comply. They were not optimistic that patients would form their own opinions and make appropriate medical choices. For example, Rush advised physicians to "yield to them [patients] in matters of little consequence, but maintain an inflexible Authority over them in matters that are essential to life" (Rush, 1786, 323). Gregory underscored that the physician must be keenly aware of the harm that untimely revelations might cause. There is no assertion of the importance of respecting rights of self-determination for patients or of obtaining consent for any purpose other than a medically good outcome (Gregory, 1772). Gregory and Rush appreciated the value of information and dialogue from the patient's point of view, but the idea of informed consent was not foreshadowed in their writings.

The Nineteenth Century

Thomas *Percival's* historic *Medical Ethics* (1803) stands in this same tradition. It makes no more mention of consent solicitation and respect for decision making by patients than had previous codes and treatises. Percival did struggle with the issue of truth telling, but he held that the patient's right to the truth must yield in the face of an obligation to benefit the patient in cases of conflict—a benevolent deception. Percival maintained that

> to a patient ... who makes inquiries which, if faithfully answered, might prove fatal to him, it would be a gross and unfeeling wrong to reveal the truth. His right to it is suspended, and even annihilated; because, its beneficial nature being reversed, it would be deeply injurious to himself, to his family, and to the public. And he has the strongest claim, from the trust reposed in his physician, as well as from the common principles of humanity, to be guarded against whatever would be detrimental to him. ... The only point at issue is, whether the practitioner shall sacrifice that delicate sense of veracity, which is so ornamental to, and indeed forms a characteristic excellence of the virtuous man, to this claim of professional justice and social duty (Percival, 1803, 165–166).

Percival was struggling against the arguments of his friend, the Rev. Thomas Gisborne, who opposed practices of giving false assertions intended to raise patients' hopes and lying for the patient's benefit: "The physician ... is invariably bound never to represent the uncertainty or danger as less than he actually believes it to be" (Gisborne, 1794, 401). From Percival's perspective, the physician does not lie or act improperly in beneficent acts of deception and falsehood as long as the objective is to give hope to the dejected or sick patient.

The American Medical Association (AMA) accepted virtually without modification the Percival paradigm in its 1847 Code (American Medical Association, 1847, 94). Many passages in Percival appear almost verbatim in this Code (AMA, 1847, "Code of Medical Ethics," see esp. Ch. I, Art. I, sect. 4). This Code, as well as most codes of medical ethics before and after, does not include rules of veracity. For more than a century thereafter, American and British medical ethics remained fundamentally under Percival's vision.

There was, however, a notable nineteenth-century exception to the consensus that surrounded Percival's recommendations. Connecticut physician Worthington Hooker was the first champion of the rights of patients to information, in opposition to the model of benevolent deception that had reigned from Hippocrates to the AMA. He and Harvard Professor of Medicine Richard Clarke Cabot may have been the only physician champions of this model prior to the second half of the twentieth century. Moreover, there may never have been a figure who swam, in regard to truth telling, so against the stream of indigenous medical tradition as Hooker.

Hooker's arguments are novel and ingenious, but do not amount to a recommendation of informed consent. Hooker was concerned with "the *general effect* of deception" on society and on medical institutions. He thought the effect disastrous. But no more in Hooker than in the AMA Code is there a recommendation to obtain the permission of patients or to respect autonomy for the sake of autonomy. Hooker's concerns were with expediency in disclosure and truth telling rather than with the promotion of autonomous decision making or informed consent. The idea that patients should be enabled to understand their situation so that they are able to participate with physicians in decisions about medical treatment was an idea whose time had yet to come (Hooker, 1859).

Although the nineteenth century saw no hint of a rule or practice of informed consent in clinical medicine, consent procedures were not entirely absent. Evidence exists in surgery records that consent seeking and rudimentary rules for obtaining consent existed since at least the middle of the nineteenth century (Pernick, 1982). However, the consents obtained do not appear to have been meaningful by standards of informed consent, as they had little to do with the patient's right to decide after being informed. Practices of obtaining consent in surgery prior to the 1950s were pragmatic responses to a combination of concerns about medical reputation, malpractice suits, and practicality in medical institutions. It is physically difficult and interpersonally awkward to perform surgery on a patient without obtaining the patient's permission. Such practices of obtaining permission, however, did not constitute practices of obtaining informed consent, although they did provide a modest nineteenth-century grounding for this twentieth-century concept.

The situation is similar in research involving human subjects. Little evidence exists that, until recently, requirements of informed consent had a significant hold on the practice of investigators. In the nineteenth century, for example, it was common for research to be conducted on slaves and servants without consent on the part of the subject. By contrast, at the turn of the century, American Army surgeon Walter Reed's yellow fever experiments involved formal procedures for obtaining the consent of potential subjects. Although deficient by contemporary standards of disclosure and consent, these procedures recognized the right of the individual to refuse or authorize participation in the research. The extent to which this principle became ingrained in the ethics of research by the mid-twentieth century remains a matter of historical controversy.

Although it has often been reported that the obtaining of informed and voluntary consent was essential to the ethics of research and was commonplace in biomedical investigation, it is unclear that consent seeking on the part of investigators was standard practice. Anecdotal evidence suggests that biomedical research often proceeded without adequate consent at least into the 1960s (Faden & Beauchamp, 1986).

Early Twentieth-Century Legal History

The legal history of disclosure obligations and rights of self-determination for patients evolved gradually. In the doctrine of legal precedent, each decision, relying on earlier court opinions, joins a chain of authority that incorporates the relevant language and reasoning from the cited cases. In this way, a few early consent cases built on each other to produce a legal doctrine. The best known and ultimately the most influential of these early cases is *Schloendorff v. Society of New York Hospitals* (1914). *Schloendorff* used rights of "self-determination" to justify imposing an obligation to obtain a patient's consent. Subsequent cases that followed and relied upon *Schloendorff* implicitly adopted its reasoning. In this way, "self-determination" came to be the primary justification for legal requirements that consent be obtained from patients.

In the early twentieth century, the behavior of physicians was often egregious in the neglect of consent, and courts did not shrink from using ringing language and sweeping principles to denounce it. The same language was then applied as precedent in later cases in which physicians' behavior was less outrageous. As the informed consent doctrine developed and problems grew more subtle, the law could have turned away from the language of self-determination, but instead increasingly relied on this rationale as its fundamental premise. The language in the early cases suggests that rights of freedom from bodily invasion contain rights of medical decision making by patients.

The 1950s and 1960s

During the 1950s and 1960s, the traditional duty to obtain consent evolved into a new, explicit duty to disclose certain forms of information and then to obtain consent. This development needed a new term, and so "informed" was tacked onto "consent," creating the expression "informed consent," in the landmark decision in *Salgo v. Leland Stanford, Jr. University Board of Trustees* (1957). The *Salgo* court suggested, without accompanying analysis, that the duty to disclose the *risks and alternatives* of treatment was not a new duty, but a logical extension of the already established duty to disclose the treatment's *nature and consequences*. Nonetheless, *Salgo* clearly introduced new elements into the law. The *Salgo* court was not interested merely in whether a recognizable consent had been given to the proposed procedures. The *Salgo* court latched tenaciously onto the problem of whether the consent had been adequately informed. The court thus created the language and the substance of informed consent by invoking the same right of self-determination that had heretofore applied to a less robust consent requirement.

Shortly thereafter, two opinions by the Kansas Supreme Court in the case of *Natanson* v. *Kline* (1960) pioneered the use of negligence in informed consent cases, rather than using battery. The court established the duty of disclosure as the obligation "to disclose and explain to the patient in language as simple as necessary the nature of the ailment, the nature of the proposed treatment, the probability of success or of alternatives, and perhaps the risks of unfortunate results and unforeseen conditions within the body." Thus, the *Natanson* court required essentially the same extensive disclosure—of the nature, consequences, risks, and alternatives of a proposed procedure—as had *Salgo*.

Not surprisingly, the number of articles in the medical literature on issues of consent increased substantially following this and other precedent legal cases. Typically written by lawyers, these articles functioned to alert physicians both to "informed consent" as a new legal development and to potential malpractice risk. How physicians reacted to these legal developments in the 1950s and 1960s is not well documented, but some empirical studies of informed consent in clinical medicine provide insights. A study done in the early to mid-1960s, conducted by the lawyer–surgeon team of Nathan Hershey and Stanley H. Bushkoff, indicates that a preoperative *consent form* was not yet a ubiquitous feature of the practice of surgery. As part of their study, Hershey and Bushkoff required that cooperating surgeons complete a "fill-in-the-blank" consent form for each of their patients. However, surgeons at several hospitals objected to the study because they were not currently using *any* kind of consent form for surgery. In the end, only 10 surgeons, representing but 3 hospitals, participated in the study. Together, these surgeons provided data on "informed consent" in 256 surgical cases. From this limited sample, Hershey and Bushkoff inferred that a consistent standard of disclosure existed among the surgeons studied and that this standard included a description of the operative procedure and its attendant risks and consequences (Hershey & Bushkoff, 1969).

Indifference to consent procedures seems to have begun to change by the late 1960s, when most physicians appear to have recognized some moral and legal duty to obtain consent for certain procedures and to provide some kind of disclosure. There is also evidence, however, that physicians' views about proper consent practices even in the late 1960s differed markedly from the consensus of opinion and convention that would begin to be fixed only 10 years later. For example, in one study, half of the physicians surveyed thought it medically proper, and 30% ethically proper, for a physician to perform a mastectomy with no authorization from the patient other than her signature on the blanket consent form required for hospital admission. Also, more than half of the physicians thought that it was ethically appropriate for a physician not to tell a cancer patient that she had been enrolled in a double-blind clinical trial of an experimental anticancer drug (Hagman, 1970).

An explosion of commentary on informed consent emerged in the medical literature of the early 1970s, but much of this commentary was negative: Physicians saw the demands of informed consent as impossible to fulfill and, at least in some cases, inconsistent with good patient care. Nonetheless, empirical studies conducted at the time suggest that there was at least enough documentable consent seeking in such areas as surgery, organ donation, and angiography to warrant empirical investigation. During this period, the procedure-specific consent form was gaining acceptance, although it was not yet universally in use. Whether in the 1960s physicians generally regarded informed consent as a legal nuisance or as an important moral problem is unclear (Faden & Beauchamp, 1986).

The histories of informed consent in research and in clinical medicine were at this time developing largely as separate pieces in a larger mosaic of biomedical ethics. These pieces have never been well integrated even when they developed simultaneously. Research ethics prior to World War II was no more influential on research practices than the parallel history of clinical medicine was on clinical practices. But events that unquestionably influenced thought about informed consent occurred at the Nuremberg trials. The Nuremberg Military Tribunals unambiguously condemned the sinister political motivation of Nazi experiments. A list of 10 principles constituted the Nuremberg Code. Principle One of the code states, without qualification, that the primary consideration in research is the subject's voluntary consent, which is "absolutely essential" (*United States* v. *Karl Brandt*, 1947).

The Nuremberg Code served as a model for some professional and governmental Codes formulated in the 1950s and 1960s. During this period, several additional incidents involving consent violations moved the discussion of Post-Nuremberg problems into the public arena. Thus began a rich and complex interplay of influences on research ethics: scholarly publications, journalism, public outrage, legislation, and case law. In the United States, one of the first incidents to achieve notoriety in research ethics involved a study conducted at the Jewish Chronic Disease Hospital (JCDH) in Brooklyn, New York. In July 1963, Dr. Chester Southam of the Sloan-Kettering Institute for Cancer Research persuaded the hospital's medical director, Emmanuel E. Mandel, to permit research involving injection of a suspension of foreign, live cancer cells into 22 patients at the JCDH. The objective was to discover whether a decline in the body's capacity to reject cancer transplants was caused by their cancer or by debilitation. Patients without cancer were needed to supply the answer. Southam had convinced Mandel that although the research was nontherapeutic, such research was routinely done without consent. Some patients were informed orally that they were involved in an experiment, but it was not disclosed that they were being given injections of *cancer* cells. No written consent was attempted, and some subjects were incompetent to give informed consent. In 1966, the Board of Regents of the State University of New York censured Drs. Southam and Mandel for their role in the research. They were found guilty of fraud, deceit, and unprofessional conduct (*Hyman v. Jewish Chronic Disease Hospital*, 1965).

Another major controversy about the ethics of research in the United States developed at Willowbrook State School, an institution for "mentally defective" children on Staten Island, New York. Beginning in 1956, Saul Krugman and his associates began a series of experiments to develop an effective prophylactic agent for infectious hepatitis. They deliberately infected newly admitted patients with isolated strains of the virus based on parental consents obtained under controversial circumstances that may have been manipulative. The issues in the Willowbrook case are more complex than those in the Jewish Chronic Disease Hospital case, and still today there are those who defend, at least in part, the ethics of these experiments. Krugman's research unit was eventually closed, but closure on the debate about the ethics of the studies conducted in the unit was never achieved (*Proceedings of the Symposium on Ethical Issues in Human Experimentation*, 1972).

The most notorious case of prolonged and knowing violation of subjects' rights in the United States was a Public Health Service (PHS) study initiated in the early 1930s. Originally designed as one of the first syphilis control demonstrations in the United States, the stated purpose of the Tuskegee Study, as it is now called, was to compare the health and longevity of an untreated syphilitic population with a nonsyphilitic but otherwise similar population. These subjects, all African American males, knew neither the name nor the nature of their disease. Their participation in a nontherapeutic experiment also went undisclosed. They were informed only that they were receiving free treatment for "bad blood," a term local African Americans associated with a host of unrelated ailments, but which the white physicians allegedly assumed was a local euphemism for syphilis (Jones, 1993).

It was remarkable that, although this study was reviewed several times between 1932 and 1970 by PHS officials and medical societies, and reported in 13 articles in prestigious medical and public health journals, it continued uninterrupted and without serious challenge. It was not until 1972 that the Department of Health, Education, and Welfare (DHEW) appointed an ad hoc advisory panel to review the study and the department's policies and procedures for the protection of human subjects. The panel found that neither the DHEW nor any other government agency had a uniform or adequate policy for reviewing experimental procedures or securing subjects' consents.

The 1970s and 1980s

These events do not, of course, explain why informed consent became the focus of so much attention in both case law and biomedical ethics. Many hypotheses can be invoked to explain these developments. The most likely explanation is that law, ethics, and medicine were all affected by issues and concerns in the wider society regarding individual liberties and social equality. These issues were made dramatic by an increasingly technological, powerful, and impersonal medical care. The issues raised by civil rights, women's rights, the consumer movement, and the rights of prisoners and the mentally ill often included health care components and helped reinforce public acceptance of rights applied to health care. Informed consent was swept along with this body of social concerns, which propelled the new bioethics throughout the 1970s.

Three 1972 court decisions stand as informed consent landmarks: *Canterbury v. Spence, Cobbs v. Grant, and Wilkinson v. Vesey*. *Canterbury* had a particularly massive influence in demanding a more patient-oriented standard of disclosure. In *Canterbury*, surgery on the patient's back and a subsequent accident in the hospital led to further injuries and unexpected paralysis, the possibility of which had not yet been disclosed. Judge Spottswood Robinson's opinion focuses on the needs of the reasonable person and the right to self-determination. As for sufficiency of information, the court holds: "The patient's right of self-decision shapes the boundaries of the duty to reveal. That right can be effectively exercised only if the patient possesses enough information to enable an intelligent choice."

Among the most important publications in the medical literature to appear during this period was a statement by the Judicial Council of the American Medical Association in 1981. For the first time, the AMA recognized informed consent as "a basic social policy" necessary to enable patients to make their own choices, even if their physician disagrees. The AMA's statement is a testament to the impact of the law of informed consent on medical ethics. The AMA's position roughly followed the language of *Canterbury v. Spence*.

The President's Commission for the Study of Ethical Problems in Medicine and Biomedical and Behavioral Research provides further evidence about the status informed consent had achieved in the 1970s and early 1980s. The President's Commission was first convened in January 1980, with informed consent as a main item on its agenda. In 1982, it produced one three-volume report that dealt directly with informed consent: *Making Health Care Decisions: The Ethical and Legal Implications of Informed Consent in the Patient-Practitioner Relationship*. The President's Commission argued that although informed consent had emerged primarily from a history in law, its requirements are essentially moral and policy oriented. It held that informed consent is based on the principle that competent persons are entitled to make their own decisions from their own values and goals, but that the context of informed consent and any claim of "valid consent" must derive from active, shared decision making. The principle of self-determination was described as the "bedrock" of the President's Commission's viewpoint.

The 1980s saw the publication of several books devoted to the subject of informed consent, as well as hundreds of journal articles and the passage of procedure-specific, informed consent laws and regulations. These events give testimony to the importance of informed consent in moral and legal thinking about medicine in the United States. By themselves, however, they tell us little about physicians' or researchers' actual consent practices or opinions, or about how informed consent was viewed or experienced by patients and subjects.

As might be expected, the empirical evidence on this subject during the 1980s is mixed, although it is clear that procedures of informed consent had taken a firm hold in some parts of medical practice. For example, routine practice encouraged the obtaining of signatures on consent forms and the disclosing of information about alternative treatments, risks, and benefits. The best data on this subject are the findings of a national survey conducted for the President's Commission by Louis Harris and Associates in 1982. Almost all of the physicians surveyed indicated that they obtained written consent from their patients before inpatient surgery or the administration of general anesthesia. At least 85% said they usually obtained some kind of consent—written or oral—for minor office surgery, setting of fractures, local anesthesia, invasive diagnostic procedures, and radiation therapy. Only blood tests and prescriptions appear to have proceeded frequently without patient consent, although about half of the physicians reported obtaining oral consent.

The overall impression conveyed by this survey is that the explosion of interest in informed consent in the 1970s had a powerful impact on medical practice. However, evidence from the Harris survey and other sources raises questions about the quality and meaningfulness of this consent-related activity. The overwhelming impression from the empirical literature and from reported clinical experience is that the actual process of soliciting informed consent often fell short of a serious show of respect for the decisional authority of patients. As the authors of one empirical study of physician–patient interactions put it, "despite the doctrine of informed consent, it is the physician, and not the patient, who, in effect, makes the treatment decision" (Siminoff & Fetting, 1991, 817).

The history of informed consent, then, indicates that medicine has undergone widespread changes under the influence of legal and moral requirements of informed consent, but it also reminds us that informed consent is an evolving process, not a set of events whose history has passed.

THE CONCEPT AND ELEMENTS OF INFORMED CONSENT

Informed consent began to play a central role in clinical and research ethics when problems of the autonomy of subjects gradually grew more insistent in twentieth-century practice and research, and when the idea of respecting autonomy gained equal recognition as a form of justification for protecting against risk. The practice of obtaining consent is a social phenomenon, and no analysis of the concept of informed consent will succeed if it ignores the contexts in which informed consent arose. Considerable vagueness has attended the term *informed consent* in these contexts, leaving a need to sharpen the concept.

Presumptions About the Concept

The claim that something is an informed consent or that an informed consent has been obtained cannot always be taken at face value. Before we can confidently infer that what appears to have been or was called an "informed consent" is a bona fide instance of informed consent, we need to know what to look for. This inquiry requires criteria of what will qualify for the label "informed consent."

If overdemanding criteria such as "full disclosure and complete understanding" are adopted, an informed consent becomes impossible to obtain. Conversely, if underdemanding criteria such as "the patient signed the form" are used, an informed consent becomes too easy to obtain and the term loses all moral significance. Many interactions between a physician and a patient or an investigator and a subject that have been called informed consents have been so labeled only because they rest on underdemanding criteria; they are inappropriately referred to as informed consents. For example, a physician's truthful disclosure to a patient has often been declared the essence of informed consent, as if a patient's silence following disclosure could add up to an informed consent. The existence of such inadequate understandings of informed consent can be explained in part by empirical information about physicians' beliefs concerning informed consent.

Contemporary Presumptions in Medicine

Some data about the meaning of informed consent are found in the aforementioned survey of physicians conducted by Louis Harris (Harris, in President's Commission, 1982, 302), which asked physicians, "What does the term informed consent mean to you?" In their answers, only 26% of physicians indicated that informed consent had anything to do with a patient giving permission, consenting, or agreeing to treatment; only 9% indicated that it involved the patient making a choice or stating a preference about his or her treatment. Similar results have been found in recent surveys of Japanese physicians' beliefs about informed consent (Hattori, 1991; Kai, 1993; Mizushima, 1990; Takahashi, 1990).

Like lawyers and courts, the overwhelming majority of these doctors appeared to recognize only disclosure as the criterion of "informed consent." That is, they view informed consent as explaining to a patient the nature of his or her medical condition together with a recommended treatment plan. But if physicians regard informed consent as nothing more than an event of conveying information to patients, rather than a process of discussion and obtaining permission from the patient, then claims that they regularly "obtain consents" from their patients before initiating medical procedures are vague and unreliable unless we know in some detail about the procedures used.

Matters may be worse than they appear: Perhaps all these physicians understand by "informed consent" is that the patient's signature has been obtained, or perhaps they mean only that some kind of disclosure has been made. This interpretation fits with the results of several studies of informed consent that have failed to find any sizeable evidence of "informed consent" in clinical medicine and that have found little evidence that the consents being obtained are meaningful exercises of informed choice by patients (Quaid, 1990, 249–259; Scherer & Reppucci, 1988, 123–141; Siminoff & Fetting, 1991, 813–818; Siminoff, Fetting, & Abeloff, 1989, 1192–1200).

The Authority of Oaths, Codes, and Treatises

Similar problems exist regarding what can be reasonably inferred from oaths, prayers, Codes of ethics, published lectures, and general pamphlets and treatises on medical conduct, usually written by individual physicians or medical societies for their colleagues. In the absence of more direct data about actual consent practices, these documents have been relied on heavily in writings on informed consent as sources that provide information about the history of informed consent and related matters of clinical medical ethics. However, it is often difficult to determine whether the statements that appear in these documents are primarily exhortatory, descriptive, or self-protective. Some writings describe, for educational purposes, conduct that was in accordance with prevailing professional standards. Other documents aim at reforming professional conduct by prescribing what should be established practice. Still others seem constructed to protect the physician from suspicions of misconduct or from legal liability.

The Elements of Informed Consent

Legal, philosophical, regulatory, medical, and psychological literatures have often tried to define or analyze informed consent in terms of its "elements." The following elements have been widely mentioned as fundamental to the concept: (1) disclosure, (2) comprehension, (3) voluntariness, (4) competence, and (5) consent (Levine, 1978, 3–9; Meisel & Roth, 1981; National Commission, 1978, 10). The postulate is that a person gives an informed consent to an intervention if and only if the person is competent to act, receives a thorough disclosure about the procedure, comprehends the disclosed information, acts voluntarily, and consents.

This definition is attractive because of its consistency with standard usage of the term *informed consent* in medicine and law. However, medical convention and malpractice law tend to distort the meaning of informed consent in ways that need correction. Analyses using the aforementioned five elements, as well as conventional usage in law and medicine, are best suited for cataloging the analytical *parts* of informed consent and for delineating moral and legal *requirements* of informed consent, not for conceptually analyzing the *meaning* of "informed consent." Neither requirements nor parts amount to a *definition*.

To take but one instance of the potential bias at work in this form of definition, the U.S. Supreme Court addressed the definition of informed consent in *Planned Parenthood of Central Missouri v. Danforth* as follows: "One might well wonder...what 'informed consent' of a patient is.... We are content to accept, as the meaning [of informed consent], the giving of information to the patient as to just what would be done and as to its consequences" (1976, 67, *n*. 8). The exclusive element of informed consent here is *disclosure*, which recalls the assumptions made by physicians in the Harris poll. However, nothing about an informed consent requires disclosure as part of its *meaning*. A patient or subject already knowledgeable about a proposed intervention could give a thorough informed consent without having received a disclosure from a second party. Similarly, other conditions in the aforementioned list of conditions are not necessary. For example, persons who are legally incompetent (see element 4) sometimes give informed consents, and in some instances even psychologically incompetent persons (also often the referent of element 4) may be able to consent meaningfully to or refuse a particular intervention. These norms delineate an *obligation to make disclosures* so that a consent can be informed, rather than a *meaning of informed consent*. Even all five of these elements merged as a set do not satisfactorily capture the meaning of "informed consent."

The following seven categories express the analytical components of informed consent more adequately than the aforementioned five categories, but this sevenfold list still does not adequately express the *meaning* of "informed consent" (Beauchamp & Childress, 1994):

I. **Threshold elements (preconditions)**
   1. Competence (to understand and decide)
   2. Voluntariness (in deciding)

II. **Information elements**
    3. Disclosure (of material information)
    4. Recommendation (of a plan)
    5. Understanding (of elements 3 and 4)

III. **Consent elements**
    6. Decision (in favor of a plan)
    7. Authorization (of the chosen plan)

The language of "material information" in element 3 is pivotal for an adequate analysis of the elements of disclosure (element 3) and understanding (element 5). Critics of legal requirements of informed consent have often held that procedures sometimes have so many risks and benefits that they cannot be disclosed and explained, but "material risks" are simply the risks a reasonable patient needs to understand in order to decide among the alternatives. Only these risks and benefits need to be disclosed and understood.

Informed consent *requirements* can be constructed to correspond to each of the aforementioned *elements*. That is, specific disclosure requirements, comprehension requirements, noninfluence requirements, competence requirements, authorization requirements, and the like can be fashioned. These requirements would specify the conditions that must be satisfied for a consent to be *valid*, but they may not provide an adequate analysis of the meaning of "informed consent."

Two Meanings of "Informed Consent"

The question "What is an informed consent?" is complicated because at least two common, entrenched, and irreducibly different meanings of "informed consent" have been at work in its history. That is, the term is analyzable in different ways because different conceptions of informed consent have emerged. In one sense, an informed consent is an *autonomous authorization* by individual patients or subjects. In the second sense, informed consent is analyzable in terms of *institutional and policy rules of consent* that collectively form the social practice of informed consent in institutional contexts (Faden & Beauchamp 1986, 276–287).

In the first meaning, an *autonomous authorization* requires more than merely acquiescing in, yielding to, or complying with an arrangement or a proposal made by a physician or investigator. A person gives an informed consent in this first sense if and only if the person, with substantial understanding and in substantial absence of control by others, intentionally authorizes a health professional to do something. A person who intentionally refuses to authorize an intervention, but otherwise satisfies these conditions, gives an *informed refusal*. This first sense derives from philosophical premises that informed consent is fundamentally a matter of protecting and enabling autonomous or self-determining choice.

In the second meaning, "informed consent" refers only to a legally or institutionally effective approval given by a patient or subject. An approval is therefore "effective" or "valid" if it conforms to the rules that govern specific institutions, whatever the operative rules may be. In this sense, unlike the first, conditions and requirements of informed consent are relative to a social and institutional context and need not be autonomous authorizations. This meaning is driven by demands in the legal and health care systems for a generally applicable and efficient consent mechanism by which responsibilities and violations can be readily and fairly assessed.

Under these two contrasting understandings of "informed consent," a patient or subject can give an informed consent in the first sense, but not in the second sense, and vice versa. For example, if the person consenting is a minor and therefore not of legal age, he or she cannot give an effective or valid consent under the prevailing institutional rules; a consent is invalid even if the minor gives the consent autonomously and responsibly. ("Mature minor" laws do sometimes make an exception and give minors the right to authorize medical treatments in a limited range of circumstances.)

"Informed consent" in the second sense, as institutional consent, has until very recently constituted the mainstream conception in the regulatory rules of federal agencies as well as in health care institutions. The documents governing consent in these contexts derive from a conception of what the rules must be in order to promote effective authorizations in these institutions, but the rules were only rarely premised on a conception of autonomous authorization that had more than a superficial quality. However, literature in bioethics has increasingly suggested that any justifiable analysis of informed consent must be rooted in autonomous choice by patients and subjects.

In principle, although less clearly in practice, the conditions of informed consent as autonomous authorization can function as model standards for fashioning the institutional and policy requirements of informed consent—a model of autonomous choice thus serving as the benchmark against which the moral adequacy of prevailing rules and practices might be evaluated.

Autonomous Choice

It has often been said that the justification of requirements of informed consent (in the first sense at least) is the principle of respect for autonomy. However, the goal of ensuring that persons make "autonomous choices" has proved to be difficult to implement. Historically, little more can be said beyond the fact that a clear societal consensus has developed that there must be adequate protection of patients' and subjects' decision-making rights, especially their autonomy rights. We therefore need to examine the meaning of "autonomy" in addition to the meaning of "informed consent."

In the literature on informed consent, "autonomy" and "respect for autonomy" are terms loosely associated with several ideas, such as privacy, voluntariness, self-mastery, choosing freely, the freedom to choose, choosing one's own moral position, and accepting responsibility for one's choices. Because of this conceptual uncertainty, the concept of autonomy and its connection to informed consent need careful analysis.

In moral philosophy, personal autonomy has come to refer to personal self-governance: personal rule of the self by adequate understanding while remaining free from controlling interferences by others and from personal limitations that prevent choice. Many issues about consent concern failures to respect autonomy, ranging from manipulative underdisclosure of pertinent information to nonrecognition of a refusal of medical interventions. To respect an autonomous agent is to recognize with due appreciation the person's capacities and perspective, including his or her right to hold certain views and to take certain actions based on personal values and beliefs. Accordingly, an informed consent based on an autonomous authorization suggests a well-informed agent with the competence to authorize or refuse authorization of a medical or research intervention.

It has sometimes been claimed that informed consent, so understood, has a mythical quality, because true informed consent is never obtained under such a high ideal. The idea is that most patients and subjects cannot comprehend enough information or appreciate its relevance sufficiently to make decisions about medical care or about participation in research. This objection, however, springs from a misunderstanding of the nature and goals of informed consent, based in part on unwarranted standards of full disclosure and full understanding. The ideal of complete disclosure of all possibly relevant knowledge needs to be replaced by a more acceptable account of how patients and subjects understand relevant information. Merely because our actions fail to be fully informed, voluntary, or autonomous is no indication that they are never adequately informed or autonomous. We would never autonomously sign contracts, have automobiles repaired, file income-tax returns, and the like if this were the case.

This argument does not deny that some individuals have a knowledge base that is so impoverished that autonomous decision making about alien or novel situations is exceedingly difficult, but even under difficult situations there may be no reason to foreclose the possibility of making an adequate decision. Successful communication of novel, alien, and specialized information to laypersons can be accomplished by drawing analogies between the information and more ordinary events with which the patient or subject is familiar. Similarly, professionals can express probabilities in both numeric and nonnumeric terms while helping the patient or subject to assign meanings to the probabilities through comparison with more familiar risks and prior experiences.

THE LAW AND ITS LIMITS

The law of informed consent has been more influential as an authoritative set of statements and source of reflection than any other body of thought on the subject. "The doctrine of informed consent," as it is sometimes called, *is* the legal doctrine; and "informed consent" has often been treated as synonymous with this legal doctrine, which derives from the common law and includes the entire body of law dealing with the obligation to obtain consent. This legal vision is focused on *disclosure* and on *liability for injury*. There are good reasons, as we shall now see, why the law turns on such a narrow basis and also why it is ill-equipped to serve beyond these boundaries.

Theory of Liability

The primary basis for the legal doctrine is tort law. A "tort" is a civil injury to one's person or property that is inflicted by another and that is measured in terms of, and compensated by, money damages. This law imposes duties on members of society, and one who fails to fulfill a legal duty is liable for compensation for the misdeed (in the civil law). The theory of liability under which a case is tried determines the duty that must be fulfilled. In recent informed consent cases, negligence is the theory of liability almost uniformly applied. However, the informed consent doctrine originally developed and flourished under battery, which is a different theory of liability. Currently, no unified legal theory underlies all informed consent cases.

Under battery theory, the defendant is held liable for any intended (i.e., not careless or accidental) action that results in physical contact for which the plaintiff has given no permission. A defendant need not have an evil intent, nor must injury result; the unpermitted contact is itself considered wrongful. Under negligence theory, by contrast, unintentional, "careless" action or omission is the source of liability. The carelessness occurs in regard to some activity in which the defendant has a duty to take care or to behave reasonably toward others, and an injury measurable in monetary terms is caused by failure to discharge the duty (*Berkey*, 1969; Meisel, 1977; *Schloendorff*, 1914).

The Duty of Disclosure

Two competing disclosure standards have evolved as attempts to resolve problems regarding the nature and amount of the information that must be disclosed: the professional practice standard and the reasonable person standard. A third standard, the subjective standard, has also been discussed in legal commentary. The professional practice standard holds that both the range of the duty to disclose and the criteria of adequate disclosure are properly determined by the customary practices of a professional community. These practices establish the standards of care for disclosure and care alike. The patient, subject, or reasonable person lacking expert knowledge is considered unqualified to decide what should be disclosed.

Although the professional practice standard remains the primary standard in informed consent law, it contains inadequacies and it may be doubted whether a customary standard of disclosure exists for much of medical practice. A basic problem is that negligent care might be perpetuated if relevant professionals throughout the profession offer inferior information, and another doubtful premise is that physicians have sufficient expertise to be able to judge in many cases which items of *information* their patients need. However, the principal objection to this standard is its failure to promote decisional autonomy, the protection of which is generally accepted as the primary function and moral justification of informed consent requirements.

In contrast to the professional practice standard, the reasonable person standard focuses on the information a "reasonable person" needs to know about procedures, risks, alternatives, and consequences. The legal test of an adequate disclosure is the "materiality," or significance, of information to the decision making of the patient. Thus, the right to decide what information is material and due is shifted away from the physician to the reasonable patient. The reasonable person standard requires a physician to divulge any fact that is material to a reasonable person's decision, but no requirement exists to meet the unreasonable demand of a patient.

This reasonable person standard is as vulnerable to criticism as the professional-based standard. It can be doubted whether the reasonable person standard serves the interests of those patients who know little about either their informational needs or the medical system. The interpretation of the standard for clinical practice is also difficult, because it specifies no precise duty for physicians. Both the concept of material information and the central concept of the reasonable person are left at an intuitive level. It can therefore be doubted whether the reasonable person standard more adequately protects the patient's right to choose than does the professional practice standard.

These arguments are not intended to eliminate standards of disclosure. In the absence of a disclosure initiated by a professional, patients or subjects often cannot formulate their concerns and ask meaningful questions. A patient or subject needs to understand what an informed professional judges to be of value for most patients or subjects as material information, and what it means for consent to be an authorization to proceed. The problem is not whether we need adequate disclosures but whether a legal vehicle can be expected to provide an adequate standard of disclosure for clinical practice and research settings. I shall return to this issue under the discussion of "the quality of consent."

The larger problem with these standards is that they will not be of major assistance in formulating a conception of informed consent for clinical medicine and research. Because courts are captivated by the context of after-the-fact resolution of narrow and concrete questions of duty, responsibility, blame, injury, and damages in specific cases, the law has no systematic way of affecting *contemporary* medical practice other than by a somewhat muted threat of prosecution for legal wrongdoing.

For all of these reasons, the heart of issues about informed consent is not legal but moral. Informed consent has less to do with the liability of professionals and more to do with the understanding and autonomous choices of patients and subjects.

THE QUALITY OF CONSENT

In discussing both autonomous choice and the limits of law, we have noted that problems about the quality and adequacy of consent probably cannot be resolved unless conventional disclosure rules are redirected toward the quality of understanding present in a "consent." This approach focuses on the need for communication, dispensing with liability-oriented discussions about proper legal standards of disclosure. The key to effective communication is to invite participation by patients or subjects in an exchange of information and dialogue. Asking questions, eliciting the concerns and interests of the patient or subject, and establishing a climate that encourages the patient or subject to ask questions seem more important for medical ethics than requirements of disclosure in law.

Without a proper climate in the consent context, a request from a professional that the patient or subject ask for information is as likely to result in silence as to elicit the desired result of a meaningful informational exchange and consent. Patients find it difficult to approach physicians with questions or concerns, and even when they do not understand their physicians, many still do not ask questions. The extent to which this passive attitude characterizes research subjects is less clear. Although still understudied, it is a good guess that relatively little educating of this quality occurs at present in either clinical practice or research in the United States.

VULNERABLE SUBJECTS AND COMPLIANT PATIENTS

Patients and subjects are entitled to expect that physicians and research investigators who request decisions will do so free of coercion and manipulation. Much discussion about the morality of asking subjects and patients to consent centers not on how *informed* the subjects are, but on how *free* they are. For example, this topic dominated the deliberations of the National Commission for the Protection of Human Subjects over the involvement of prisoners in drug research. The National Commission raised the question of "whether prisoners are, in the words of the Nuremberg Code, 'so situated as to be able to exercise free power of choice.'" The National Commission answered that "although prisoners who participate in research affirm that they do so freely, the conditions of social and economic deprivation in which they live compromise their freedom. The Commission believes, therefore, that the appropriate expression of respect consists in protection from exploitation" (National Commission, 1976, 5–7).

The National Commission went on to recommend a ban on drug research with prisoners, on grounds that in coercive institutions free choice would be too often compromised. Six years later this argument continued: Robert Levine, who had served on the staff of the National Commission, argued—as had a minority of commissioners—that prisoners are actually better off, not worse off, by their involvement in research and that exclusion from research was a deeper restriction of free choice than allowing inclusion in the research (Levine, 1982, 6). Many were dubious, however, that such abstract statements take account of the realities of manipulation and coercion in the prison (Dubler, 1982, 10).

A similar controversy occurred in the 1980s when Dr. Mortimer Lipsett at the National Institutes of Health (National Institute of Child Health and Human Development) explored the question of whether phase I clinical trials of cancer chemotherapies involve a special class of subjects deserving special protections. He presented the problem as follows:

> The President's Commission for the Study of Ethical Problems in Medicine and Biomedical and Behavioral Research developed and extended the concept of the vulnerable subject in medical research. Children, prisoners, and the mentally disabled were defined as vulnerable because a variety of constraints and inducements effectively removed their capacity to function autonomously. Similarly, patients with advanced cancer are faced with inducements that may sway their judgment of the risk-benefit ratio. Should such patients be treated as vulnerable research subjects necessitating extraordinary supervision by third parties? (Lipsett, 1982, 941–942)

Lipsett answered that every patient entering such a therapeutic trial is vulnerable by virtue of the disease state and the unique opportunity to receive a promising drug, but he maintained that the problem could be and was being overcome by "painstaking consultation and preparation" involving families, institutional review boards, third-party consultation, and the like. He concluded that, as conducted, phase I clinical trials of "cancer chemotherapies are ethical and necessary" (Lipsett, 1982, 941–942).

Some published responses to Lipsett were less sanguine: Alexander Capron, who had been staff director of the President's Commission, as well as Terrence Ackerman and Carson Strong, argued that the notion of therapeutic intent in the trials is easily subject to misunderstanding by patients, who may be misled by the hope of a favorable effect, especially when the prospect for therapeutic efficacy is as remote as it often is at the dosage level offered. They maintained that patients should be given a realistic picture of how they are contributing to medical knowledge and noted the dangers of "manipulating" subjects and of subjecting them to "affective" factors that impair understanding and judgment. In general, they challenged the view that present safeguards are sufficient to preclude exploitation (Ackerman & Strong, 1983, 883; Capron, 1983, 882–883).

Underlying these discussions is a theoretically difficult and partially unresolved set of problems about free choice, coercion, and manipulation. Certain forms of withholding information, playing on emotion, or presenting constraints can rob an autonomous person of the capacity of free choice through manipulation or coercion. Deceptive and misleading statements limit freedom by restricting the range of choice and by getting a person to do what the person otherwise would not do (cf. Bok, 1992, 1118–1119). The National Commission was worried about *coercion* in the case of prisoners; by contrast, those engaged in the discussion of phase I trials and cancer chemotherapies were interested in *manipulation*.

A continuum of controlling influences is present in our daily lives, running from coercion, which is at the most controlling end of the continuum (compare the National Commission's model of prisoners), to persuasion and education, which are not controlling at all, even though they are influences. For an action to be classified as either voluntary or nonvoluntary, cut-off points on the continuum of control to noncontrol are required. To fix the point of voluntariness, only a *substantial* satisfaction of the condition of noncontrol is needed. The line between the substantial and the insubstantial can be fixed in light of specific objectives of decision making. These lines will be influenced by moral views of when it is appropriate to respect a person's decision as substantially voluntary, but this connection need not be pursued here.

Influence does not necessarily imply constraint, governance, force, or compulsion, although these concepts are essential to certain kinds of influence. Important decisions are usually made in contexts replete with influences in the form of competing claims and interests, social demands and expectations, and straight-forward or devious attempts by others to bring about the outcome they desire. Some of these influences are unavoidable, and some may be desirable. Not all of them interfere with or deprive persons of autonomous belief and action, as when patients are persuaded by sound reasons to do something.

Coercion that involves a threat of harm so severe that a person is unable to resist acting to avoid it is always completely controlling. It entirely negates freedom because it entirely controls action. Persuasion, by contrast, is the intentional and successful attempt to induce a person, through appeals to reason, to freely accept the beliefs, attitudes, values, intentions, or actions advocated by the persuader. Like informing, persuading is entirely compatible with free choice.

The most sweeping and difficult area of influence is manipulation, a broad, general category that runs from highly controlling to altogether noncontrolling influences. The essence of manipulation is getting people to do what the manipulator intends without resort to coercion or to reasoned argument. In a paradigm case of manipulation in contexts of informed consent, information is closely managed to bring about the "choice" by a patient that the physician wants the patient to make, and the patient does not know what the manipulative physician intends. Whether such uses of information necessarily compromise or restrict free choice is an unresolved and untidy issue, but one plausible view is that some manipulations (e.g., the use of rewards such as reduced medical fees for being involved in research) are compatible with free choice, whereas others (e.g., deceptive offers of hope of a cure where there is none) are not compatible with free choice.

In informed consent contexts, the central question is not whether we are entirely free of manipulative influences, but whether we are *sufficiently* free to remain autonomous—free to perform our own actions—as opposed to controlled by the actions of another. The thorniest of all problems about autonomy and manipulation is not that of punishment and threat, but the effect of rewards and offers. This category refers to the intentional use of offers of rewards to bring about a desired response. For example, during the Tuskegee Syphilis experiments, various methods were used to stimulate and sustain the interest of subjects in continued participation. They were offered free burial assistance and insurance, free transportation, and a free stop in town on the return trip. They were also rewarded with free medicines and free hot meals on the days of the examination. The deprived socioeconomic condition of these subjects made them easily manipulable by those means.

This general range of problems is compounded further by what is sometimes called the problem of "coercive situations," but is better formulated as "constraining situations." Most accounts of coercion require that coercion be intentional by the coercer, but constraining situations suggest nonintentional "coercion" where the person is controlled by the situation, not by the design of another person.

Sometimes people unintentionally make other persons feel "threatened," and sometimes situations of illness and economic necessity present "threats" of serious harm that a person feels compelled to prevent at all costs. The earlier example of using prisoners in experimentation is again applicable if we assume that a prisoner is left without any viable alternative to participation in research because of the risks of the alternatives in the circumstance or because of what may appear to be threats presented by prison officials. As Alvin Bronstein, director of the National Prison Project, once put the problem for informed consent, "You cannot create... [a prison] institution in which informed consent without coercion is feasible" (Bronstein, 1975, 130–131).

Beyond the prison, in circumstances of severe physical or health deprivation, a person might accept an offer or sign a contract that the person would refuse under less stringent circumstances. Cancer patients provide good examples: The prospect of death if an objectionable toxic drug is rejected seems to "coerce" a choice of the drug no less than an intentional threat. The psychological effect on the person forced to choose may be identical, and the person can appropriately say in both cases, "There was no real choice; I would have been crazy to refuse." But if, as we usually believe, a contract signed under another person's threat is invalid (and the consent behind the signing an invalid consent), can we not say that a person who agrees to drug experimentation in a constraining situation has made an invalid contract (and given an invalid consent)?

It is a mistake to suppose that persons in such constraining situations cannot act *autonomously*. A loss of alternatives cannot be equated with coercion. It is, then, a confusion to move from a correct claim about a loss of options caused by desperate circumstances to the conclusion that there has been a loss of autonomy because of a constraining situation. Nevertheless, even if knowledgeable intent to threaten is not present, one may feel just as forced to a choice and may just as heartily wish to avoid it. Such perceptions are why the issues are often presented in the language of "vulnerable subjects." Their situation does make them vulnerable, even desperately vulnerable, and may subject them to "control" by their emotions and anxieties to an abnormal degree.

Despite the tense and pressured nature of such circumstances, most patients have the ability to consent freely and will do so if properly managed. What may be doubted is how often a free informed consent does in fact occur.

COMPETENCE TO CONSENT

I observed earlier that competence is commonly considered a necessary condition of informed consent. In legal and policy contexts, reference to competent persons is far more common than reference to autonomous persons. Competence judgments function as a gatekeeping device for informed consent. That is, competence judgments function to distinguish persons from whom consent should be solicited from those from whom consent need not or should not be solicited. In health care, competence judgments distinguish the class of individuals whose autonomous decisions must be respected from those individuals whose decisions need to be checked and perhaps overridden by a surrogate (Buchanan & Brock, 1989, 26–27; Faden & Beauchamp, 1986, 287–292).

Competence can be either a factual or a categorical determination. Minors, for example, are incompetent in law, whereas adults can generally be declared legally incompetent only on the basis of some factual determination. The issue of legal capacity is more complex for adult patients, for whom an individual determination normally must be made. If a person is incompetent, the physician is usually required, absent an emergency, to secure some form of third-party consent from a guardian or other legally empowered representative. Placement of the label "incompetent" on a patient or subject automatically introduces the possibility of coercive treatment and the presumption that there is no need to obtain consent. "Competence" commonly functions to denote persons whose consents, refusals, and statements of preference will be accepted as binding, while "incompetence" denotes those who are to be placed under the guidance and control of another.

JUSTIFICATIONS FOR NOT OBTAINING CONSENT

Several standard exceptions to requirements of informed consent exist in law and ethics. All courts passing judgment on the issue have ruled that a patient's right to self-determination is not absolute. Five exceptions to the informed consent requirement are generally recognized: the public health emergency, the medical emergency, the incompetent patient, the therapeutic privilege, and the patient waiver (Meisel, 1979). All but the therapeutic privilege have been widely accepted in law and ethics. However, the therapeutic privilege has elicited a particularly furious exchange over whether autonomy rights can be validly set aside.

The therapeutic privilege allows a physician to withhold information based on a sound medical judgment that to divulge the information would be potentially harmful to a depressed, emotionally drained, or unstable patient. Several harmful outcomes have been cited, including endangering life, causing irrational decisions, and producing anxiety or stress (*Canterbury v. Spence*, 1972, 785–789; van Oosten, 1991, 31–41). In clinical settings, this privilege has long been used to justify not obtaining consent. If framed broadly, the therapeutic privilege can permit physicians to withhold information if disclosure would cause *any* countertherapeutic deterioration, however slight, in the physical, psychological, or emotional condition of the patient. If framed narrowly, it can permit the physician to withhold information if and only if the patient's knowledge of the information would have serious health-related consequences—for example, by jeopardizing the success of the treatment or harming the patient psychologically by impairing decision making.

The narrowest formulation is that the therapeutic privilege can be validly invoked only if the physician has good reason to believe that disclosure would render the patient incompetent to consent to or refuse the treatment—that is, would render the decision nonautonomous. To invoke the therapeutic privilege under such circumstances does not conflict with respect for autonomy, because an autonomous decision could not be made. However, broader formulations of the privilege that require only "medical contraindication" do operate at the expense of autonomy. These formulations may unjustifiably endanger autonomous choice, as when use of the privilege is based on the belief that an autonomous patient would refuse an indicated therapy for medically inappropriate reasons.

Unless the therapeutic privilege is tightly and operationally formulated, the medical profession can use it to deprive the unreasonable but competent patient of the right to make decisions, especially if the physician sees his or her commitment to the patient's best interest as the overriding consideration. Loose standards can permit physicians to climb to safety over a straw bridge of speculation about the psychological consequences of information. In short, there is a significant potential for abuse of the privilege because of its inconsistency with the patient's rights to know and to decline treatment (Faden & Beauchamp, 1986, 38).

In 1986, U.S. Supreme Court Justice Byron White vigorously attacked the idea that concerns about increasing a person's anxiety about a procedure provide grounds for an exception to rules of informed consent: "It is the very nature of informed consent provisions that they may produce some anxiety in the patient and influence her in her choice. This is in fact their reason for existence, and . . . it is an entirely salutary reason" (*Thornburgh v. American College of Obstetricians*, 1986, 2199–2200). White is suggesting that the legal status of the doctrine of therapeutic privilege is no longer as secure as it once was.

In addition to the five standard exceptions to informed consent, several circumstances are encountered in contemporary medicine and research that suggest a need to relax requirements of informed consent. For example, in observational studies that examine behavior without the subject's knowledge and in secondary-data analysis, we often need only to avoid invasions of privacy and the presentation of significant risk to subjects, without procuring consents. Some vital research in epidemiology could not be conducted if consent were needed to obtain access to records. Use of records without consent is not necessarily an ethical violation. Research may be the first stage of an investigation to determine whether one needs to trace and contact particular individuals and obtain their permission for further participation in a study. In other cases, third-party consent is sometimes acceptable when access to a subject is impractical or the subject is incompetent. In some cases of low-risk research, subjects of research need not be contacted at all, and occasionally disclosures and warnings may be substituted for obtaining explicit informed consents. Thus, disclosures and warnings may sometimes justifiably be substituted for informed consents.

Finally, it does not follow from the great social importance of the rules and practices of informed consent that institutional policies of informed consent must rank the protection of decision making above all other values. The preservation of autonomous choice is the first, but not the only, institutional commitment. For example, a patient's need for education and counseling must be balanced against the interests of other patients and of society in maintaining a productive and efficient health care system. Accordingly, institutional policies must consider what is fair and reasonable to require of health care professionals and researchers and what the effect would be of alternative consent requirements on efficiency and effectiveness in the delivery of health care and the advancement of science.

CONCLUSION

Jay Katz has argued that the history of the physician–patient relationship from ancient times to the present reveals how inattentive physicians have been to their patients' rights and needs. Katz is equally unrelenting in his criticisms of court decisions and legal scholarship. He regards the declarations of courts as filled with overly optimistic rhetoric. The problem, in his view, is that the law has little to do with fostering real communication in the clinic and tends to line up with the professional judgments of physicians in the crucial test cases (Katz, 1984, 2–4, 28, 49–50, 79; 1987).

Katz is correct in judging that informed consent has always been an alien notion in the history of medicine and medical ethics and that informed consent requirements have still not deeply modified forms of communication between physicians and their patients. At the same time, the scene in medicine throughout the world is undergoing what may prove to be an extensive transformation through the implementation of the idea of informed consent. Patients are giving more "informed consents" and more attention is being paid in institutions to the quality of those consents. It is indisputable that research ethics and policies have been dramatically affected by requirements of informed consent.

Before we condemn the defects in the writings and practices of the past, we should remember that the history of informed consent is still unfolding and that our failures may be no less apparent to future generations than are the failures that we find with the past.

References

Ackerman, Terrence F., and Carson M. Strong. In "Letters." *Journal of the American Medical Association* 249 (Feb. 18, 1983): 882–883.

American Medical Association, *Proceedings of the National Medical Conventions*. Held in New York, May 1846, and in Philadelphia, May 1847. Adopted May 6, 1847, and submitted for publication in Philadelphia, 1847.

Beauchamp, Tom L., and James F. Childress. *Principles of Biomedical Ethics*. 4th ed. New York: Oxford University Press, 1994 (and later editions).

Berkey v. Anderson, 1 Cal. App. 3d 790, 82 Cal. Rptr. 67 (1969).

Bok, Sissela. "Informed Consent in Tests of Patient Reliability." *Journal of the American Medical Association* 267, no. 8 (Feb. 26, 1992): 1118–1119.

Bronstein, Alvin. "Remarks." In *Experiments and Research with Humans: Values in Conflict*, National Academy of Sciences, 130–131. Washington, DC: National Academy, 1975.

Buchanan, Allen E., and Dan W. Brock. *Deciding for Others: The Ethics of Surrogate Decision Making*. Cambridge: Cambridge University Press, 1989.

Canterbury v. Spence, 464 F.2d 772 (D.C. Cir. 1972).

Capron, Alexander M. In "Letters." *Journal of the American Medical Association* 249 (Feb. 18, 1983): 882–883.

Cobbs v. Grant, 104 Cal. Rptr. 505, 502 P.2d 1 (1972).

Dubler, Nancy. "The Burdens of Research in Prisons." *IRB* 4 (November 1982): 9–10.

Faden, Ruth R., and Tom L. Beauchamp. *A History and Theory of Informed Consent*. New York: Oxford University Press, 1986.

Gisborne, Thomas. *An Enquiry into the Duties of Men in the Higher and Middle Classes of Society in Great Britain, resulting from their Respective Stations, Professions, and Employments*. London: B. & J. White, 1794.

Gregory, John. *Lectures on the Duties and Qualifications of a Physician*. London: W. Strahan and T. Cadell, 1772.

Hagman, D. B. "The Medical Patient's Right to Know: Report on a Medical-Legal-Ethical, Empirical Study," *U.C.L.A. Law Review* 17 (1970): 758–816.

Harris, Louis, et al. "Views of Informed Consent and Decisionmaking: Parallel Surveys of Physicians and the Public." In *Making Health Care Decisions*, Vol. 2, President's Commission for the Study of Ethical Problems in Medicine and Biomedical and Behavioral Research (as below).

Hattori, Hiroyuki, et al. "The Patient's Right to Information in Japan—Legal Rules and Doctor's Opinions." *Social Science and Medicine* 32 (1991): 1007–1016.

Hershey, Nathan, and Bushkoff, Stanley H. *Informed Consent Study*. Pittsburgh, PA: Aspen Systems Corporation, 1969.

Hippocrates. In *Hippocrates*, 4 vols., translated by W.H.S. Jones, 1923-1931. Cambridge, MA: Harvard University Press.

Hooker, Worthington. *Physician and Patient; or a Practical View of the Mutual Duties, Relations and Interests of the Medical Professions and the Community*. New York: Baker and Scribner, 1859.

Hyman v. Jewish Chronic Disease Hospital, 251 N.Y. 2d 818 (1964), 206 N.E. 2d 338 (1965).

Jones, James H. *Bad Blood*. 2nd ed. New York: Maxwell Macmillan, 1993.

Kai, Ichiro, et al. "Communication between Patients and Physicians about Terminal Care: A Survey in Japan." *Social Science and Medicine* 36 (1993): 1151–1159.

Katz, Jay. "Physician-Patient Encounters 'On a Darkling Plain.'" *Western New England Law Review* 9 (1987): 207–226.

Katz, Jay. *The Silent World of Doctor and Patient*. New York: The Free Press, 1984.

Levine, Robert J. "The Nature and Definition of Informed Consent in Various Research Settings." *The Belmont Report*. Appendix: Vol. I. Washington, DC: DHEW Publication No. (OS) 78-0013, 1978, (3-1)–(3-91).

Levine, Robert J. "Research Involving Prisoners: Why Not?" *IRB* 4 (May 1982): 6.

Lipsett, Mortimer B. "On the Nature and Ethics of Phase I Clinical Trials of Cancer Chemotherapies." *Journal of the American Medical Association* 248 (Aug. 27, 1982): 941–942.

Meisel, Alan. "The 'Exceptions' to the Informed Consent Doctrine: Striking a Balance Between Competing Values in Medical Decisionmaking." *Wisconsin Law Review* 1979 (1979): 413–488.

Meisel, Alan. "The Expansion of Liability for Medical Accidents: From Negligence to Strict Liability by Way of Informed Consent." *Nebraska Law Review* 56 (1977): 51–152.

Meisel, Alan, and Loren H. Roth. "Toward an Informed Discussion on Informed Consent: A Review and Critique of the Empirical Studies." *Arizona Law Review* 25 (1983): 265–346.

Meisel, Alan, and Loren Roth. "What We Do and Do Not Know About Informed Consent." *Journal of the American Medical Association* 246 (November 1981): 2473–2477.

Mizushima, Yutaka, et al. "A Survey Regarding the Disclosure of the Diagnosis of Cancer in Toyama Prefecture, Japan." *Japanese Journal of Medicine* 29 (1990): 146–155, esp. 146.

National Commission for the Protection of Human Subjects of Biomedical and Behavioral Research. *The Belmont Report*. Washington, DC: DHEW Publication No. (OS) 78-0012, 1978.

National Commission for the Protection of Human Subjects. *Research Involving Prisoners*. Washington, DC: DHEW Publication No. (OS) 76-131, 1976.

Percival, Thomas. *Medical Ethics; or a Code of Institutes and Precepts, Adapted to the Professional Conduct of Physicians and Surgeons*. Manchester, England: S. Russell, 1803. The most available edition is *Percival's Medical Ethics*, edited by Chauncey D. Leake. Huntington, NY: Robert E. Krieger Publishing Company, 1975.

Pernick, Martin S. "The Patient's Role in Medical Decisionmaking: A Social History of Informed Consent in Medical Therapy." In *Making Health Care Decisions*, Vol. 3, President's Commission for the Study of Ethical Problems in Medicine and Biomedical and Behavioral Research. Washington, DC: U.S. Government Printing Office, 1982.

Planned Parenthood of Central Missouri v. Danforth, 428 U.S. 52 (1976).

President's Commission for the Study of Ethical Problems in Medicine and Biomedical and Behavioral Research. *Deciding to Forego Life-Sustaining Treatment*. Washington, DC: U.S. Government Printing Office, March 1983.

President's Commission for the Study of Ethical Problems in Medicine and Biomedical and Behavioral Research. *Making Health Care Decisions*, Vols. 1–3. Washington, DC: U.S. Government Printing Office, 1982.

Proceedings of the Symposium on Ethical Issues in Human Experimentation: The Case of Willowbrook State Hospital Research. Urban Health Affairs Program. New York: University Medical Center, 1972.

Quaid, Kimberly A., et al. "Informed Consent for a Prescription Drug: Impact of Disclosed Information on Patient Understanding and Medical Outcomes." *Patient Education and Counselling* 15 (1990): 249–259.

Rush, Benjamin. *Medical Inquiries and Observations*, Vol. 2, 2nd ed. Philadelphia: Thomas Dobson, 1794. Published as a single essay entitled *An Oration . . . An Enquiry into the Influence of Physical Causes upon the Moral Faculty.* Philadelphia: Charles Cist, 1786.

Salgo v. Leland Stanford Jr. University Board of Trustees, 317 P.2d 170 (1957).

Scherer, David G., and N. D. Reppucci. "Adolescents' Capacities to Provide Voluntary Informed Consent." *Law and Human Behavior* 12 (1988): 123–141.

Schloendorff v. Society of New York Hospitals, 211 N.Y. 125, 105 N.E. 92 (1914).

Siminoff, L. A., and J. H. Fetting. "Factors Affecting Treatment Decisions for a Life-Threatening Illness: The Case of Medical Treatment for Breast Cancer." *Social Science and Medicine* 32 (1991): 813–818.

Siminoff, L. A., J. H. Fetting, and M. D. Abeloff. "Doctor-Patient Communication about Breast Cancer Adjuvant Therapy." *Journal of Clinical Oncology* 7 (1989): 1192–1200.

Takahashi, Yoshimoto. "Informing a Patient of Malignant Illness: Commentary from a Cross-Cultural Viewpoint." *Death Studies* 14 (1990): 83–91.

Thornburgh v. American College of Obstetricians, 106 S.Ct. 2169 (1986) (White, J., dissenting).

United States v. Karl Brandt, Trials of War Criminals Before the Nuremberg Military Tribunals under Control Council Law No. 10, Vols. 1 and 2, "The Medical Case," Military Tribunal I, 1947. Washington, DC: U.S. Government Printing Office, 1948–1949.

van Oosten, F. F. W. "The So-Called 'Therapeutic Privilege' or 'Contra-Indication': Its Nature and Role in Non-Disclosure Cases." *Medicine and Law* 10 (1991): 31–41.

Wilkinson v. Vesey, 295 A.2d 676 (R.I. 1972).

5

WHO DESERVES AUTONOMY AND WHOSE AUTONOMY DESERVES RESPECT?

"Autonomy," "respect for autonomy," and "rights of autonomy" are strikingly different notions. "Respect for autonomy" and "rights of autonomy" are moral notions, but "autonomy" and "autonomous person" are not obviously moral notions. Indeed, they seem more metaphysical than moral. However, this distinction between the metaphysical and the moral has fostered precarious claims such as these: (1) analysis of autonomy is a conceptual, metaphysical project, not a moral one; (2) a theory of autonomy should not be built on moral notions, but on a theory of mind, self, or person; and (3) the concept of autonomy is intimately connected to the concept of person, which anchors the concept of moral status.

I will be assessing these claims with the objective of determining who qualifies as autonomous and what sort of autonomy deserves our respect. I will argue that moral notions—in particular, respect for autonomy—should affect how we construct theories of autonomous action and the autonomous person. However, theories of autonomy should only be *constrained* by the principle of respect for autonomy, not wholly *determined* by it.

CONCEPTS AND THEORIES OF AUTONOMY

Autonomy is generally understood as personal self-governance: personal rule of the self free of controlling interferences by others and free of personal limitations that prevent choice. Two basic conditions of autonomy, therefore, are (1) *liberty* (independence from controlling influences) and (2) *agency* (capacity for intentional action). However, disagreement exists over how to analyze these conditions and over whether additional conditions are needed. Each notion is indeterminate until further specified, and each can be used only as a rough guide for philosophers in the construction of a theory of autonomy.[1]

Some available theories of autonomy feature traits of the *autonomous person*, whereas others focus on *autonomous action*. Theories of the autonomous person are theories of a kind of agent. For example, the autonomous person is portrayed in some theories as consistent, independent, in command, resistant to control by authorities, and the source of his or her basic values and beliefs. These theories are structured in terms of virtues and persistent ideals. My analysis of autonomy is not focused on such traits of the person, but on actions. My interest is on choice rather than general capacities for governance. Until the final section in this essay, I will not be concerned with conditions of personhood. I assume that autonomous persons sometimes fail to act autonomously because of temporary constraints caused by illness or depression, circumstantial ignorance, coercion, or other conditions that restrict options. An autonomous person who signs a contract or consent agreement without understanding the document and without intending to agree to its conditions is qualified to act autonomously, but fails to do so. Similarly, a man who is threatened with death by a thief and who hands over his wallet because he does not wish to suffer the threatened consequences does not act autonomously, even if he is an autonomous person.

Conversely, some persons who are generally incapable of autonomous decision making make some autonomous choices. For example, some patients in mental institutions who are unable to care for themselves and are legally incompetent make autonomous choices such as ringing for a nurse, stating preferences for meals, and making telephone calls to acquaintances. These persons act autonomously even if they fail critical conditions of the autonomous person.

THE ROLE OF THE PRINCIPLE OF RESPECT FOR AUTONOMY

To maintain coherence with fundamental principles of morality, a theory of autonomy should be kept consistent with the substantive assumptions about autonomy implicit in the principle of respect for autonomy. To respect an autonomous agent is to recognize with due appreciation that person's capacities and perspective, including the right to control his or her affairs, to make certain choices, and to take certain actions based on personal values and beliefs. Autonomous agents are entitled to determine their own destiny, and respect requires noninterference with their actions. Respect involves acknowledging decision-making rights and enabling persons to act, whereas disrespect involves attitudes and actions that ignore, insult, or demean others' rights of autonomy. This thesis does not entail that, from the moral point of view, we are to respect only the morally good intentions and actions of agents. Many acts of individual autonomy are morally neutral, yet are owed respect.

Making Theory Conform to Moral Principle

Some theories of autonomy do not presume that a principle of respect for autonomy provides a substantive basis for the theory. They do not mention the principle or attempt to conform the theory to its assumptions. This matter is of the first importance because a theory that distinguishes nonautonomous acts from autonomous ones teaches us what it is that we are to respect, and opens up the possibility of disrespecting certain "choices" that are of penetrating importance to the agent, on grounds that these choices are nonautonomous. Any theory that classifies acts as not autonomous that are of the greatest importance to us in the basic governance of our affairs is morally dangerous and conceptually dubious. If, for example, a theory declares *nonautonomous* the acts of average persons in opening a bank account, writing a will, selling a house, or refusing an offered surgical procedure, the theory is unacceptable. To declare these choices nonautonomous is to imply that another person may legitimately serve as guardian and decision maker. On this basis a will could be invalidated or a surgical procedure authorized against the person's wish. As Onora O'Neill has cautioned in her work, standards of autonomy so high that we cannot live up to them will have the devastating effect of inappropriately classifying "a far larger proportion of the patient population as lacking competence."[2]

An instructive example of the moral perils that a theory of autonomy can pose is found in the work of Julian Savulescu on decisions to limit choices for or against life-sustaining treatments. In developing his account, Savulescu realizes that he must set out the conditions of autonomy in just the right way in order to get morally justified outcomes. If he fails in the theory of autonomy, the choices of patients will be inappropriately limited or reversed. Savulescu sharply distinguishes autonomous and nonautonomous acts using a distinction between *mere desires* and *rational desires*. Autonomous actions are only those performed from rational desires. Savulescu argues that health care professionals and guardians are only required to respect the actions of a patient that are done from rational desire; an *expressed desire* is not sufficient. He argues that many choices (e.g., a Jehovah's Witness's decision to refuse a blood transfusion) can and should be judged not rational, and therefore not autonomous, and therefore lacking in moral weight.[3]

The theory of autonomy that I present in this essay presumes the cardinal moral importance of protecting everyday choices by consulting the principle of respect for autonomy. I am assuming that everyday choices of ordinary persons are paradigm cases of autonomous choices. A critical test of the adequacy of any theory of autonomy, then, is whether it coheres with the moral requirement that we respect everyday choices such as opening bank accounts, purchasing goods in stores, and authorizing an automobile to be repaired.

I am not asserting either that ordinary persons never fail to choose autonomously or that we are morally required to respect all autonomous choices by not interfering with them. Certain behaviors "performed" or "willed" by individuals are clearly not autonomous (e.g., giving up one's wallet when coerced and attempting to fly off a balcony when in a drug-induced state); and we are just as certainly not required to respect all choices of thieves, religious zealots who spew hatred, persons who act with conflicts of interest, and the like.

A Typical Example

As an example of the choices of ordinary persons having status as autonomous, consider the refusal of a blood transfusion by a Jehovah's Witness who has never reflectively questioned whether he should be a member of his faith or asked whether he wants to be the kind of person who refuses blood transfusions. Throughout his life he has been a firmly committed Jehovah's Witness, but now his religious commitments conflict with the healing commitments of health care professionals who are urging a transfusion. His life is on the line, and he adheres to the doctrines of his faith.

One could challenge the proposition that this Jehovah's Witness is acting autonomously on grounds that his beliefs are unreflective assumptions instilled by authoritarian dogma or what Savulescu calls irrational desires, but this challenge seems to me conceptually and empirically doubtful and, as a matter of theory and policy, fraught with danger. That we adopt beliefs and principles deriving from forms of institutional authority does not prevent them from being our beliefs and principles. Individuals autonomously accept moral notions that derive from many forms of cultural tradition and institutional authority. If the Witness's decision can be legitimately invalidated on grounds of acting nonautonomously, so may a great many institutionally guided choices. I hypothesize that a theory of autonomy that conflicts with this assumption is an unacceptable and morally problematic theory.

A CONCISE THEORY OF THE CONDITIONS OF AUTONOMOUS ACTION

I will be assuming in this article an account of autonomous choice that I have elsewhere set out in terms that I believe to be compatible with the constraints on theory that I just outlined.[4] That is, this account of autonomy is designed to be coherent with the assumptions that we must make when we insist that the choices of ordinary persons be respected. In this account, I analyze autonomous action in terms of normal choosers who act (1) intentionally, (2) with understanding, and (3) without controlling influences. What follows is a brief statement of these conditions, omitting their subtleties.

The Condition of Intentionality

Intentional actions require plans in the form of representations of the series of events proposed for the execution of the action. For an act to be intentional, it must correspond to the actor's conception of the act in question, although a planned outcome might not materialize as projected. Unintended acts, such as a pediatrician's dropping of a newborn infant during delivery, are nonautonomous, but the agent may still be held responsible for what occurs. Imagine that Professor X intends to read a paper that he has written on a toxic chemical and intends thereby to win first prize at a convention. His paper is on toxic chemical A. Professor X's plan entails executing a sequence of actions, chief of which is a particular set of arguments about A that he believes will be well received by this audience. However, in preparing to travel to the convention, Professor X accidentally packs the wrong paper, which is on the subject of toxic chemical B. The professor is forgetful and does not realize when he reads his paper at the convention that it is the wrong paper. Despite this lapse, he wins first prize for the best paper. Professor X has read a paper on a toxic chemical and won first prize, which he intended, yet he did not do so intentionally in the way the action was performed. His reception by the audience and his winning the prize were, as it turns out, not brought about according to his plan of action.

In a theory of autonomy (and of informed consent), we need to decide whether special kinds of wants or desires are necessary conditions of intentional action. It might be thought that foreseen acts that the actor does not want and does not desire to perform are not intentional. Alvin Goldman uses the following example in an attempt to prove that agents do not intend merely foreseen effects.[5] Imagine that Mr. G takes a driver's test to prove competence. He comes to an intersection that requires a right turn and extends his arm to signal for a turn, although he knows it is raining and that he will get his hand wet. According to Goldman, Mr. G's signaling for a turn is an intentional act. By contrast, his wet hand is an unintended effect, or "incidental by-product," of his hand signaling. However, as I see it, getting the hand wet *is* part of an intentional action. It is willed in accordance with a plan and is neither accidental, inadvertent, nor habitual. There is nothing about intentional acts, as opposed to accidental occurrences, that rules out aversions. One's motivation for getting one's hand wet may reflect *conflicting* wants and desires, and clearly the driver does not want a wet hand, but this fact does not render the act of getting the hand wet less than intentional or autonomous.

Some intentional acts are wanted or desired for their own sake, and not for the sake of something else. For example, someone who loves to swim may want to swim for the sake of swimming, as may not be the case for another person who swims for the sake of a tanned or fit body. The desire to perform an act for its own sake is *intrinsic* wanting. Wanting for the sake of something else is *instrumental* wanting. When a surgeon cuts into the body of the patient, the patient has consented to the cutting and the cutting is part of the plan, but it is for the sake of better function or health. In such cases, the actor believes the action is the means to a goal wanted in the primary sense. Goldman would only consider an act intentional if at least one of these two forms of wanting is involved.

However, other intentional acts are not wanted in either of these two senses. An actor may view these acts as, *ceteris paribus*, undesirable or unwanted. They are performed only because they are entailed in the doing of other acts that are wanted. Such acts are foreseen and wanted acts in the sense that the actor wants to perform them in the circumstances more than he or she wants not to perform them. It is suitable in such cases to discard the language of "wanting" and to say that foreseen but not desired effects are "tolerated."[6] These effects are not so undesirable that the actor would choose not to perform the act in the first place. The actor includes them as a part of his or her plan of intentional action.

Accordingly, I use a model of intentionality based primarily on what is *willed* rather than what is *wanted*. Intentional actions include any action and any effect specifically willed in accordance with a plan, including merely tolerated effects.[7] In this conception, a physician can desire not to do what he intends to do, in the same way that one can be willing to do something but reluctant to do it, or even detest doing it. Consider Mr. X, who has become convinced that there is no meaningful way that he can both undergo facial surgery and avoid the scarring involved. After considering the alternative of refusing surgery, Mr. X intentionally consents to surgery, and in so doing he intentionally consents to being scarred by surgery. Although his consenting to a facial scar is a toleration of and not a desire for the scarring, the intentional act of consenting to the scarring is no less Mr. X's own act than is his consenting to surgery. Mr. X, then, intentionally consents to being scarred by surgery.

Under this account, the distinction between what agents do intentionally and what they merely foresee in a planned action is not viable.[8] For example, if a man enters a room and flips a switch that he knows turns on both a light and a fan, but desires only to activate the light, he cannot say that he activates the fan unintentionally. Even if the fan made an obnoxious whirring sound that he does not want, it would be incorrect to state that he unintentionally brought about the obnoxious sound by flipping the switch. Here and in the other examples mentioned previously, one might introduce a distinction between what an agent intends and an intentional action. Perhaps the agent does not intend the effect of a screeching fan and does not intend it as the goal of his action even though it is an intentional action. Likewise, one might be said to consent intentionally to being scarred in surgery while not intending to be scarred. In short, what it means for an act to be intentional need not be equated with what the agent of the action intends. However, I will not further pursue the merits of this distinction between what is intentional and what is intended, because I am concerned only with analysis of what it means for an action to be intentional, and especially the relationship between intentional action and autonomous choice.

The Condition of Understanding

An action is not autonomous if the actor has no appropriate understanding of it. Here we need a way of analyzing the question, "Do you understand what you are doing?" Starting with the extreme of *full* or *complete* understanding, a person understands an action if the person correctly apprehends all of the propositions that correctly describe the nature of the action and the foreseeable consequences or possible outcomes that might follow as a result of performing or not performing the action. This full understanding does not amount to omniscience, because the criterion demands only foreseeability. Less complete understanding occurs by degrees, with no understanding at the end of the continuum.

There are several reasons why limited understanding can occur in a process of deliberative choice and consent. Some patients and subjects are calm, attentive, and eager for dialogue, whereas others are nervous or distracted in ways that impair or block understanding. Conditions that limit their understanding include illness, irrationality, and immaturity. Deficiencies in the communication process also often hamper understanding. A breakdown in a person's ability to accept information as true or untainted, even if he or she adequately comprehends the information, can compromise decision making. For example, a seriously ill patient who has been properly informed about the nature of the illness and has been asked to make a treatment decision might refuse the proposed treatment while under the false belief that he or she is not ill. Even if the physician recognizes the patient's false belief and adduces conclusive evidence to prove to the patient that the belief is mistaken, and the patient comprehends the information provided, the patient still may go on believing that what has been (truthfully) reported is false.

The so-called "therapeutic misconception" occurs when subjects in research fail to distinguish between clinical care and research and fail to understand the purpose and aim of research, misconceiving their participation as therapeutic in nature.[9] Such a therapeutic misconception may invalidate the subject's consent to research. Some participants understand that they are involved in research, and not clinical care, but overestimate the therapeutic possibilities and probabilities—that is, the odds that a participant will benefit.[10] This overestimation may render a choice insufficiently autonomous and invalidate a consent.

Autonomous actions require only a basic understanding of the action, not a full understanding. An account of understanding that required an extremely high level of understanding would be oppressive if made a condition of autonomy. Many years ago when I decided to become a philosopher, I did not well understand the profession or its demands. However, I did know something about the writings of philosophers, I did know a few graduate students in philosophy, and I did have a reasonably good idea of my abilities as a student of philosophy. To say that my decision to be a philosopher was nonautonomous because I lacked relevant information about the profession would be inaccurate, even if such information was relevant to the choice made.

The Condition of Noncontrol, or Voluntariness

The third of the three conditions constituting autonomy is that a person, like an autonomous political state, must be free of controls exerted either by external sources or by internal states that rob the person of self-directedness. *Influence* and *resistance to influence* are basic concepts for this analysis. Not all influences are controlling. Many influences are resistible, and some are even trivial in their impact on autonomy. The category of influence is broad enough to include acts of love, threats, education, lies, manipulative suggestions, and emotional appeals, all of which can vary dramatically in their impact on persons. My analysis will focus on three categories of influence: persuasion, coercion, and manipulation.[11]

Persuasion is here understood as rational persuasion. A person comes to believe something through the merit of reasons another person advances. This is the paradigm of an influence that is not controlling and also warranted. If a physician presents reasons that persuade the patient to undergo a procedure when the patient is reluctant to do so, then the physician's actions influence, but do not control. In health care settings, there is often a problem of distinguishing emotional responses from cognitive responses and of determining whether the cognitive or the emotional is the primary factor in a decision. Some informational approaches that rationally persuade one patient overwhelm another whose fear or panic short-circuits reason.

Coercion occurs if and only if one person intentionally uses a credible and severe threat of harm or force to control another.[12] If a physician orders a reluctant patient to undergo a diagnostic examination and coerces the patient into compliance through a threat of abandonment, the physician's influence controls the patient. The threat of force used by some police, courts, and hospitals in acts of involuntary commitment for psychiatric treatment is coercive. Some threats will coerce virtually all persons (e.g., a credible threat to imprison a person), whereas others might succeed in coercing only a few persons (e.g., a parent's threat to cut off funding for a son in college unless the son consents to the donation of one of his kidneys to his sister).

Compliance merely because a person *feels* threatened, when no threat has been issued, is not coercion. Coercion occurs only if a credible and intended threat disrupts and reorders a person's self-directed course of action. Under these coercive conditions, even intentional and well-informed actions can be nonvoluntary. Handing over one's wallet to a thief with a gun is both intentional and well informed, though nonvoluntary. Being coerced does not entail that the person coerced lacks voluntary decision-making capacity in complying with a threat. It also does not entail that the person did not choose to perform the action or that the coercion involved always invalidates consent. The point is only that the action was not voluntary.

Manipulation is a term for several forms of influence that are neither persuasive nor coercive. It involves getting people to do what the manipulator wants through a nonpersuasive means that alters a person's understanding of a situation and motivates the person to do what the agent of influence intends. In health care and research, the most likely forms of manipulation are informational manipulation that nonpersuasively alters a person's understanding and offers of rewards or potential benefits. Critics of various recruiting practices in biomedical research have suggested that there is often informational manipulation through withholding critical information about risks together with a misleading exaggeration of benefits. Other critics have said that offers of compensation and health care are manipulative when made excessively attractive.

Nevertheless, it is easy to inflate the threat of control by manipulation beyond its significance in health care. We typically make decisions in a context of competing influences such as familial constraints, legal obligations, offers of rewards, and institutional pressures. These influences usually do not control decisions to a morally questionable degree. In biomedical ethics we need only establish general criteria for the point at which influence threatens autonomous choice, while recognizing that in many cases no sharp boundary separates controlling and noncontrolling influences.

I have concentrated in this section on *external* controlling influences—usually attempts by one person to influence another. No less important are *internal* influences on the person, such as those caused by mental illness. These conditions can also be voluntariness depriving. However, I will not here pursue problems of lack of internal control. I simply stipulate that an adequate theory of voluntariness must take account of both internal and external controlling influences.

Degrees of Autonomy and Substantial Autonomy

The first of the aforementioned three conditions of autonomy, intentionality, is not a matter of degree: Acts are either intentional or nonintentional. However, acts can satisfy both the conditions of understanding and absence of controlling influences to a greater or lesser extent. For example, threats can be more or less severe, and understanding can be more or less complete. Actions are autonomous by degrees, as a function of satisfying these conditions to different degrees. For both conditions, a continuum runs from fully present to wholly absent. For example, children exhibit different degrees of understanding at various ages, as well as different capacities of independence and resistance to influence attempts. This claim that actions are autonomous by degrees is an inescapable consequence of a commitment to the view that two of the necessary conditions of autonomy are satisfied by degrees.

For an action to be classified as either autonomous or nonautonomous, cut-off points on these continua are required. To fix these points, only a *substantial* satisfaction of the conditions of autonomy is needed, not a full or categorical satisfaction of the conditions. The line between what is substantial and what is insubstantial may seem arbitrary, but thresholds marking substantially autonomous decisions can be carefully fixed in light of specific objectives of decision making, such as deciding about surgery, buying a house, choosing a university to attend, making a contribution to charity, driving a car, and hiring a new employee.

Problems of Adequacy and Completeness

One can, and should, raise questions about whether the theory I have outlined contains an adequate set of conditions for a theory of autonomy. This theory looks to be what, in other philosophical literature, might be called a theory of free will or free agency. Free agency has often been analyzed in terms of (*1*) a condition of persons through which intentional actions are willed (a condition absent in contrastive cases such as dreaming and unintentional word-slips) and (2) the absence of internal and external controls (compulsion, constraint, etc.) that determine the choice of actions. This theory of free choice is similar to the one I am proposing for the analysis of autonomy.

However, if my theory reduces to a theory of free agency, it may have missed its target of *autonomy*. To test this hypothesis, I now look at a type of theory that proposes one or more conditions different from those that I have proposed.

SPLIT-LEVEL THEORIES OF AUTONOMY

Several philosophers maintain that autonomy consists of the capacity to control and identify with one's first-order desires or preferences by means of higher-level (second-order) desires or preferences through processes of deliberation, reflection, or volition. Harry Frankfurt's theory of the freedom of persons and Gerald Dworkin's theory of autonomy are widely discussed examples. I will closely follow the language of Dworkin's theory, since Frankfurt's theory of *persons* is not explicitly presented as a theory of *autonomy*.[13] However, I give neither theory a priority status.

An autonomous person, in this theory, is one who has the capacity to accept, identify with, or repudiate a lower-order desire or preference, showing the capacity to change (or maintain) one's preference structure or one's configuration of the will. All and only autonomous persons possess such distanced self-reflection, in which second-order mental states have first-order mental states as their intentional objects and considered preferences are formed about first-order preferences and beliefs. For example, a long-distance runner may have a first-order desire to run several hours a day, but also may have a higher-order desire to decrease the time to one hour. If he wants at any given moment to run several hours, then he wants at that moment what he does not truly want. Action from a first-order desire that is not endorsed by a second-order volition is not autonomous and is typical of animal behavior.

Frankfurt argues that it is essential to *being a person* that the second-order desires or volitions be such that the individual "wants a certain desire to be his will."[14] These second-order desires or volitions he calls "second-order volitions." Since they are essential to being a *person*, any individual lacking these volitions is not a person. Dworkin offers a "content-free" definition of *autonomy* as a "second-order capacity of persons to reflect critically upon their first-order preferences, desires, wishes, and so forth and the capacity to accept or attempt to change these in the light of higher-order preferences and values."[15] The language of *capacity* strongly suggests that this theory is one of autonomous *persons*, not a theory of autonomous *actions*.

Problems with the Theory

Several problems haunt this theory. First, there is nothing to prevent a reflective acceptance, preference, concern, or volition at the second level from being caused by and assured by the strength of a first-order desire. The individual's acceptance of or identification with the first-order desire would then be no more than a causal result of an already formed structure of preferences. Frankfurt writes that "whether a person identifies himself with [his] passions, or whether they occur as alien forces that remain outside the boundaries of his volitional identity, depends upon what he himself wants his will to be."[16] The problem is that the identification with one's passions may be governed by the strength of the first-order passion, not by an independent identification. If a person's identification (from what "he himself wants his will to be") at any point is itself the result of a process of thoroughgoing conditioning or lower-level passion, then the identification is never sufficiently independent to qualify as autonomous.

For example, the alcoholic with a passion for red wine who identifies with drinking seems nonautonomous if his second-level volition or desire to drink red wine is causally determined by a first-level desire. Suppose the alcoholic forms, as a result of the strength of first-order desire, a second-order volition to satisfy his strongest first-order desire, whatever it is. This behavior seems nonautonomous, but looks as if it would satisfy Frankfurt's conditions. Moreover, an alcoholic can reflect at ever-higher levels on lower-level desires without achieving autonomy if identification at all levels is causally determined by initial desires.

To make this split-level theory plausible as an account of autonomy, a supplementary theory would have to be added that distinguished influences or desires that rob an individual of autonomy from influences or desires consistent with autonomy.[17] Frankfurt seems to address these problems with the thesis that "truly autonomous choices" require "being satisfied with a certain desire" and having preexisting "stable volitional tendencies."[18] However, this analysis does not rescue the split-level theory. Anomalous actions can derive from choices that are out of character as a result of surrounding events that are unprecedented in the actor's experience, such as serious disease. These acts can be well planned, intentional, and free from the control of other persons. The actors may be unaware of the motivational or conditioning history that underlies and prompts their actions and may have made no reflective identification with the origins of their actions. This fact does not supply a sufficient reason to declare them nonvoluntary or nonautonomous.

Second, this theory risks running afoul of the criterion of coherence with the principle of respect for autonomy mentioned earlier. If reflective identification with one's desires or second-order volitions is a necessary condition of autonomous action, then many ordinary actions that are almost universally considered autonomous, such as cheating on one's spouse (when one truly wishes not to be such a person) or selecting tasty snack foods when grocery shopping (when one has never reflected on one's desires for snack foods), would be rendered non-autonomous in this theory. Requiring reflective identification and stable volitional patterns unduly narrows the scope of actions protected by a principle of respect for autonomy.

Frankfurt's theory runs this risk in its treatment of persons who have a "wanton" lack of concern about "whether the desires that move him are desires by which he wants to be moved to act." Such an individual, says Frankfurt, is "no different from an animal."[19] Indeed, "insofar as his desires are utterly unreflective, he is to that extent not genuinely a person at all. He is merely a wanton."[20] This theory needs more than a convincing account of second-order desires and volitions; it needs a way to ensure that ordinary choices qualify as autonomous even when persons have not reflected on their preferences at a higher level and even when they are hesitant to identify with one type of desire rather than another.

Depending on how "reflection," "volition," and the like are spelled out in this theory, few choosers and few choices might turn out to be autonomous because few would fail to engage in higher-order reflection. Often the agents involved will not have reflected on whether they wish to accept or identify with the motivational structures that underlie such actions. Actors will in some cases be unaware of their motivational or conditioning histories and will have made no reflective identifications. Actions such as standing up during a religious service, lying to one's physician about what one eats, and hiding one's income from the Internal Revenue Service might on this basis turn out to be nonautonomous. The moral price paid in this theory is that individuals who have not reflected on their desires and preferences at a higher level deserve no respect for actions that derive from their most deep-seated commitments, desires, and preferences. There is a danger that they will be classified as no different than animals.[21]

Conversely, if one relaxes the standards of higher-order reflection, then many acts will become autonomous that these theorists wish to exclude from the realm of autonomy. For example, some actions of nonhuman animals will be autonomous. I will return to this problem in the final section of this essay.

Converting the Theory to Nonrepudiated Acceptance

The defender of a split-level theory could shift ground and require as a condition of autonomous action only *nonrepudiation* in the values underlying choice, not *reflective acceptance* of them—a move occasionally suggested, obliquely, by Frankfurt.[22] This position is negative rather than positive: Values, motives, and actions are autonomous if the agent does not reflectively repudiate or abjure them, and not autonomous if they are repudiated. This set of repudiated actions would presumably not be large, but would include important cases of weakness of the will, such as acts of taking drugs and acts of infidelity in which the person repudiates the driving desire or value while nonetheless acting on it: "I was seduced in a weak moment." This position does not seem to make the mistake of rendering nonautonomous most of our ordinary actions that are intentional and informed.

Intriguing illustrations of this thesis come from clinical examples of repudiated phobic and compulsive behavior such as the repudiation of a compulsive hand washer. I concede the attractiveness of the theory for these examples, but I push beyond them to more commonplace examples of repudiated action to see if the theory remains attractive. What should we say about a corporate executive who sincerely repudiates her characteristic avarice and greed? She repeatedly, but unsuccessfully, tries to become more spiritual and less material in her desires. She goes on being an aggressive corporate executive of the sort that she wishes she were not, but is. Are her actions nonautonomous because repudiated? Her repudiation is an insufficient reason to withhold classification of her acts as autonomous. The perpetual dieter who continuously repudiates eating carbohydrates but goes on eating carbohydrates anyway is a similar case. These agents may not be acting autonomously, but, if not, nonautonomy seems to derive from some form of involuntariness (e.g., uncontrollable desire), not from a failure to conform to a repudiation of desire.

There are related problems about allowing a person's actions to qualify as autonomous when values and motives are *not* repudiated. For example, in the case of the compulsive hand washer, suppose that, instead of repudiating desires for or the choice of hand washing, the hand washer has never reflectively considered his or her desires or motives. It is implausible to describe compulsive actions of hand washing as autonomous. Again, we have a problem of external noncontrol, not internal nonrepudiation. Similar questions can be raised about Frankfurt's unwilling addict who identifies himself through a second-order volition as desiring not to be an addict but goes on being one because he is in the hold of the addiction. Frankfurt argues that this addict is a person, not a wanton, but that his actions of drug intake are not of his own free will.[23] I agree that he is a person who is not acting freely, but is he acting autonomously? Frankfurt never answers this question, but the analysis suggests (whether or not this conclusion is intended) that the addict "acts" unfreely but autonomously.

It will not be easy to construct a split-level theory using second-order identification or nonrepudiation as a criterion. These conditions are not clearly needed for a theory of autonomous action or the autonomous person. The condition of noncontrol (as analyzed previously) is a more promising way to fill out a theory of both autonomous choice and the autonomous person.

AUTONOMOUS PERSONS AND THE PROBLEM OF MORAL STATUS

Thus far I have concentrated on autonomous choice, although the most plausible interpretation of split-level theories (and other theories of autonomy) is that they are theories of autonomous persons. Setting aside how best to interpret particular theories, I proceed in this section to autonomous persons in order to address questions of moral status.

It is often assumed in philosophical literature on persons that they are essentially autonomous; all persons are autonomous, and all autonomous individuals are persons. However, not all theories make such an assumption. Some maintain that fetuses, young children, advanced Alzheimer's patients, and even the irreversibly comatose are persons, but ones who lack autonomy. I will not pursue this controversy. My concern is with theories that find autonomy or some feature of autonomy (e.g., intention, rationality, or second-level identification) to be constitutive of personhood. When I use the term *person* hereafter, it refers exclusively to autonomous persons.

I said earlier that a theory with demanding conditions of autonomy (e.g., requiring full understanding, no external or internal constraint on the agent, or second-level reflective identification) will reach the conclusion that many of our presumed choices are not *autonomous* choices. This conclusion likewise applies to persons; the more demanding the conditions in a theory of persons, the fewer the number of individuals who satisfy the conditions, and therefore the fewer who qualify for the moral status conferred by being persons. The conditions in the theory can then be built into how we should interpret the principle of respect for autonomy (or, perhaps, respect for persons). As the quality or level of required mental skill is reduced in a theory, the number of individuals who qualify for protection under the principle will increase. As the quality or level of mental activity is increased (made more demanding), the number of individuals who qualify for protection under the principle will decrease.

If a theory demands a high threshold of mental capacity and a robust personal history of reflective identification with values, then various individuals normally regarded as autonomous will be deemed nonautonomous, or at least many of their preferences and choices will be rendered nonautonomous. For example, many decisions by hospital patients about their care will be classified as nonautonomous.[24] Correlatively, if a theory demands only a low threshold of mental skills (modest understanding, weak resistance to manipulation, etc.), then many individuals who are normally regarded as *nonautonomous* will be deemed autonomous—for example, certain nonhuman animals. This problem underlies and motivates my discussion of moral status in this section.

Metaphysical and Moral Theories

Some theories of autonomous persons are *metaphysical*, others *moral*.[25] As I draw the distinction, autonomous persons in a metaphysics of persons are identified by a set of psychological (not moral) properties. Properties found in various theories include intentionality, rationality, self-consciousness (of oneself as existing over time), free will, language acquisition, higher-order volition, and possibly various forms of emotion.[26] The metaphysical goal is to identify a set of psychological properties possessed by all and only autonomous persons. Morally autonomous persons, by contrast, are capable of moral agency. In principle, an entity could satisfy all the properties requisite for being a metaphysically autonomous person and lack all the properties requisite for being a morally autonomous person.

Unfortunately, most theories of persons cannot easily be distinguished into one of these two types. These theories are not attentive to the distinction between metaphysical and moral persons. For three decades, and arguably for several centuries, the dominant trend in the literature has been to delineate properties of individuals in a metaphysical account from which conclusions can be drawn about their moral status. Most philosophical accounts attempt to remain faithful to the commonsense concept of person, which is, roughly speaking, identical to the concept of human being. However, there is no warrant for the assumption that only properties distinctive of the human species count toward personhood or autonomy, or that species membership has anything to do with moral status. Even if certain properties that are strongly correlated with membership in the human species qualify humans for moral status more readily than the members of other species, these properties are only contingently connected to being human. The properties could be possessed by members of nonhuman species or by entities outside the sphere of natural species such as the great apes and genetically manipulated species.[27]

What Have Metaphysical Theories to Do with Moral Theories?

Proponents of metaphysical theories often spread confusion by moving from a metaphysical claim about persons to one about moral status or moral worth. This move can be baffling, because metaphysical properties have no moral implications. A metaphysical-to-moral connection can be made only through a correlative appeal to a moral principle such as a principle of respect for persons or respect for autonomy. The principle must be defended independently of the metaphysical theory and given some suitable content and relationship to the theory. If individual X acts autonomously, rationally, self-consciously, and the like, how is moral autonomy or any form of moral status established by this fact? No moral conclusions follow merely from the presence of these properties.

Many philosophers, including Aristotle and Kant, hold that animals have minds but lack critical human properties such as rationality, language use, or dignity. Kant judged that human dignity—which he closely linked to moral autonomy—places humans in a privileged position in the order of nature; humans have properties that confer upon them a moral status not held by nonhuman animals.[28] Whatever the merits of Kant's view in particular, the belief persists generally in philosophy, religion, and popular culture that some special property—perhaps autonomy or a property connected to it—confers a unique moral status or standing on human persons. In philosophy, it is commonly asserted that nonhuman animals lack properties such as self-awareness, a sense of continuity over time, the capacity to will, the capacity to love, and/or autonomy, and therefore lack personhood (or its functional equivalent), and therefore lack moral status.[29]

However, it is not demonstrated in these theories that nonhuman animals in fact lack the relevant property. I have not seen a philosophical theory that argues the point by reference to available empirical evidence. A typical statement by philosophers is the following thesis of Frankfurt's:

> It is conceptually possible that members of novel or even of familiar non-human species should be persons.... It seems to be peculiarly characteristic of humans, however, that they are able to form what I shall call "second-order desire".... Many animals appear to have the capacity for what I shall call "first-order desires".... No animal other than man, however, appears to have the capacity for reflective self-evaluation that is manifested in the formation of second-order desires.[30]

Philosophical theories typically ignore striking evidence of types and degrees of self-awareness of nonhuman animals, not to mention the pervasive presence of intentionality in animals and the findings in comparative studies of the brain. In some studies, language-trained apes appear to make self-references, and many animals learn from the past and then use their knowledge to forge intentional plans of action.[31] These animals distinguish their bodies and interests from those of the bodies and interests of others. In play and social life, they understand assigned functions and either follow designated roles or decide for themselves what roles to play.[32]

These abilities of nonhuman animals have rarely been taken seriously in contemporary philosophy, and yet they provide plausible reasons to attribute elementary self-consciousness and some degree of autonomy to nonhuman animals. Their abilities seem to admit degrees of just the properties that I identified previously. Any theory similar to the one I presented there must allow for the possibility (I think inevitability) that some nonhuman animals are at a higher level of autonomy (or, possibly, personhood) than some humans. Some measure of autonomy can be gained or lost over time by both humans and some nonhuman animals as critical capacities are gained, enhanced, or lost.

The fact that humans will generally exhibit higher levels of cognitive capacities under these criteria than other species of animals is a contingent fact, not a necessary truth about the human species. A nonhuman animal may overtake a human whenever the human loses a measure of mental abilities after a cataclysmic event or a decline of capacity. If, for example, the primate in training in a language laboratory exceeds the deteriorating human, the primate may achieve a higher level of autonomy (or, perhaps, personhood), and may thereby be positioned to gain a higher moral status, depending on the precise connection asserted in the theory. (Even if animals such as the great apes fail to qualify as autonomous *persons*, it does not follow that they have no capacities of autonomous *choice*.)

Criteria of Morally Autonomous Persons

The category of *morally* autonomous persons is relatively uncomplicated by comparison to the category of *metaphysically* autonomous persons. I will not attempt an account of the necessary and sufficient conditions, but it seems safe to assume that X is a morally autonomous person if (1) X is capable of making moral judgments about the rightness and wrongness of actions and (2) X has motives that can be judged morally. Being a morally autonomous person, unlike being a metaphysically autonomous person, is sufficient for moral status. Moral agents are paradigm bearers of moral status. Any morally autonomous person is a member of the moral community and qualifies for its benefits, burdens, protections, and punishments. Nonhuman animals are not, on current evidence, plausible candidates for classification as morally autonomous persons, though some evidence suggests that the great apes, dolphins, and other animals with similar properties could turn out to be exceptions. I will not defend this view, but I will mention a conclusion of Charles Darwin's that I accept.[33] He denied that animals make moral judgments, but affirmed that some animals display moral emotions and dispositions. Though they do not make genuine judgments of moral blame when they punish their peers for misbehavior, they do display genuine love, affection, and generosity toward their peers. However difficult it is to prove this thesis, it is no less difficult to disprove it.

Finally, if being morally autonomous is the sole basis of moral status (a view I do not hold), then many humans lack moral status—and precisely for the reasons that nonhuman animals do. Fetuses, newborns, psychopaths, severely brain-damaged patients, and various dementia patients are candidate cases. These humans are in the same situation as many nonhumans: Moral status for them is grounded in something other than being morally autonomous. However, this topic of moral status will have to be the subject of another paper aimed at showing that certain *noncognitive* and *nonmoral* properties, such as emotions and affective responses, are sufficient to confer some form or level of moral status.

CONCLUSION

Theories of autonomy, like many theories in philosophy, develop from pretheoretical, considered judgments. Considerable vagueness surrounds the ordinary concept of autonomy, and philosophical theories of autonomy that attempt to give the notion substance should be welcomed. These theories are interesting in their own right, and practically, they may be of assistance in helping us understand what it is that we are to respect when we respect another's autonomy. At the same time, in the development of these theories we should not stray from our pretheoretical judgments about what deserves respect when willed or chosen by another. The moral value of respect for autonomy precedes and is not the product of a philosophical theory, and no theory is acceptable if it threatens this value.

Notes

1. Cf. treatments of the concept of autonomy in Joel Feinberg, *Harm to Self*, Vol. III in *The Moral Limits of the Criminal Law* (New York: Oxford University Press, 1986), chaps. 18–19; and Thomas E. Hill, Jr., *Autonomy and Self-Respect* (Cambridge: Cambridge University Press, 1991), chaps. 1–4. Individual (by contrast to political) autonomy is a recent concept lacking a significant history of philosophical analysis. When the eight-volume *Encyclopedia of Philosophy* (Macmillan) was published in 1967, it offered no indexed mention of "autonomy." (Its sole reference is to "autonomous idiolects"; the entries under "self-determination" are scarcely more informative.) In its current non-Kantian uses, the term came into vogue in philosophy shortly after this *Encyclopedia* went to press.

2. O'Neill, *Rethinking Informed Consent in Bioethics* (Cambridge: Cambridge University Press, 2007), 25, 189. See also her *Autonomy and Trust in Bioethics* (Cambridge: Cambridge University Press, 2002), sect. 7.6, 154–160.

3. Julian Savulescu, "Rational Desires and the Limitation of Life-Sustaining Treatment," *Bioethics* 8 (1994): 191–222; and Savulescu and Richard Momeyer, "Should Informed Consent Be Based on Rational Beliefs?" *Journal of Medical Ethics* 23 (1997): 282–288. I am not asserting that Savulescu's conclusions could never be warranted; obviously a Jehovah's Witness could be acting nonautonomously. I am pointing to the profound practical consequences to which a theory of autonomy may be put and suggesting a different starting point than the one used by Savulescu.

4. Ruth R. Faden and Tom L. Beauchamp, *A History and Theory of Informed Consent* (New York: Oxford University Press, 1986), chap. 7; Tom L. Beauchamp and James Childress, *Principles of Biomedical Ethics* (New York: Oxford University Press, 2001), chap. 3. Some writers committed to a feminist perspective have argued that my theory is not entirely compatible with the constraints on theory that I have proposed, or at least that my theory needs adjustments. See Carolyn Ells, "Shifting the Autonomy Debate to Theory as Ideology," *Journal of Medicine and Philosophy* 26 (2001): 417–430; and Anne Donchin, "Autonomy and Interdependence," in *Relational Autonomy*, ed. C. Mackenzie and N. Stoljar (New York: Oxford University Press, 2000), 236–258.

5. Alvin I. Goldman, A Theory of Human Action (Englewood Cliffs, NJ: Prentice-Hall, 1970), 49–85.

6. Hector-Neri Castañeda, "Intensionality and Identity in Human Action and Philosophical Method," *Nous* 13 (1979): 235–260, esp. 255.

7. This analysis draws from Faden and Beauchamp, *A History and Theory of Informed Consent,* chap. 7.

8. I follow John Searle in thinking that we cannot reliably distinguish, in many situations, among acts, effects, consequences, and events. Searle, "The Intentionality of Intention and Action," *Cognitive Science* 4 (1980): esp. 65.

9. This now widely used label seems to have been coined by Paul S. Appelbaum, Loren Roth, and Charles W. Lidz in "The Therapeutic Misconception: Informed Consent in Psychiatric Research," *International Journal of Law and Psychiatry* 5 (1982): 319–329. For evidence that the misconception is enduring, see Appelbaum, Lidz, and Thomas Grisso, "Therapeutic Misconception in Clinical Research: Frequency and Risk Factors," IRB: *Ethics and Human Research* 26 (2004): 1–8. See, further, W. Glannon, "Phase I Oncology Trials: Why the Therapeutic Misconception Will Not Go Away," *Journal of Medical Ethics* 32 (2006): 252–255.

10. See Sam Horng and Christine Grady, "Misunderstanding in Clinical Research: Distinguishing Therapeutic Misconception, Therapeutic Misestimation, & Therapeutic Optimism," *IRB: Ethics and Human Research* 25 (January–February 2003): 11–16.

11. See the original formulation of this view in Faden and Beauchamp, *A History and Theory of Informed Consent,* chap. 10.

12. This formulation is indebted to Robert Nozick, "Coercion," in *Philosophy, Science and Method: Essays in Honor of Ernest Nagel,* ed. Sidney Morgenbesser, Patrick Suppes, and Morton White (New York: St. Martin's Press, 1969), 440–472; and Bernard Gert, "Coercion and Freedom," in *Coercion: Nomos XIV,* ed. J. Roland Pennock and John W. Chapman (Chicago: Aldine, Atherton Inc., 1972), 36–37. See also Alan Wertheimer, *Coercion* (Princeton, NJ: Princeton University Press, 1987).

13. Dworkin, *The Theory and Practice of Autonomy* (New York: Cambridge University Press, 1988), chaps. 1–4; Harry G. Frankfurt, "Freedom of the Will and the Concept of a Person," *Journal of Philosophy* 68 (1971): 5–20, as reprinted in *The Importance of What We Care About* (Cambridge: Cambridge University Press, 1988): 11–25. See also Laura W. Ekstrom, "A Coherence Theory of Autonomy," *Philosophy and Phenomenological Research* 53 (1993): 599–616; and Gary Watson, "Free Agency," *Journal of Philosophy* 72

(1975): 205–220. Although it is far from clear that Frankfurt holds a theory of autonomy, see his uses of the language of "autonomy" in his *Necessity, Volition, and Love* (Cambridge: Cambridge University Press, 1999), chaps. 9, 11. Frankfurt's early work was on *persons* and *freedom of the will*. In his later work, he seems to regard the earlier work as providing an account of autonomy, which is a reasonable estimate even if it involves some creative reconstruction.

14. Frankfurt, "Freedom of the Will and the Concept of a Person," in *The Importance of What We Care About*, 16. Frankfurt has, in his later philosophy, modified his early theory of identification. See his "The Faintest Passion," in *Necessity, Volition, and Love*, 95–107, esp. 105–106.

15. Dworkin, *The Theory and Practice of Autonomy*, 20

16. Frankfurt, "Autonomy, Necessity, and Love," in *Necessity, Volition, and Love*, 137.

17. Problems of this sort were first called to my attention by Irving Thalberg, "Hierarchical Analyses of Unfree Action," *Canadian Journal of Philosophy* 8 (1978): 211–226.

18. "The Faintest Passion" and "On the Necessity of Ideals," in *Necessity, Volition, and Love*, 105, 110.

19. "Freedom of the Will and the Concept of a Person," in *The Importance of What We Care About*, 18.

20. "The Faintest Passion," in *Necessity, Volition, and Love*, 105–106.

21. There are more demanding theories than these second-order theories. Some theories require extremely rigorous standards in order to be autonomous or to be persons. For example, they demand that the autonomous individual be authentic, consistent, independent, in command, resistant to control by authorities, and the original source of values, beliefs, rational desires, and life plans. See Stanley Benn, "Freedom, Autonomy and the Concept of a Person," *Proceedings of the Aristotelian Society* 76 (1976): 123–130, and *A Theory of Freedom* (Cambridge: Cambridge University Press, 1988): 3–6, 155f, 175–183; R. S. Downie and Elizabeth Telfer, "Autonomy," *Philosophy* 46 (1971): 296–301; Christopher McMahon, "Autonomy and Authority," *Philosophy and Public Affairs* 16 (1987): 303–328.

22. "The Faintest Passion," in *Necessity, Volition, and Love*, 104–105. See esp. the account of satisfaction. A nuanced version of this theory of nonrepudiated acceptance (using the language of *nonresistance*) seems to be held by John Christman, "Autonomy and Personal History," *Canadian Journal of Philosophy* 21 (1991): 1–24, esp. 10ff.

23. Frankfurt, "Freedom of the Will and the Concept of a Person," in *The Importance of What We Care About*, 18.

24. See Savulescu, "Rational Desires and the Limitation of Life-Sustaining Treatment": 202ff (summarized at 221–222).

25. Other philosophers have used this or a similarly worded distinction, but not as I analyze the distinction. See Daniel Dennett, "Conditions of Personhood," In *The Identities of Persons*, ed. Amelie O. Rorty (Berkeley: University of California Press, 1976), 175–196, esp. 176–178; Joel Feinberg and Barbara Baum Levenbook, "Abortion," in *Matters of Life and Death: New Introductory Essays in Moral Philosophy*, 3rd edition, ed. Tom Regan (New York: Random House, 1993), 197–213; Stephen F. Sapontzis, *Morals, Reason, and Animals* (Philadelphia: Temple University Press, 1987), 47ff.

26. See Michael Tooley, *Abortion and Infanticide* (Oxford: Clarendon Press, 1983); Harry Frankfurt, "On the Necessity of Ideals," in *Necessity, Volition, and Love*, 113–115, and "Freedom of the Will and the Concept of a Person," in *The Importance of What We Care About*, ch. 2, esp. 12; Dennett, "Conditions of Personhood": 177–179; Mary Anne Warren, *Moral Status* (Oxford: Oxford University Press, 1997), chap. 1; H. Tristram Engelhardt, Jr. *The Foundations of Bioethics*, 2nd edition (New York: Oxford University Press, 1996), chaps. 4, 6; Loren Lomasky, *Persons, Rights, and the Moral Community* (Oxford: Oxford University Press, 1987); Lynne Rudder Baker, *Persons and Bodies* (Cambridge: Cambridge University Press, 2000), chaps. 4, 6.

27. On the relevance and plausibility of robots and physical-mental systems that imitate human traits, see John Pollock, *How to Build a Person* (Cambridge, MA: MIT Press, 1989), and Ausunio Marras, "Pollock on How to Build a Person," *Dialogue* 32 (1993): 595–605.

28. For Kant, a person's dignity—indeed, "sublimity"—comes from being his or her own moral lawgiver, that is, from being morally autonomous. Kant, *Foundations of the Metaphysics of Morals*, Lewis White Beck, trans. (Indianapolis: Bobbs-Merrill Company, 1959), 58. Kant added that the dignity deriving from this capacity is of a priceless worth that animals do not have: "[Each person] possesses a dignity (an absolute inner worth) whereby he exacts the respect of all other rational beings.... The humanity in one's person is the object of the respect which he can require of every other human being." Kant, *The Metaphysical Principles of Virtue*, pt. I, James W. Ellington, trans., in Kant, *Ethical Philosophy* (Indianapolis, IN.: Hackett Publishing Co., 1983), 97–98.

29. As is asserted, more or less, by Harry Frankfurt, "Autonomy, Necessity, and Love," in his *Necessity, Volition, and Love*, 131, n. 2, and his "Freedom of the Will and the Concept of a Person," in *The Importance of What We Care About*, 16–17; Allen Buchanan and Dan Brock, *Deciding for Others: The Ethics of Surrogate Decision Making* (Cambridge: Cambridge University Press, 1989), 197–199; John Harris, *The Value of Life* (London: Routledge, 1985), 9–10; Dworkin, *The Theory and Practice of Autonomy*, esp. chap. 1.

30. Frankfurt, "Freedom of the Will and the Concept of a Person," in *The Importance of What We Care About*, 12.

31. See Donald R. Griffin, *Animal Minds* (Chicago: University of Chicago Press, 1992); and Rosemary Rodd, *Ethics, Biology, and Animals* (Oxford: Clarendon Press, 1990), esp. chaps. 3, 4, 10.

32. Cf. Gordon G. Gallup, "Self-Recognition in Primates," *American Psychologist* 32 (1977): 329–338; David DeGrazia, *Taking Animals Seriously: Mental Life and Moral Status* (New York: Cambridge University Press, 1996), esp. 302.

33. Charles Darwin, *The Descent of Man and Selection in Relation to Sex* (Detroit: Gale Research Co., 1974), chaps. 3, 4.

6

THE CONCEPT OF PATERNALISM IN
BIOMEDICAL ETHICS

The idea that paternalism has a positive role to play in medicine and public health descends from ancient ideas about the duties and virtues of physicians. Traditional notions of the physician's obligations have been expressed primarily in terms of principles of beneficence and nonmaleficence: "As to disease, make a habit of two things—*to help, or at least to do no harm.*"[1] Until the recent rise of literature on medical paternalism, medical tradition placed little significance in a principle of respect for the autonomy of patients. However, as medicine confronted cultural claims of patients' rights to make independent judgments about their medical fate, paternalism loomed ever larger.

In biomedical ethics today, paternalism has been both defended and attacked in clinical medicine, public health, health policy, and government agencies. Unfortunately, it is unclear in much of this literature what paternalism is and which types of paternalism, if any, are justified. The closest thing to consensus in this literature seems to be that so-called strong (or hard) paternalism is not justified. In this paper I will argue that despite the preponderance of opinion in the literature on paternalism, so-called strong paternalism can be justified. I will also argue that it is the only interesting form of paternalism.

THE IDEA OF AN AUTONOMY-LIMITING PRINCIPLE

In philosophy, the history of criticism of paternalism can be traced to John Stuart Mill's attack on paternalism in his theory of a person's liberty rights and whether they can be justifiably limited. Although he does not use today's favored term *autonomy,* he defends a personal and community ideal of "the *free development of individuality,*" which is the functional equivalent for him of the development of personal autonomy.[2] Mill argues that our liberty rights are sometimes justifiably overridden because they conflict with other values that we treasure, such as health and welfare. For example, in a welfare state, people are legitimately taxed against their will—a deprivation of their liberty to spend their money—in order to benefit those who need assistance in the form of health care, job insurance, food, child care, and the like. Such conflicts between the value of liberty and other goods present a need to establish the proper limits on autonomous choice and action for individuals, groups, and institutions. Various principles, generally assumed to be *moral* principles, have been proposed to justify the limitation of individual human liberties.

In closely tracking Mill's arguments in *On Liberty,* Joel Feinberg called these principles "liberty-limiting principles" and "coercion-legitimizing principles."[3] The issue is the proper moral justification for limiting liberty. I will refer to these principles as "autonomy-limiting" principles. These principles allegedly state valid restrictions of an autonomous agent's liberty. The principles are said by their proponents to provide a good reason for interference with autonomy and for any corresponding use of coercion necessary for the interference. The following are the four most commonly discussed autonomy-limiting principles in the model proposed by Feinberg:

1. *The harm principle*: A person's autonomy is justifiably restricted to prevent harm to others caused by that person.
2. *The principle of paternalism*: A person's autonomy is justifiably restricted to prevent harm to self caused by oneself, irrespective of whether harm is caused to others.
3. *The principle of legal moralism*: A person's autonomy is justifiably restricted to prevent that person's immoral behavior, irrespective of whether that person's conduct is harmful or offensive.
4. *The offense principle*: A person's autonomy is justifiably restricted to prevent hurt or offense (as contrasted to harm or injury) to others caused by that person's behavior.

Mill defended the first principle while rejecting the others. He delivered the following compelling attack on the principle of paternalism in his monograph *On Liberty*:

The only purpose for which power can be rightfully exercised over any member of a civilized community, against his will, is to prevent harm to others. His own good, either physical or moral, is not a sufficient warrant. He cannot rightfully be compelled to do or forbear because it will be better for him to do so, because it will make him happier, because in the opinions of others, to do so would be wise, or even right. These are good reasons for remonstrating with him, or reasoning with him, or persuading him, or entreating him, but not for compelling him.... In the part which merely concerns himself his independence is, of right, absolute.[4]

Mill thus regarded true paternalism as always unjustified (and not merely prima facie unjustified). His arguments, though presented as utilitarian, seem to rest on additional premises. Purely utilitarian grounds rarely, if ever, warrant absolute restrictions. Mill's own formulations of utilitarianism seem insufficient for the conclusion that even if society can know the best interests of individuals, it should not advance them by compulsion. Mill seems, in the end, more compelled by the idea that we have an absolute right not to have our liberty overridden, whether or not the benefits outweigh the risks.

To move now beyond Mill, paternalism as a philosophical problem arises from this general theoretical problem of justifying principles that provide grounds for the limitation of autonomy. There are several distinguishable issues, two being the chief issues. The first is how we should understand the concept of paternalism. The second is whether paternalism should be excluded from consideration as a valid autonomy-limiting principle. I will take them up in turn, starting with how to formulate the concept of paternalism and the notion of a principle of paternalism.

THE DEFINITION OF PATERNALISM

In ordinary discourse, by contrast to theoretical discussion of a system of valid autonomy-limiting principles, the term *paternalism* dates from the principle and practice of paternal administration, especially government in the model of paternal benevolence. The analogy presupposes that a father acts beneficently toward his children and makes decisions about his children's welfare without allowing the child's preferences to be the determinative consideration. In health care and public health, this analogy builds on the idea that a professional has superior training, knowledge, and insight and is thus in an authoritative position to determine the best interests of those under his or her care and administration. The nature of paternalism thus begins in analogy, but what, more precisely, is the meaning of the term *paternalism,* and how broad is its scope?

The Autonomy-Limiting Definition

"Paternalism" could be understood as referring to acts or practices that restrict the autonomy of individuals without their consent even though they have the capacity to act autonomously. This conception leads to the following definition, which I will call the *autonomy-limiting definition*: Paternalism is the intentional limitation of the autonomy of one person by another, where the person who limits autonomy justifies the action exclusively by the goal of helping the person whose autonomy is limited.[5] Following this definition, paternalism seizes decision-making authority by overriding a person's autonomous choice on grounds of providing the person with a benefit—in medicine, a medical benefit. Here an act of paternalism overrides the principle of respect for autonomy on grounds of the welfare of the person whose autonomy is overridden.

Examples of paternalism in medicine in this strong sense include court orders for blood transfusions when patients have refused them, involuntary commitment to institutions for treatment, intervention to stop rational suicides, resuscitating patients who have asked not to be resuscitated, withholding medical information that patients have requested, denial of an innovative therapy to someone who wishes to try it, and government-enforced efforts to promote health. Other health-related examples include laws requiring motorcyclists to wear helmets and motorists to wear seat belts and the regulations of governmental agencies that prevent people from purchasing possibly harmful or inefficacious drugs and chemicals. The motivation in these cases is the beneficent promotion of health and welfare of those whose autonomous choice is overridden.

The Preference-Limiting Definition

Some writers object to the boldness of autonomy restriction in this autonomy-limiting definition of paternalism. They judge that it fails to grasp the subtleties of the term as it has descended from common usage and legal precedent. The notion is linked in these literatures to guardianship, surrogate decision making, and government intervention to protect the vulnerable or unwary. The root sense of paternalism is joined with the law's wide-ranging use of terms such as *parens patriae* to produce a broad meaning of paternalism that includes interventions with both autonomous actions and questionably autonomous actions. In this conception, even if a person's plans or actions do not derive from a substantially autonomous choice, overriding them can still be paternalistic.[6] For example, if a patient still groggy from surgery attempts to get out of bed, it is paternalistic to prevent him from doing so despite the fact that he has not made a substantially autonomous choice.

Those who follow this broader conception recommend the following definition, which I will call the *preference-limiting definition*: Paternalism is the intentional overriding of one person's known preferences by another person, where the person who overrides justifies the action by the goal of benefiting the person whose will or preference is overridden. Under this second definition, if a person's stated preferences do not derive from a substantially autonomous choice, the act of overriding his or her preferences is still paternalistic. The main condition of a paternalistic action is that a beneficent treatment is the reason for overriding a known preference, whether or not the preference is formed autonomously.[7]

A Final Definition

These two definitions are both entrenched in current literature, but neither dominates the literature. I will follow the more limited and far more interesting commitments of the first definition because of its fidelity to the core problem of the limitation of autonomy. There are compelling reasons for resisting the second (preference-limiting) definition on grounds that paternalism originates in ethical theory as an issue about the valid limitation of autonomy (or liberty), and the second definition does not require substantial autonomy. To include cases involving persons who lack substantial autonomy such as drug addicts and the mentally handicapped broadens the term in a way that obscures the central issue, which is how, whether, and when autonomy can be justifiably limited.

It might be doubted that the first definition is adequate on grounds that it is not a necessary condition of paternalism that autonomy be *overridden*. Perhaps autonomy is simply not *consulted* in the sense that a paternalist can act without caring what the wishes are of the person toward whom he or she acts beneficently.[8] For example, suppose a doctor thinks he knows best and does not consult the patient's wishes; he does not know or have any belief about the patient's choices or intentions. The doctor simply acts in the patient's best medical interests. Such an action is authoritarian and beneficent, but it seems conceptually dubious that these conditions render the action paternalistic. They conform more to the idea of good medical care than they do to medical paternalism. Consider the analogous case in which a father pays his 21-year-old son's taxes without consulting his son's wishes in the matter. Nothing in this act smacks of paternalism; the father has always paid his son's taxes and merely acts in a parental role in his son's best interests. In short, unless a specific desire or choice of a person is overridden, an action falls short of paternalism.

Accordingly, the definition of paternalism I will follow hereafter is this: Paternalism is the intentional overriding of one person's autonomous choices or actions by another person, where the person who overrides justifies the action by appeal to the goal of benefiting or of preventing or mitigating harm to the person whose choices or actions are overridden. A person's choices or actions must be substantially autonomous to qualify as paternalistic under this definition. Later in this chapter I will make some qualifications on this notion of "one person ... by another" in light of some important issues about the large populations that confront persons responsible for public policies governing all motorcyclists, all institutions that screen for disease, and the like.

My definition is value neutral in the sense that it does not presume whether paternalism is justified. The term *paternalism*, following this definition, has neither a negative nor a positive valence and leaves questions of justification open. The definition assumes an act of beneficence analogous to parental beneficence, but it does not prejudge whether the beneficent act is justified, obligatory, or misplaced.

WEAK (SOFT) PATERNALISM AND STRONG (HARD) PATERNALISM

Acceptance of this final definition instead of the broader preference-limiting definition will play an important role in determining whether one accepts a type of paternalism often distinguished in the literature as weak paternalism, also called "soft" paternalism (a distinction owing much to Feinberg).[9] I do not regard weak (or soft) paternalism as a true type of paternalism, but many do so regard it, and it is important to see what is at stake.

In *weak paternalism,* a paternalistic actor "has the right to prevent self-regarding conduct only when it is substantially nonvoluntary or when temporary intervention is necessary to establish whether it is voluntary or not."[10] Permissible limitations of autonomy are confined to substantially nonautonomous behaviors, usually conditions of compromised ability or even dysfunctional incompetence. Conditions that can significantly compromise the ability to act autonomously include the influence of psychotropic drugs, painful labor while delivering a child, and a blow to the head that affects memory and judgment. A physician who overturns the preferences of a substantially nonautonomous patient in the interests of medical welfare acts paternalistically and justifiably by the standards of weak paternalism. Given the reasonableness of the claim that nonautonomous preferences can be validly overridden, the conclusions of weak paternalism have been generally accepted in law, medicine, and moral philosophy. However, the reasonableness of weak paternalistic interventions does not make it an interesting or conceptually coherent form of paternalism. As Feinberg has pointed out, weak paternalism is a rather uninteresting type, because it is not clearly a liberty-limiting principle independent of the harm principle.[11] The final definition I proposed earlier rules it out as a form of paternalism. Moreover, the idea that paternalism is justified "only when it is substantially nonvoluntary" will be shown later in this essay to be dubious.

Strong paternalism, by contrast to weak, supports interventions that protect competent adults by restricting substantially autonomous behaviors. For example, refusing to release a competent hospital patient who will die outside the hospital but requests the release knowing the consequences is an act of strong paternalism. Strong paternalism usurps autonomy by either restricting the information available to a person or overriding the person's informed and voluntary choices. These choices need not be *fully* autonomous or voluntary (a notion that may be empty, perhaps even meaningless), but in order to qualify as strong paternalism, the choices of the beneficiary of paternalistic intervention must be substantially autonomous or voluntary. For example, a strong paternalist might prevent a patient capable of making reasoned judgments from receiving diagnostic information if the information would lead the patient to a state of depression and a decision to commit suicide.

Under the final definition I have supported, only strong paternalism qualifies as paternalism. Accordingly, weak paternalism will hereafter not be under discussion. Whether strong paternalism is justified will of course need close consideration.

PATERNALISM IN POLICY, PATERNALISTIC INTENT, AND PATERNALISTIC EFFECT

Those who frame a policy in public policy and public health contexts often seek to avoid harm to or to benefit persons without directly consulting them. Often it is known that some percentage of the population would not agree to provisions in the policy that restrict choice. The policymakers will know that some members of the group affected regard the policy as autonomy depriving, whereas others strongly approve of the policy. In effect, the policy is intended to benefit all members of a population without consulting the autonomous preferences of individuals, though with the knowledge that many individuals would reject the control the policy exerts over their lives. Policy contexts, by contrast to clinical situations in the patient–physician relationship, commonly present this situation.

These policies are paternalistic in intent and commonly will be paternalistic in their effect on some members of the population, which points to the importance of a distinction between paternalistic intent and paternalistic effect. A term such as *paternalistic action* generally carries the meaning of both intent and effect (or outcome), but the two should be distinguished. Mere paternalistic intent is insufficient for paternalistic effect; and it muddies the waters to speak only of "paternalistic action." For example, a physician may intend to override a patient's choice while misunderstanding that the patient has already chosen what the physician wants; and a policymaker may formulate a paternalistic health policy, such as a prohibition of a certain kind of fat in marketed food products, only to find that no one actually wants that type of fat in food products.

In his work on paternalism, Cass Sunstein has maintained that "The idea of libertarian paternalism might seem to be an oxymoron, but it is both possible and desirable for private and public institutions to influence behavior while also respecting freedom of choice."[12] "Libertarian paternalism" is indeed an oxymoron on the conceptual account of paternalism I have proposed. However, we can make sense of, and accept, Sunstein's proposal by using the distinction between paternalistic intent and paternalistic effect. Suppose that the available evidence establishes that smokers psychologically discount the risks of smoking because of an "optimism bias"; it does not thereby seem correct to say, Sunstein argues, "that government would violate their autonomy" through programs intended to turn their biases around—even if these efforts involve manipulative television advertisements that graphically present the suffering that occurs from smoking.[13] This claim is premised on the view that people have a bounded rationality that creates a limitation on their capacity to act autonomously. Autonomous persons would value health over the ill health caused by smoking, and in this sense one's deepest autonomous commitment is to be a nonsmoker. Accordingly, we are justified *on autonomy grounds* in arranging choice situations for populations in a way likely to correct for cognitive biases and bounded rationality. This strategy favors the manipulation of people into doing what is good for them. So interpreted, Sunstein's position is paternalistic (possibly even a hard paternalism), depending on the nature of the manipulation and the nature of smokers' choices. The exact measure of paternalism, if any, will have to be ascertained in the context of each specific case.

Those who make decisions and formulate policies may have a paternalistic intent, such as that of reversing the autonomous choices of smokers to smoke, and may act accordingly, but the result may or may not be paternalism in a meaningful sense. Suppose the smokers, though they every day choose to smoke cigarettes, would welcome rather than reject or even resist manipulative efforts to change behavior. In that event, no autonomy is overridden, and the action taken is not paternalistic even though a paternalistic intent motivates the action. This paternalism presumably reflects values that individuals would recognize or realize themselves if they did not encounter internal limits of rationality and control. If such paternalistically motivated plans and policies face no opposition from the targeted group, they have no paternalistic effect, despite the paternalistic intent.

Some paternalistic policies appear to be based entirely on the value of the predicted outcomes for the beneficiary, without consideration of whether a person's autonomy is diminished and without knowledge of the person's preferences. If the intervention is based on evidence that people are not rational decision makers in the relevant sphere of action, a major part of the appeal is to limited autonomy or perhaps nonautonomy, in which case it may turn out to be a form of weak paternalism or no paternalism at all.

THE PROBLEM OF JUSTIFICATION AND THE PRINCIPLE OF PATERNALISM

The *definition* or *conceptual analysis* of paternalism—the center of the discussion thus far—should be kept distinct from the *justification* of paternalism. Questions of justification return us to the philosophical theory deriving from Mill with which we began: Can a principle of paternalism be justified as an autonomy-limiting principle, or is it an invalid autonomy-limiting principle? If it is an invalid principle, then paternalism cannot be justified.

How, then, might strong paternalism be justified? This paternalism might be justified as a "social insurance policy" that fully rational persons endorse.[14] That is, one might attempt to justify it by the conditions to which an impartial rational agent would consent if he or she were to appreciate that he or she might be tempted at times to make decisions to commit acts such as suicide that are potentially dangerous and irreversible. In this conception a paternalistic act protects the deepest kind of autonomy by protecting a person's deepest values and preferences. A physician might lie to a patient, for example, in order to prevent a suicide, where the physician knows that the patient at the deeper level wants to live.[15]

This proposed justification fails to clarify the central issues about the justification of strong paternalism. Why do we need the indirect device of rational approval? Would a hypothetically consented-to arrangement even be paternalistic? Most important, if the paternalist's true objective is to protect or improve the welfare of another person, then the intervention finds its justification in the harm avoidance or benefit production that constitutes welfare promotion, as is the case in the justification of the root notion of parental actions that override the wishes of their children. If people should be handled paternalistically, it is not because they hypothetically would or ultimately will consent or would have consented were they rational, but because they will be better off. This justification rests on providing for the welfare of another, not on respecting the other's autonomy.

The Challenge of Antipaternalism

Some philosophers believe that paternalism is never justified. The most influential argument to this effect is that rightful authority resides in the individual because of the strict demands of the principle of respect for autonomy. Since (hard) paternalistic interventions necessarily display disrespect toward autonomous agents and fail to treat them as moral equals, they override (and, some would say, necessarily *violate*) the agents' right to be an independent chooser of their own good. If others impose their conception of the good, they deny the respect owed us, even if they have a better conception of our needs than we do and act to benefit us. In effect, the argument is that individuals have a right of autonomy that is absolute and can never be overridden on grounds merely of welfare interests.

Mill often seems to embrace such a strident antipaternalism, despite the fact that his philosophy (utilitarianism) is centrally one of balancing different welfare interests so as to maximize overall value. This theory seems to reach directly out to an embrace of paternalism, but this is not Mill's view. He maintains only that we can permissibly restrict a person's autonomy temporarily to ensure that the person is acting autonomously, and therefore acting with adequate knowledge of the consequences of his or her action. Once warned, the person must be allowed, Mill says, to choose whatever course he or she desires. Like Mill, virtually all antipaternalists permit a temporary infringement of autonomy in the belief that persons who have a well-formed, autonomous resolution to do something harmful to themselves will eventually have an opportunity to perform the action after the temporary intervention. This position is akin to an appeal to a precautionary principle that provides an opportunity to determine whether an action would be paternalistic. It justifies caution, not paternalism.

However, in a theory that is more strongly committed to balancing benefits, risks, and values such as self-development, on what conceivable grounds could paternalism be prohibited? The only grounds would be that, on balance, autonomy always outweighs all other interests. But what argument would anchor such a position? Perhaps a theory of rights might, but rights theories are not usually so grounded. Such theories in the end will face the same problem: An individual's rights will have to be balanced against the rights of others and also against a variety of interests such as public welfare. Defense of absolute autonomy rights is an unpromising possibility.

The Justification of Paternalism

The main question about the justification of paternalism, then, is whether conditions can be specified that are reasonable and allow for some range of justifiable limitations of autonomy without opening up a heavy medical paternalism or state paternalism. A paternalist might propose various conditions with the goal of keeping paternalism to a minimum, yet without absolutizing antipaternalism. For example, the paternalist might maintain that interventions are justified only if there are circumstances in which no acceptable alternative to the paternalistic action exists, a person is at risk of serious harm, risks to the person introduced by the paternalistic action itself are not substantial, projected benefits to the person outweigh risks to the person, and any infringement of the principle of respect for autonomy is minimal. The thesis is that these conditions are necessary conditions of any justified paternalistic action.

The most plausible justification of paternalistic actions places benefit on a scale with autonomy interests and balances both: As a person's interests in autonomy increase and the benefits for that person decrease, the justification of paternalistic action becomes less plausible. Conversely, as the benefits for a person increase and that person's autonomy interests decrease, the justification of paternalistic action becomes more plausible. From this perspective, preventing minor harms or providing minor benefits while deeply disrespecting autonomy will lack plausible justification, but actions that prevent major harms or provide major benefits while only trivially disrespecting autonomy may be justified paternalistic actions.

The claim is that as the risk to a patient's welfare increases or the likelihood of an irreversible harm increases, the likelihood of a justified paternalistic intervention correspondingly increases.[16] For example, if a dying patient who will live for one month in the most extreme form of pain refuses pain medication on grounds that he might become addicted to the medication, it is plausibly justified for a physician to administer an undetectable pain medication without informing the patient of the decision. It would not be difficult to generate a large body of cases in which benefits are major and risks minor (even effectively zero) and it is appropriate to act with a minor autonomy offense. Such hypothetical cases might seem contrived and less than convincing. Accordingly, in the remainder of this article I propose to test the hypothesis of a justified paternalism by considering a range of practical problems in medicine and public policy. Justified paternalism can be found in some of these cases, whereas in others it cannot.

THE PLACE OF PATERNALISM IN BIOMEDICAL ETHICS

I will consider seven common problems of paternalism in biomedical ethics, some of which involve policies and laws and some of which do not. In each I will indicate the values that need to be balanced when making a judgment about whether a paternalistic intervention is justified.

Reporting and Preventing Suicide Attempts

Many policies and laws about reporting, preventing, or intervening in suicide are paternalistic—either paternalistic in intent or in effect, or both. It has often been said that a principle of respect for life creates an obligation to prevent suicide that overrides obligations of respect for autonomy. A weaker account relies on Mill's strategy of temporary paternalism: Intervention is justified to establish autonomy in the person, but after it is determined that the person's decisions are substantially autonomous, further intervention would be unjustified. However, the most straightforward account of laws and policies that allow or promote suicide intervention is the following paternalistic thesis: Preventing suicide is justified by the goal of preventing a person from doing serious self-harm. This rationale is grounded in the view that other persons do sometimes know our best interests with more insight and foresight than we do, even when we act autonomously.

A related view that supports paternalism in suicide intervention is that friends and health care professionals are relieved of (i.e., excused from) duties of confidentiality when they report suicide threats. Some writers and policymakers even defend a paternalistic *obligation* to report suicide threats.[17]

Involuntary Hospitalization of Persons Harmful to Themselves

A vast literature surrounds the involuntary hospitalization of persons who have never harmed others or themselves, but now stand in danger of harming themselves (or at least are vulnerable to harms that might occur to them, as is not infrequently the case with homeless persons). Part of the contemporary rationale for use of police powers for the emergency detention and civil commitment of those dangerous to themselves is a paternalism supported by the knowledge that treatment has often helped persons over a momentary crisis. These interventions can involve a double paternalism: a paternalistic justification for commitment and a paternalistic justification for forced therapy (e.g., psychotherapy) after commitment.

On the one hand, it is difficult to justify the view that institutionalization involves only a minor harm. On the other hand, if the benefit were sufficiently large, it might, on balance, outweigh the harm done, especially if institutionalization is of a short duration. Consider the classic case of Catherine Lake, who suffered from arteriosclerosis, which caused temporary confusion and mild loss of memory, interspersed with times of mental alertness and rationality. All parties agreed that Lake never harmed anyone or presented a threat of danger. Still, she was committed to a mental institution because she often seemed in a confused and defenseless state as she walked city streets. Her condition was interspersed with periods of mental alertness and rationality in which she clearly could make autonomous judgments. At a court trial, while rational and capable of making autonomous choices, she testified that she knew the risks of living outside the hospital and preferred to assume those risks rather than remain in the hospital. The court of appeals denied her petition, arguing that she was "mentally ill," a "danger to herself," and "not competent to care for herself." In its legal justification, the court cited a statute that "provides for involuntary hospitalization of a person who is 'mentally ill and, because of that illness is likely to injure himself.' "[18] The court interpreted the law as having paternalistic intent, and in Lake's case it also had a paternalistic effect.

Antipaternalists argue that since Lake did not harm others and understood the dangers under which she placed herself, her freedom should not have been restricted. However, this case could and probably should be viewed very differently if there were a strong promise that Lake would be cured during the course of a brief hospitalization, despite her resistance to the hospitalization. From this perspective, a paternalistic intervention is justified by the intent to benefit and the likelihood of benefit, which outweighs obligations to respect autonomous choice.

The Risks and Benefits of Treatment Refusal

Should a beneficial medical procedure be withheld or withdrawn because the patient autonomously refuses the procedure? The right to refuse treatment is often treated in the literature of biomedical ethics as absolute, that is, as a right that cannot legitimately be balanced against other considerations. Justifications for overruling a patient's refusal need not be paternalistic, but they often are paternalistic because their objective is to prevent harm that would be caused by the patient's refusal. The issue is not whether a physician in fact knows what is best for the patient, but whether the patient has a right to refuse treatment irrespective of what the physician knows. The patients here envisioned are competent to refuse therapy, because otherwise the act would presumably not be paternalistic.

A commonplace example of justified paternalism that overrides an autonomous refusal appears in the following case:

> After receiving his preoperative medicine, C, a 23-year-old male athlete scheduled for a hernia repair, states that he does not want the side rails up [on his bed]. C is of clear mind and understands why the rule is required; however, C does not feel the rule should apply to him because he is not the least bit drowsy from the preoperative medication and he has no intention of falling out of bed. After considerable discussion between the nurse and patient, the nurse responsible for C's care puts the side rails up. Her justification is as follows: C is not drowsy because he has just received the

preoperative medication, and its effects have not occurred. Furthermore, if he follows the typical pattern of patients receiving this medication in this dosage, he will become drowsy very quickly. A drowsy patient is at risk for a fall. Since there is no family at the hospital to remain with the patient, and since the nurses on the unit are exceptionally busy, no one can constantly stay with C to monitor his level of alertness. Under these circumstances the patient must be protected from the potential harm of a fall, despite the fact that he does not want this protection.... The nurse restricted this autonomous patient's liberty based on ... protection of the patient from potential harm ... and *not* as a hedge against liability or for protection from criticism.[19]

Medical interventions of this sort present minor risks and offer substantial protection. Their commonness in hospitals is by itself no justification of such actions, but the lowered risk makes such actions plausible candidates for status as justified in the circumstances.

Withholding Information

Physicians and families sometimes maintain that a potentially devastating diagnosis or prognosis should not be disclosed to a patient. The concern is that bad news will adversely affect the patient's health or lead the patient to commit suicide. If the patient asks for the information or expects a truthful disclosure, it is paternalistic to withhold the truth, and it is also paternalistic to not disclose the information if the patient has a right to the information. Similarly, genetic counselors who use potential marital conflict for a patient as a reason not to disclose a condition such as nonpaternity deprive a patient of information that was itself generated in part by materials the patient provided.

In one case a physician obtains the results of a myelogram (a graph of the spinal region) following examination of a patient. The test yields inconclusive results and needs to be repeated, but also suggests a serious pathology. When the patient asks for detailed information, the physician decides to withhold potentially negative information, knowing that the patient would be highly distressed by the information. The physician is also confident that nondisclosure will not affect the patient's consent to another myelogram. However, the physician is committed to being completely truthful with the patient in the future about the results of the second test and about needed procedures. This physician's act of nondisclosure seems warranted even though paternalistic.[20]

Government Paternalism in Health Policy

Some government bureaus function in ways that follow a model of paternalistic guardianship. They are illustrative of acting with paternalistic intent, though sometimes with little or no paternalistic effect on the targeted population. The Food and Drug Administration (FDA) in the United States is an example, because the agency was chartered to restrict persons from purchasing foods, drugs, and medical devices that are unsafe or inefficacious even if they wish to purchase them. A controversial decision by the FDA in 1992 to severely restrict the use of silicone-gel breast implants exemplifies paternalistic controversies that have beset the FDA. Women had elected to use implants for over 30 years, either to augment their breast size or to reconstruct their breasts following mastectomies. Over 2 million women in the United States had had the implants (3 million worldwide) when, in April 1992, the FDA restricted the use of silicone-gel breast implants until additional studies could be conducted. Concerns centered on the implants' longevity, rate of rupture, and causal link to various diseases. Those who defended this restriction contended that no woman should be allowed to take a risk of unknown, but potentially serious, magnitude, because her consent could not be informed. The FDA defended a restrictive policy, rather than prohibition, because it held that patients with breast cancer and others have a legitimate need for breast reconstruction. The FDA distinguished sharply between reconstruction candidates and augmentation candidates, arguing that the favorable risk–benefit ratio is confined to reconstruction candidates.[21]

This decision has deservedly been criticized as inappropriately paternalistic. The sweeping character of the decision suggests that the government crossed the line into an unjustified paternalism by overreacting to what were probably overstated risks, and there had been inadequate consultation with those who would experience the risks. The government failed to duly consider whether the subjective benefits for many women outweigh the identified risks. At the time opinion surveys indicated that most women receiving the implants were satisfied with them. In light of this result, the most defensible policy would seem to be to permit use of silicone-gel breast implants while demanding that adequate disclosure be provided about risks. Raising the level of disclosure standards is usually a more appropriate approach than raising the level of paternalistic restraints on choice.

It does not follow that the only adequate policy is one of better disclosure or that paternalism is never justified in such a case. If there were a targetable group of particularly vulnerable women with high risk of harm from silicone implants, a paternalistic prohibition might well be an adequate policy for this particular group. As with other cases, the best policy is one that carefully weighs the benefits and risks, and then weighs the result against patients' rights to information and choice.

Risk in the Formulation of Health Policy

Paternalism in health policy has played a well-known role in the prohibition or punishment of smoking, drinking, and hazardous recreational activities such as hang gliding, mountain climbing, and whitewater rafting. Extreme paternalistic prohibitions are usually avoided in health policy, but minor-risk paternalistic interventions are common in these policies. Two classic cases in American law involve requirements that helmets be worn when riding motorcycles. In one case, a judge relied extensively on Mill's views about autonomy limitation. He argued that requiring motorcyclists and their passengers to wear crash helmets for paternalistic reasons was an instance of reasoning that could lead to unlimited state paternalism. He acknowledged that highway safety is a relevant reason for legal restrictions, but not where the *cyclist alone* is at risk. This legal opinion reads almost as if it were a direct application of Mill's philosophy.[22] By contrast, a judge in a different case argued that "we ought to admit frankly that the purpose of the helmet [requirement] is to preserve the life and health of the cyclist"—and not to promote public health or highway safety. The judge saw justifiable paternalism.[23] This judgment is reasonable. The cost for the cyclist is minimal, and the potential benefit for the cyclist is life as a healthy person. Only a legal system of absolute rights would force us to a different conclusion.

Research Ethics: The Use of Prisoners and Vulnerable Groups in Research

Problems in research ethics only infrequently raise issues of paternalism, but there are exceptional cases. An example appears in biomedical research involving prisoners. This case is interesting for its illustration of how an action may appear to be paternalistic when in fact it is nonpaternalistic, but could easily have been paternalistic.

In its report on research involving prisoners, the National Commission for the Protection of Human Subjects of Biomedical and Behavioral Research argued that the closed nature of prison environments creates a potential for abuse of authority and therefore invites the exploitation and coercion of prisoners.[24] Although a study authorized by the National Commission indicated that most prisoners wanted to accept the research opportunity and believed that neither coercion nor undue influence would compromise their consent to research, the National Commission argued that prisons' coercive and exploitative possibilities justify regulations prohibiting the use of prisoners in research, even if they volunteer to participate.

This restriction at first sight seems paternalistic, but closer analysis in this particular case shows that it was not presented paternalistically in the Natonal

Commission's report. The National Commission used a hypothetical to argue that if a prison environment were not exploitative or coercive (and if a few other conditions were met), then prisoners should be allowed to choose to participate in research. The National Commission's justifying ground was that we cannot predict or control whether prisoners will be exploited in settings that render them vulnerable, and that society should prohibit even research to which prisoners *might validly consent* in some prisons because society cannot adequately monitor whether the subjects' consent is, in fact, valid and what the subsequent conditions of participation will be.

A variety of circumstances in biomedical ethics suggest a need to examine whether so-called vulnerable classes of persons, including prisoners, are being exploited. Restrictions placed on members of these classes may or may not be paternalistic. For example, healthy, nonrelated organ donors and cancer patients solicited for research are sometimes treated in a manner similar to the prisoners just mentioned. Protective requirements aimed at the protection of their welfare may or may not be paternalistic. There is no reason why a balance of considerations might not justify a paternalistic policy in these cases. In some cases the justification of an act, policy, or practice of nonacquiescence or intervention in a person's preferences may be *partially*, but not purely, paternalistic because it is intermixed with nonpaternalistic reasons, such as protection of third parties. Such impure or mixed paternalism is common in public policy debates.

CONCLUSION

Many paternalistic interventions are unjustified. It does not follow that they all are. I have argued that it is an open question whether reasonably minor offenses to autonomy, such as withholding certain forms of information, are justified in light of critical medical goals, such as the administration of lifesaving therapies and the prevention of suicide. It will well serve moral reflection if we do not follow Mill in the banishment of a principle of strong paternalism.

I have not argued that it is part of the justification of medical paternalism that physicians are explicitly authorized to take care of patients. However, the fact that physicians are positioned to make sound and caring decisions from a position of authority merits special consideration when judging whether paternalism in medicine is warranted. In biomedical ethics we are accustomed to thinking of the right to authorize as belonging exclusively to patients and their surrogates. This way of thinking about the conduct of physicians is short-sighted.

Notes

1. *Epidemics* 1, 11, in: Jones, W. H. S. (ed.) (1923): *Hippocrates*, I, Cambridge, MA: Harvard University Press, 165.

2. Mill, J. S. (1977): *On Liberty*, 4th ed., in: *Collected Works of John Stuart Mill*, vol. XVIII, Toronto: University of Toronto Press, 261.

3. See Feinberg (1986-v4) in his four-volume work *The Moral Limits of the Criminal Law*, principally the final volume, *Harmless Wrongdoing*, New York: Oxford University Press, 9. The schema of principles outlined here is heavily indebted to Feinberg's work.

4. Mill, J. S (1977): On Liberty, 223.

5. Dworkin, G. (1992): "Paternalism," in: Becker, L. (ed.): *Encyclopedia of Ethics*, New York: Garland Publishing, 939–942; Arneson, R. (1980): "Mill versus Paternalism," *Ethics* 90, 470–489; Archard, D. (1990): "Paternalism Defined," *Analysis* 50, 36–42; Beauchamp, T.L., McCullough, L.B. (1984): *Medical Ethics: The Moral Responsibilities of Physicians*, Englewood Cliffs, NJ: Prentice-Hall.

6. See VanDeVeer, D. (1986): *Paternalistic Intervention: The Moral Bounds on Benevolence*, Princeton, NJ: Princeton University Press, 16–40; Kleinig, J. (1983): *Paternalism*, Totowa, NJ: Rowman and Allanheld, 6–14.

7. VanDeVeer, D. (1986); Kleinig, J. (1983).

8. Feinberg (1986-v3), *Harm to Self* (in the four-volume work on *The Moral Limits of the Criminal Law*), 5; Seana Shiffrin (2000): "Paternalism, Unconscionability Doctrine, & Accommodation," *Philosophy and Public Affairs* 29, 205–251.

9. Feinberg (1986-v3).

10. Feinberg, J. (1971): "Legal Paternalism," in: *Canadian Journal of Philosophy* 1, 105–124, esp. 113, 116. Revised (1973) in *Social Philosophy*, Englewood Cliffs, NJ: Prentice-Hall; and later restated in *Harm to Self*, Chapter 17.

11. Feinberg, (1971): "Legal Paternalism," 113, 124. Though some say that weak paternalism is the only form of justified paternalism, I believe that it is easy to justify the conclusions of weak paternalism independent of any mention of a principle of paternalism. Everyone supports altruistic beneficence directed at confused cardiac patients, ignorant consumers, frightened clients, and young persons who know little about the dangers of alcohol, smoking, drugs, and motorcycles. No caring person would leave these individuals unprotected, and no reasonable philosopher would defend a normative thesis that permits such outcomes. The knotty problems about the justification of paternalism lie not in these behaviors. They lie exclusively in strong paternalism, which takes over and overrides autonomy.

12. Cass R. Sunstein and Richard H. Thaler, "Libertarian Paternalism is Not an Oxymoron," *University of Chicago Law Review* 70 (2003): 1159–1202, esp. 1159.

13. Christine Jolls and Cass R. Sunstein, "Debiasing through Law," *The Journal of Legal Studies* 33 (2006): 232.

14. Dworkin, G. (1972): "Paternalism," in: *The Monist* 56, 64–84, esp. 65.

15. Dworkin (1972); see also VanDeVeer (1986) and Kleinig (1983).

16. Compare Kleinig's similar conclusion in *Paternalism*, 76.

17. Bloch, K.E. (1987): "The Role of Law in Suicide Prevention: Beyond Civil Commitment—A Bystander Duty to Report Suicide Threats," in: *Stanford Law Review* 39, 929–953.

18. See Katz, J., Goldstein, J., and Dershowitz, A.M. (eds.) (1967): *Psychoanalysis, Psychiatry, and the Law*. New York: The Free Press, 552–554, 710–713; and Burt, R.A. (1979): *Taking Care of Strangers: The Rule of Law in Doctor-Patient Relations*, New York: The Free Press, chap. 2.

19. Silva, M.C. (1989): *Ethical Decision-making in Nursing Administration*, Norwalk, CT: Appleton and Lange, 64.

20. Beauchamp, T.L., and Childress, J.F. (2009): *Principles of Biomedical Ethics*, 6th ed., New York: Oxford University Press, 215.

21. Kessler, D.A. (1992): "Special Report: The Basis of the FDA's Decision on Breast Implants," in: *New England Journal of Medicine* 326, 1713–1715.

22. *American Motorcycle Association v. Department of State Police* 158 N.W. 2d 72. Mich. App (1968).

23. *Florida v. Eitel* 227 So. 2d 489 (Fla. 1969).

24. National Commission for the Protection of Human Subjects of Biomedical and Behavioral Research (1976): *Report and Recommendations: Research Involving Prisoners*, Washington, DC: DHEW Publication No. OS 76-131.

7

WHEN HASTENED DEATH IS NEITHER KILLING NOR LETTING DIE

There are two fundamental moral issues about physician-assisted hastening of death: Are physicians morally justified in complying with requests by patients who ask for assistance? Is there an adequate moral basis to justify the legalization of physician-assisted hastening of death at the patient's request? Legal developments in the United States have encouraged us to frame virtually all moral questions as ones of legalization. As important as legalization is, the question of whether physicians are morally justified in complying with requests for aid in dying presents the more fundamental moral issue. Accordingly, my concern is primarily with the moral justification of individual acts of hastening death.

The thesis that physician-assisted hastening of death is morally prohibited has commonly been grounded in the premises that there is a defensible and relevant distinction between letting die and killing and that physicians may let patients die but cannot kill them. I do not reject the distinction between killing and letting die; indeed, I offer an analysis that makes sense of it. Nonetheless, this distinction is fatally deficient and flawed as a means of treating the major problems of physician-assisted death that face medicine and society today. Physician-assisted hastening of death need not involve either killing or letting die; and even if an act is one of killing or letting die, it must be shown whether the act is justified or unjustified. The categories of "killing" and "letting die" therefore need to be redirected to the key moral issue that should drive discussions of physician-assisted death, which is the liberty to choose and the justification (if any) for limiting that liberty.[1]

THE CONCEPTUAL FOUNDATION OF THE DISTINCTION BETWEEN
KILLING AND LETTING DIE

In examining the conceptual foundation of the distinction between killing and letting die, the first question is whether physicians kill patients by causing their deaths either through interventions or through intentional noninterventions. In medical tradition, the term *killing* has understandably carried meanings of wrongfulness and blameworthiness. However, in contexts external to traditional medical morality, "killing" does not imply wrongful behavior; it refers only to causal action that brings about another's death. In settings both within and outside medicine, "letting die" refers to intentionally not intervening so that disease, system failure, injury, or circumstance causes death.

In ordinary discourse, medicine, and law, these conceptions are conspicuously vague. Some cases of letting die count also as acts of killing, thereby undermining the hypothesis that these terms distinguish two different sets of cases. For example, health professionals kill patients—that is, cause patients to die—when they intentionally let them die in circumstances in which a duty exists to keep the patients alive, such as a patient with pneumonia who could easily be cured and wants to be cured but is "allowed to die" by a physician who chooses not to "intervene." In much of the literature of medical ethics, it is unclear how to distinguish killing from letting die so as to avoid even this elementary problem of cases that satisfy the conditions of both categories.

A widely accepted account of letting die holds that intentionally forgoing a medical technology qualifies as letting die, rather than killing, only if an underlying disease or injury is intentionally allowed to cause death when death might be delayed by employing that technology.[2] According to this view, if a medical technology is intentionally withdrawn or withheld, a natural death occurs when natural conditions do what they would have done had the technology never been initiated (i.e., when existing conditions take their natural, undeterred course). By contrast, killing occurs if an act of a person or persons, rather than natural conditions, causes an ensuing death.

This account misses its mark unless other conditions are added to it, but additional conditions threaten to undermine the very point of the account. One condition that must be added is that any withholding or withdrawing of a medical technology must be justified; an unjustified withholding or withdrawing that releases natural conditions is a killing. This condition brings a moral consideration of justified action into the heart of the conceptual analysis of letting die. To see why this condition of justified withholding or withdrawing must be added, consider the case of a physician who either mistakenly (through negligence) or maleficently (through ill intent) removes a life-sustaining medical technology from a patient who wants to continue living. This action lacks justification. We could not reasonably say, "The physician did not cause the patient's death; he only allowed the patient to die of an underlying condition." In this case, the physician did cause the death, and the physician did "let the patient die" in the sense normally meant in medical morality.

Now, change the patient's wishes. Suppose that the patient autonomously refused the technology that sustains life. In this circumstance, it would not be correct to say that the physician caused the death. Whether the physician did or did not cause death is determined in these circumstances by whether the act was validly authorized. If the act is validly authorized, it is a letting die; if it is not validly authorized, it is a killing. The reason for forgoing a medical technology is therefore the key condition in conceptually distinguishing killing and letting die in cases of withholding or withdrawing life-sustaining interventions. A physician lets a patient die if he or she has valid authorization for withholding or withdrawing treatment. "Letting die" is validly authorized nonintervention in circumstances in which patients die (when and in the precise manner they do) as a result. By contrast, a comparable action or inaction is a killing if:

- the physician had a duty to treat,
- the physician withheld or withdrew a life-sustaining technology without authorization, and
- the patient subsequently died for lack of that technology.

Here a physician is the relevant cause of death and kills a patient if he or she has no valid authorization for withholding or withdrawing treatment, but the physician lets the patient die if he or she does have valid authorization for withholding or withdrawing treatment. Of course, physicians also may kill in so-called active ways. I confront this problem in due course.

LETTING DIE BASED ON MEDICAL FUTILITY

Thus far I have argued that the following are conceptually (rather than causally) sufficient conditions of letting die in medicine:

1. the patient validly refused a medical technology that is essential to the patient's continued existence,
2. the physician withheld or withdrew the refused life-sustaining technology, and
3. the patient subsequently died for lack of the technology.

To say that these conditions are conceptually sufficient for letting die is not to say that they are either necessary conditions or the only set of sufficient conditions. Withdrawing or withholding a medically futile technology can be the main reason why we categorize an action as one of letting die. Accordingly, the following conditions form a second set of (conceptually) sufficient conditions of letting die in medicine:

1. a medical authority appropriately judged that a medical technology is futile to achieve the goals for which it was initiated (though it has to this point kept the patient alive),
2. the physician withheld or withdrew the futile technology, and
3. the patient subsequently died for lack of the technology.

A common, but incorrect, thesis is that letting die occurs in medicine only if "ceasing useless medical technologies" eventuates in the patient's death.[3] This account rightly connects letting die to futility (as in 1' through 3') but wrongly assumes that in the circumstance of letting die, technologies must be futile. As demonstrated in the previous section, medical futility is not a necessary condition of letting die. A patient's valid refusal of a medical technology makes a circumstance one of letting die even if the technology is not futile.

In the case of 1' through 3', the physician's intention may also need to be of one type rather than another to qualify as letting die, but I will not here pursue this question about proper intention. What does need an additional comment is the language in 1' of "a medical authority appropriately judged that." As the previous analysis suggests, in the medical context letting die is conceptually tied to acceptable acts, where acceptability derives either from a well-substantiated judgment of the futility of a technology or from a valid refusal of the technology. In the case of a valid refusal, there exists no problem about responsibility for the death because the refusal itself justifies the physician's conduct; the refusal nullifies what would otherwise be an injury or maltreatment and makes the case one of letting die. A judgment of futility does not as transparently provide justification, but a well-substantiated judgment of futility can be the basis of a justified act of withholding or withdrawing a technology.

The language of letting die is used in medical contexts to express a moral judgment. A letting die is a justified act; it is not morally neutral or unjustified. Despite this general feature of medical discourse, it is an open question whether physicians kill or let die when they nonnegligently make a mistaken judgment about a patient's condition (after which the patient refuses treatment) or about the futility of a treatment. Assessment of such hard cases is likely to turn on special features of the cases. For present purposes, suffice it to say that a conscientious and knowledgeable physician who makes a reasoned and justifiable determination of futility in light of all the information that could be gained in the circumstances lets the patient die and does not kill the patient, even if the judgment of futility turns out to have been mistaken.

DO PHYSICIANS KILL PATIENTS WHEN THEY ASSIST IN HASTENING DEATH?

A necessary condition of killing a patient is that the actions or inactions of the physician cause the patient's death. However, the criteria of causing death in the medical setting need clarification. The conscientious and informed physician who either makes a justifiable determination of futility or follows a patient's valid refusal does not cause the patient's death even if, in the circumstances, the technology withdrawn or withheld is causally necessary for the patient's continued existence. The physician's act of withholding or withdrawing is a necessary (or "but for") condition of the patient's death as the death occurred, but the physician is not *the cause* in the pertinent sense, which is that of being *causally responsible*. A physician is not responsible for the consequences of withholding or withdrawing a technology the patient has refused, even if the physician is a contributing cause of those consequences. By contrast, the previously mentioned physician who maleficently removed a medical technology from a patient who wanted to continue living is *the cause* of death, is *causally responsible* for the outcome, and indeed *killed* the patient.

Why is the first physician not the cause, whereas the second is the cause? "The cause" judgments (or singular causal judgments) are relative to the prevailing criteria in a given context of investigation. In the circumstance of physician-caused death, judgments of causation (and, derivatively, of killing) turn on whether a physician intervened in an unwarranted manner in a course of events that could reasonably have been expected to take place. When the physician has specific warrant for action or inaction (e.g., when the physician has a valid authorization from a patient) and the patient's death is a consequence of acting or not acting, the physician is not the cause of death. Rather, the cause is disease, injury, system failure, or perhaps the decision of another party who authorized the physician's conduct.

To illustrate these abstract points and make them more transparent, consider the following thought experiment: Two patients occupy a semiprivate hospital room, both having the same illness and both respirator dependent. One has refused the respirator; the other wishes to remain on the respirator. A physician intentionally flips a master switch that turns off both respirators; the physician is aware that both respirators will shut down. The two patients die in the same way at the same time of the same physical causes and by the same physical action of the physician. (Thus, all variables are held constant except that one patient authorized the physician's action and the other did not.) Although the two patients die of the same physical causes, they do not die of the same causes of interest to law, medicine, and morality, because the proximate cause—that is, the cause responsible for the outcome—is not the same in the two otherwise identically situated patients. Consistent with the analysis provided previously, this thought experiment shows that a valid authorization transforms what would be a maleficent act of killing into a nonmaleficent act of letting die.

From both a legal and a moral point of view, one reason why physicians do not injure, maltreat, or kill patients when they withhold or withdraw medical technology is that a physician is morally and legally obligated to respect a valid refusal. Since a valid refusal of treatment binds the physician, it would be unacceptable to hold that these legal and moral duties require physicians to cause the deaths of their patients and thereby to kill them.

Quite apart from killing by means of withholding or withdrawing a treatment, killing can and occasionally does occur through a physician-initiated "active" means to death. Here is a conceptually clear case: Paul Mills was a patient in the Queen Elizabeth II Health Sciences Center in Halifax, Nova Scotia. Mills had undergone 10 unsuccessful operations for throat cancer. He was dying, and a life-support system had been withdrawn at the request of his family. It was thought that he would die a natural death within a few hours. However, the heavy sedation he had been given was not having its intended effect. Mills was suffering from infection and experiencing "tremendous discomfort" and "excruciating pain," according to hospital officials. On November 10, 1996, Nancy Morrison, Mills's physician, administered to Mills a dose of potassium chloride. Mills died shortly thereafter. His family was unaware of the injection. On May 6, 1997, Dr. Morrison was indicted for first-degree murder; these charges were thrown out on February 27, 1998, for lack of legal evidence sufficient to sustain the charge of first-degree murder.[4]

Dr. Morrison did not, and would not, describe her act as "killing," let alone as "murder." She viewed it as a compassionate act of assistance in dying. It may indeed have been an act of this description. However, Dr. Morrison had no specific authorization for her act of injecting potassium chloride, and she was the cause of Mills's death in the way and at the time that his death occurred; she was causally responsible for the death, and she killed Mills. Whether she killed him *justifiably* is another matter, and one I will now consider.

IS KILLING BY PHYSICIANS MORALLY PERMISSIBLE?

I have proposed that in cases of killing a patient the physician is causally responsible (a proximate cause), and in cases of letting die the physician is not causally responsible (not the proximate cause). This proposal so far conforms to legal and medical traditions. Now, however, I depart from those traditions.

It does not follow from the fact that a physician kills a patient that the physician acts unjustifiably. Outside of traditional thinking about medical morality, it is clear that to correctly apply the label "killing" or the label "letting die" to a set of events cannot determine whether one type of action is better or worse than the other or whether either is acceptable or unacceptable.[5] Rightness and wrongness in killing depend exclusively on the merit of the justification underlying an act of killing, not on the type of action it is.

Outside of (and independent of) medical tradition, there are several generally accepted justifications for killing, including killing in self-defense, killing to rescue a person endangered by another person's immoral acts, and killing by misadventure (accidental, nonnegligent killing while engaged in a lawful act). These excusing conditions establish that we cannot prejudge an action as wrong merely because it is a killing.[6] I hereafter assume this morally neutral sense of "kill" to see where it can and should take us in contexts of physician-hastened death.

Even though medical tradition has condemned physician killing, it is conceptually and morally open to physicians (and society) to reverse tradition and come to the conclusion that medicine and the social context have changed and that it is time to permit certain forms of assisted death including some forms that involve killing.[7] Medical morality has never been self-justifying, and traditional practices and standards in medicine may, in the face of social change, turn out to be indefensible limits on the liberty to choose. Even if, in medicine, killing is usually wrong and letting die only rarely wrong, this outcome is contingent on the features of the cases that typically appear in medicine. The general wrongness of killing and the general rightness of letting die are not surprising features of the moral world inasmuch as killings are rarely authorized by appropriate parties and cases of letting die generally are validly authorized. Be that as it may, the frequency with which one kind of act is justified, by contrast to the other kind of act, is not relevant to the moral (or legal) justification of either kind of act.

The justifiability of any particular type or instance of killing is therefore an open question, and we cannot assert without looking at a particular case (or type of case) that killing is morally worse than allowing to die. The way to decide whether killing is wrong in the medical circumstance of a request for hastened death is to determine what makes it wrong in general. Causing a person's death is wrong, when it is wrong, not simply because someone is the responsible (or proximate) cause but because an unjustified harm or loss to the deceased has occurred—for example, the person has been deprived of opportunities and goods that life would otherwise have afforded. A person must unjustifiably suffer a setback to personal interests (a harm) that the person would not otherwise have experienced.[8]

It is a complicated question whether patient-authorized killing by physicians involves any form of harm to the patient, but we can here circumvent this question. It is a generally accepted principle even in Hippocratic medicine that physicians may, under various conditions, legitimately harm patients to avoid graver or more burdensome harms. Invasive surgery that requires recuperation is a paradigm case. Because death is sometimes the more inviting of two unwelcome outcomes, physicians may have sound reasons to help their patients by causing the lesser harm.[9] If a patient chooses death as a release from a desperate and harmful circumstance, then killing at that patient's request involves no clear wrong even if it does involve a harm. Shortening life can avoid a state of burdens to a patient that is virtually uncompensated by benefits.[10]

This form of aid to patients might harm society by setting back its interests, and this harm might constitute a sufficient reason not to legalize physician-hastened death. However, this consequence would not change the status of the act as a legitimate form of physician assistance to a patient.

THE PLACE OF AUTONOMOUS REQUESTS

A request by a competent patient for assistance in hastening death does not have the same moral authority and binding force as a competent refusal of technology that would sustain life. Patients have a right to refuse and, correlatively, physicians have an obligation to comply with the refusal; but there is no comparable right or obligation in the case of a request. Autonomous refusals by patients compel physician nonintervention, but autonomous requests by patients do not necessarily compel physician intervention. Nonetheless, it does not follow that requests from patients fail to justify acts of physician assistance in hastened death.

In many circumstances in medicine, a request by patients for aid authorizes assistance by a physician. For example, a request for help in reducing pain warrants interventions to meet the request. Why is a favorable response by a physician to a request for assistance in facilitating death by hastening it different from a favorable response to requests for assistance in facilitating death by easing it? The two acts of physician assistance appear to be morally equivalent as long as there are no other differences in the cases. That is, if the disease is relevantly similar, the request by the patient is relevantly similar, the desperateness of the patient's circumstance is relevantly similar, and so on, then responding to a request to provide the means to hasten death (thought of by some as killing) is morally equivalent to responding to a request to ease death by withdrawing treatment, sedating to coma, and the like (thought of by many as letting die).

In cases of requested active assistance, requested passive nonintervention, and various borderline cases between the active and the passive (e.g., administering fatal medication when the intended goal is to ease pain or to terminally sedate), a patient is seeking the best means to quit a life of unrelieved misery. In all such cases, persons reach a judgment that lingering in life is, on balance, worse than death. The person who hastens death by ingesting fatal medication, the person who forgoes nutrition and hydration, the person who requests terminal sedation, and the person who forgoes life-sustaining technologies may each be selecting what for him or her is the best means to the end of unrelievable burdens.

Denial of help to a patient in these bleak circumstances renders life more burdensome from the patient's perspective—or, in the case of not prescribing a fatal medication, takes the decision away from the patient. It is not important that these acts are of a certain type (suicide, say) but only that they are acts of a type that can be justified.

The issue is not whether valid requests by patients place a *duty* on physicians to hasten death.[11] The question is whether valid requests render it *permissible* for a physician to lend aid in hastening death. A physician with a professional commitment to help a patient die as the patient chooses has made a moral commitment that differs from the commitment made by a physician who draws the line in opposition to all forms of assistance in hastening death. There are intermediate forms of physician commitment, as well. A physician who, in principle, accepts the permissibility of assistance may still refuse to honor a particular request by a patient for assistance in a particular case on grounds that the patient's condition has not reached a point beyond which standard measures of palliative support are adequate to relieve the patient's suffering or distress. Even a sympathetic physician who is willing to assist a patient at a specific point in the evolution of his or her condition may justifiably refuse a patient's premature request for a hastened death.

IS THE DISTINCTION BETWEEN KILLING AND LETTING DIE RELEVANT TO PHYSICIAN-ASSISTED DEATH?

Many assume that the distinction between killing and letting die is relevant to contemporary issues of physician-assisted death. This assumption is suspect. Some forms of physician-assisted hastening of death do not involve either killing or letting die. A physician who prescribes a lethal medication at a patient's request is not the cause (the proximate cause) of the patient's death and so does not kill the patient. Nor does this physician let the patient die. Neither the condition of killing nor that of letting die is satisfied. Since the prescription of fatal medication dominates much of the current discussion about hastened death, the irrelevance to these actions of the distinction between killing and letting die merits more discussion than it has received.

The fundamental ethical issue about physician-assisted hastening of death is whether it is morally acceptable for physicians to help seriously ill, injured, or suffering persons reach their goals in a manner that both the patient and the physician find appropriate. Of course, a decision to hasten death is not justified merely because a patient and a physician believe that it is justified. Moral justification of acts of hastening death requires more than patient requests and agreements between patients and their physicians. Acts of hastening death lack justification if a physician has inattentively misdiagnosed the case, if the patient's capacity to make autonomous judgments is significantly impaired, if manipulative family pressures are profoundly influencing either the physician or the patient, and the like.

If no such invalidating condition exists and the physician and the patient both act autonomously, then the choice of a hastened death is justified. One way to express this thesis is that unless a valid liberty-limiting principle warrants intervention to prevent an act of hastened death, there is no moral basis for condemning or punishing the envisioned autonomous acts of patients and their willing physicians. The question of the morality of physician-assisted hastening of death is fundamentally the question of which, if any, liberty-limiting principle justifiably prevents such choices from being effected. Although I have not considered whether there is any such valid liberty-limiting principle, I would be pleased if I had prepared the way for this question to become the central issue—freeing us from the burden of the unproductive and overvalued distinction between killing and letting die.

Elsewhere in these *Collected Essays* I further discuss valid liberty-limiting principles, with a brief reference to problems of physician-hastened death. See the essay entitled "The Concept of Paternalism in Biomedical Ethics."

Notes

1. The line between killing and letting die is relied on in the codes and guidelines of numerous professional associations; see American Medical Association, Council on Ethical and Judicial Affairs, "Physician-Assisted Suicide," Report 59, December 1993. A version of this report was published as "Physician-Assisted Suicide," *Journal of the American Medical Association* 267 (1992): 2229–2233. See also "Physician-Assisted Suicide," Current Opinions, H-270.965; "Euthanasia," *Current Opinions*, E-2.21; "Decisions Near the End of Life," *Current Opinions*, H-140.966; "Voluntary Active Euthanasia," *Current Opinions*, H-140.987 (updated June 1996); Canadian Medical Association, *Code of Ethics*, secs. 18–20 (approved

October 15, 1996); Canadian Medical Association, Policy Statement, "Euthanasia and Assisted Suicide" (June 19, 1998), which replaces the previous policy entitled "Physician-Assisted Death" (1995); World Medical Association, *Resolution on Euthanasia* (Washington, DC: World Medical Association, 2002), reaffirming the *Declaration of Euthanasia* (Madrid: World Medical Association, 1987).

In the formulations of these professional bodies, as in most nations and, effectively, in all traditions of medical ethics, killing is prohibited and letting die permitted under specified conditions. Despite this remarkable convergence of opinion, a cogent and pertinent analysis of the distinction between killing and letting die relevant to medicine remains elusive; see D. Orentlicher, "The Alleged Distinction Between Euthanasia and the Withdrawal of Life-Sustaining Treatment: Conceptually Incoherent and Impossible to Maintain," *University of Illinois Law Review* 3 (1998): 837–859; T.L. Beauchamp, ed., *Intending Death* (Upper Saddle River, NJ: Prentice Hall, 1996); J. McMahan, "Killing, Letting Die, and Withdrawing Aid," *Ethics* 103 (1993): 250–279; L.O. Gostin, "Drawing a Line Between Killing and Letting Die: The Law, and Law Reform, on Medically Assisted Dying," *Journal of Law, Medicine and Ethics* 21 (1993): 94–101; H.M. Malm, "Killing, Letting Die, and Simple Conflicts," *Philosophy and Public Affairs* 18 (1989): 238–258; B. Steinbock and A. Norcross, eds., *Killing and Letting Die*, 2nd ed. (New York: Fordham University Press, 1994).

2. F. Cohn and J. Lynn, "Vulnerable People: Practical Rejoinders to Claims in Favor of Assisted Suicide," in *The Case against Assisted Suicide: For the Right to End-of-Life Care*, edited by K. Foley and H. Hendin (Baltimore, MD: Johns Hopkins University Press, 2002), 230–260, esp. 246–247; D. Callahan, *The Troubled Dream of Life* (New York: Simon and Schuster, 1993), chap. 2; and various articles in *By No Extraordinary Means*, edited by J. Lynn (Bloomington: Indiana University Press, 1986), 227–266.

3. W. Gaylin, L.R. Kass, E.D. Pellegrino, and M. Siegler, "Doctors Must Not Kill," *Journal of the American Medical Association* 259 (1988): 2139–2140 (emphasis added). See also L.R. Kass, "Neither for Love nor Money: Why Doctors Must Not Kill," *Public Interest* 94 (1989): 25–46. It is sometimes added, as a condition, that patients must be dependent upon life-support systems; see R.E. Cranford, "The Physician's Role in Killing and the Intentional Withdrawal of Treatment," in *Intending Death*, edited by T.L. Beauchamp (Upper Saddle River, NJ: Prentice Hall, 1996), 150–162, esp. 160.

4. The facts about this case have been drawn from several articles that appeared from 1996 to 1999 in Canadian newspapers and medical journals. Some parts of the case rely on reports provided to me by Canadian physicians who investigated the case.

5. In effect, this proposal is made in J.R. Rachels, "Active and Passive Euthanasia," *New England Journal of Medicine* 292 (1975): 78–80; and D.W. Brock, "Voluntary Active Euthanasia," *Hastings Center Report* 22, no. 2 (1992): 10–22.

6. Compare Rachels, "Active and Passive Euthanasia"; J.R. Rachels, "Killing, Letting Die, and the Value of Life," in *Can Ethics Provide Answers? And Other Essays in Moral Philosophy*, by J.R. Rachels (Lanham, MD: Rowman and Littlefield, 1997), 69–79; R.W. Perrett, "Killing, Letting Die and the Bare Difference Argument," *Bioethics* 10 (1996): 131–139; Brock, "Voluntary Active Euthanasia."

7. Compare H. Brody and F.G. Miller, "The Internal Morality of Medicine: Explication and Application to Managed Care," *Journal of Medicine and Philosophy* 23 (1998): 384–410, esp. 397; G. Seay, "Do Physicians Have an Inviolable Duty Not to Kill?" *Journal of Medicine and Philosophy* 26 (2001): 75–91.

8. Compare A. Buchanan, "Intending Death: The Structure of the Problem and Proposed Solutions," in *Intending Death*, edited by T.L. Beauchamp (Upper Saddle River, NJ: Prentice Hall, 1996), 34–38; M. Hanser, "Why Are Killing and Letting Die Wrong?" *Philosophy and Public Affairs* 24 (1995): 175–201; and reflections on the roles of intention and the "right not to be killed" in D.W. Brock, "A Critique of Three Objections to Physician-Assisted Suicide," *Ethics* 109 (1999): 519–547, esp. 537.

9. F.M. Kamm, "Physician-Assisted Suicide, Euthanasia, and Intending Death," in M.P. Battin, R. Rhodes, and A. Silvers, eds., *Physician-Assisted Suicide: Expanding the Debate* (New York: Routledge, 1998), 26–49; T. Nagel, "Death," in *Mortal Questions*, by T. Nagel (Cambridge: Cambridge University Press, 1979); and F.M. Kamm, *Morality, Mortality*, vol. 1 (New York: Oxford University Press, 1993), chap. 1

10. See Kamm, "Physician-Assisted Suicide, Euthanasia, and Intending Death," and some later formulations in her "Physician-Assisted Suicide, the Doctrine of Double Effect, and the Ground of Value," *Ethics* 109 (1999): 586–605, esp. 588ff.

11. Although I am not here raising this question, Kamm has presented an "argument for a duty of a physician"; see Kamm, "Physician-Assisted Suicide, the Doctrine of Double Effect, and the Ground of Value," 589.

8

THE EXPLOITATION OF THE ECONOMICALLY DISADVANTAGED IN PHARMACEUTICAL RESEARCH

Many media reports, books, articles, and government documents serve up searing criticisms of the power and influence of the pharmaceutical industry. The industry as a whole stands accused of a sea of injustices and corruptions, including aggressive and deceptive marketing schemes, exploitative uses of research subjects, a corrupting influence on universities, a shameful use of lobbying, suppression of vital data, bias and amateurism in the presentation of data, conflicts of interest that bias research investigators, and corruption of the clinical judgment of medical students and practicing physicians.[1]

Each of these charges derives from concern about some form of unjust *influence* exerted by pharmaceutical companies. I cannot here consider the full array of alleged forms of influence. I telescope to one area: the recruitment and enrollment in clinical research of vulnerable human subjects, in particular the economically disadvantaged. I focus on the charge that subjects in clinical trials are exploited by manipulative and unfair payment schemes. I treat three problems. The first is the problem of whether the economically disadvantaged constitute a vulnerable group. I argue that classification as a "group" is a misleading characterization that may cause paternalistic overprotection. The second problem is whether the vulnerable poor are exploited by payments that constitute either an undue influence or an undue industry profit. I argue that such assessments should be made situationally, not categorically. The third problem is whether the poor give "compromised" or nonvoluntary consents. I argue that this third problem, like the second, is nuanced but practically manageable, and therefore that pharmaceutical research involving the poor and vulnerable can be carried out in an ethically responsible manner. Whether the research is so conducted is another matter—an empirical problem beyond the scope of my argument.

Some writers seem to argue that these problems are pseudo-problems in developed countries because the research oversight system for clinical research protects subjects against excessive risk and exploitation while demanding good science and clinical promise. If the system fails, this argument goes, then the system should be repaired, thereby resolving concerns about exploitation.[2] This approach is understandable and tempting, but overly sanguine. There is no evidence that research oversight systems have a firm grasp on problems of exploitation of the economically disadvantaged, let alone that these problems can safely be dismissed. Moreover, I intend my argument to apply globally, in all contexts of pharmaceutical research, irrespective of a country's system of oversight. Accordingly, I assume nothing about the adequacy of oversight systems.

VULNERABILITY AND ECONOMIC DISADVANTAGE

Some commentators have maintained that we should not use humans as research subjects under any circumstances; others have said that human research subjects should be volunteers only, not persons induced by rewards to participate. I will assume that neither view is defensible and that, under specifiable conditions, it is permissible to involve humans as research subjects and to pay them for their time and inconvenience. However, I do not presume anything about the involvement of persons who are particularly vulnerable to abuse or exploitation, or anything about levels of acceptable risk. Special protections may be needed for some subjects, and sometimes it is inappropriate to use such subjects at all. There may also be a need for strict control of the level of risk allowed.

I will here consider only economically disadvantaged, decisionally competent persons. Several issues arise: Are these subjects vulnerable to morally objectionable enticement into pharmaceutical research? If so, what renders them vulnerable? Do they lack a mental capacity of resistibility to influence? Is the worry that their inability to gain access to health care forces them to accept research? Is it that offers of money or health care are made that are too good to be refused? Is there something about the level of risk of harm that renders subjects vulnerable? Answers to these questions are understandably controversial.

Vulnerabilities and Vulnerable Groups

Everyone agrees that ethical research requires impartial review to safeguard the rights and welfare of all subjects and that some research involving vulnerable subjects needs special scrutiny. Less clear is which populations, if any, should be classified as vulnerable to inappropriate influences. Discussion of issues about the vulnerability of research subjects, commonly referred to as "vulnerable groups," has primarily focused on embryos, fetuses, prisoners, children, psychiatric patients, the developmentally disabled, those with dementia, and the like. Until recently little attention has been paid to populations of persons who possess the *capacity* to consent, but whose consent to participation in research might nonetheless be compromised, invalid, or unjust. Prisoners have been the paradigm class, but the economically distressed provide a comparable example.

My concern is with persons who are impoverished, may lack significant access to health care, may be homeless, may be malnourished, and yet do have the mental capacity to volunteer in safety and toxicity (phase I) drug studies sponsored by or managed by pharmaceutical companies. They possess the basic competence to reason, deliberate, decide, and consent. Data suggest that somewhere between 50% and 100% of subjects who are healthy volunteers self-report that financial need or financial reward is the primary motive for volunteering.[3] Persons of this description are certainly involved in some pharmaceutical research in North America, though the extent of their use is not well understood.[4] It is also known that the poor are used in other parts of the world, sometimes in developing countries, but the scope of their use is even less well studied and reported. I will not distinguish between the economic conditions in diverse countries in which research is conducted, but I will distinguish between circumstances in which it is reasonable to expect that basic health care is available to subjects outside of contact with research teams and circumstances in which basic health care is fundamentally unavailable to research subjects.

It is often assumed that the economically disadvantaged are more vulnerable to exploitation by pharmaceutical companies than subjects with stable economic resources.[5] This claim is intuitively attractive, but no data specific to pharmaceutical research support it, and some data in nonpharmaceutical research cast doubt on it.[6] Nonetheless, I will assume its plausibility. What cannot be assumed is that there is a clear connection between economically disadvantaged groups and vulnerability or between vulnerability and exploitation by pharmaceutical companies.

The class of the economically disadvantaged who are vulnerable has sometimes been treated in the literature as narrow, at other times as broad. Those so classified may or may not include individuals living on the streets, low-income persons who are the sole financial support of a large family, persons desperately lacking access to health care and physicians, and persons whose income falls below a certain threshold level. These individuals could have been in their current situation for many years, but they could also be temporarily unemployed, enduring a family disruption, working through bankruptcy, or fighting a short-term illness.

The notion of a "vulnerable group" has lost much of its historical significance in bioethics and health policy since it was first established in the 1970s, because so many groups have been declared vulnerable—from the infirm elderly, to the undereducated, to those with inadequate resources, to pregnant women, to whole countries whose members lack rights or are subject to exploitation. The language of "vulnerable groups" suggests that all members of a vulnerable group—all prisoners, all poor people, all pregnant women, and the like—are by category vulnerable, and perhaps incompetent to make their own decisions. The problem is that for many groups a label covering all members of the group overprotects, stereotypes, or even disqualifies members who are capable of making their own decisions.[7] "Vulnerable" is an inappropriate label for any class of persons when some members of the class are not vulnerable. For example, pregnant women as a class are not vulnerable, though some pregnant women are. Accordingly, I will not speak of the economically disadvantaged—"the poor"—as a categorically vulnerable group, though they have often been so categorized.[8]

However, I will speak of *vulnerabilities*. As necessary, I will focus on the forms, conditions, and properties of vulnerability. Ideally, research ethics will some day supply a schema of forms and conditions of vulnerability, rather than a list of vulnerable groups. These forms and conditions would be composed of the properties and circumstances that render a person vulnerable as a research subject—for example, incompetence to consent, misunderstanding the objectives of research, increased risk, and socioeconomic deprivation that breaks down one's resistance to influence attempts.[9]

The Concept of Vulnerability

"Vulnerability" is poorly defined and analyzed in literature on the subject. Many point to incapacities to give an informed consent, whereas others point to unequal relationships of power and resources, such as those between the economically disadvantaged and research sponsors or investigators. The notion of vulnerability in research requires some form of influence either by a second party or by some condition that renders the person susceptible to a harm, loss, or indignity.[10] "Harm" and "loss" are here to be understood in terms of a thwarting, defeating, or setting back of some party's interests.[11] "Harm" is sometimes constructed broadly to include actions that cause discomfort, offense, indignity, or annoyance. Narrower accounts view harms as setbacks to bodily and mental health. Whether a broad or a narrow construal is preferable is not a matter I need to decide. Everyone agrees that significant bodily harms and comparable setbacks to significant nonbodily interests are paradigm instances of harm, and I will restrict myself to these arenas.

The economically disadvantaged are vulnerable in several ways to influences that introduce a significant risk of harm. Their situation leaves them lacking in critical resources and forms of social power, especially access to economic resources and government programs that might be brought to bear on their behalf. They may not be able to resist or refuse acceptance of the risk involved, requiring trade-offs among their interests.[12] What, then, should be done to protect the interests of those who might be abused or exploited in pharmaceutical research?

CATEGORICAL EXCLUSION OF THE ECONOMICALLY DISADVANTAGED

A tempting strategy is to exclude economically disadvantaged persons categorically, even if they are not categorically vulnerable and even if they meet all conditions for participation in clinical trials. This remedy would eliminate the problem of their unjust exploitation in pharmaceutical research, but it would also deprive subjects of the freedom to choose and would often be economically harmful to them.

Nothing about economically disadvantaged persons justifies such an exclusion, as a group, from participation in pharmaceutical research, just as it does not follow from their status as disadvantaged that they should be excluded from participation in any legal activity. There is an increased risk of taking advantage of the economically distressed, but to exclude them altogether would be an inexcusable form of discrimination. Exclusionary protections of competent, disadvantaged persons may only serve to further marginalize, deprive, stigmatize, or discriminate against them. Many economically disadvantaged persons believe that participation in research is a worthy and personally satisfying social contribution as well as a means to the reduction of their economic plight. To them, research provides an opportunity to earn money in exchange for short-term and unskilled effort, whereas exclusion from participation is an unjust deprivation of liberty and an offensive form of paternalism.

Consider the weakly analogous case of prisoners, who have long been the paradigm of competent persons who are categorically excluded from phase I clinical trials. The right to volunteer as a research subject is denied to prisoners in U.S. federal policy on grounds of the potential for manipulation or coercion in penal institutions. Were this same potential to exist for economically disadvantaged persons, the same categorical exclusion might be appropriate. However, this problem needs to be examined in each context to see if persons who have the capacity to give an informed consent are nonetheless not able to consent freely in that context.

Assume, for the moment, both that we can obtain consents that are adequately informed and voluntary and that the research is welcomed by subjects as a source of income and possibly also as a source of contact with health care authorities. Under these conditions, a subject's situation of economic disadvantage is irrelevant. These subjects will be more advantaged by research participation than would other potential subjects, because the money earned and the access to health authorities will be more significant to them. To exclude voluntary subjects from participation would doubly disadvantage them, depriving them of money in their already economically disadvantaged circumstance.

PAYMENT AS INDUCEMENT: PROBLEMS OF UNDUE INFLUENCE AND UNDUE PROFIT

Payments and rewards such as free health care offered to potential pharmaceutical research subjects present issues about the acceptability of inducements in exchange for services. Problems of voluntariness are prominent.

Voluntariness and Types of Influence

A person acts voluntarily if he or she wills an action without being under the controlling influence of another person or condition. Of course not all influences are *controlling*, and not all controlling influences are *unwarranted*. What, then, are we to say about payments to potential subjects? Are they controlling? Are they warranted?

Three categories of influence need to be distinguished: persuasion, manipulation, and coercion.[13] In *persuasion*, a person believes in something through the merit of reasons another person advances. This is the paradigm of an influence that is *not* controlling and that is warranted. *Manipulation*, by contrast, involves getting people to do what the manipulator wants through a means other than coercion or persuasion. In recruitment for clinical studies, the most likely forms of manipulation are (1) informational manipulation that nonpersuasively alters a person's understanding and (2) offers of rewards. Critics of pharmaceutical company recruiting practices have accused companies of informational manipulation through withholding critical information and through misleading exaggeration. Other critics have said that offers of money and health care are excessively attractive. Finally, *coercion* occurs if and only if one person either intentionally and physically compels another or intentionally uses a credible and severe threat of harm or force to control another.[14] Some threats will coerce virtually all persons, whereas others will coerce only a few persons. Coercion itself is probably rare in the setting of clinical research, but a sense of being left without any significant alternatives other than acceptance of an offer that one would prefer to decline may not be uncommon. I turn now to that problem.

Constraining Situations

Subjects do sometimes report feeling heavily pressured to enroll in clinical trials, even though their enrollment is classified as voluntary.[15] These individuals may be in desperate need of some form of medication or research may be a vital source of income. Attractive offers such as free medication, in-clinic housing, and money can leave a person with a sense of having no meaningful choice but to accept research participation. Influences that many individuals easily resist are felt by these potential subjects as constraining them to a particular choice.

In these constraining situations—sometimes misleadingly called *coercive* situations—there is no coercion, strictly speaking, because no one has physically compelled another or intentionally issued a threat in order to gain compliance. A person feels controlled by the constraints of a situation such as severe illness or lack of food and shelter, rather than by the design or threat of another person. Sometimes people unintentionally make other persons feel "threatened" by their actions, and sometimes illness, powerlessness, and lack of resources are perceived as threats of harm that a person feels compelled to prevent. No doubt these situations are significant constraints on choice, though not ones that involve compulsion or threats.

The prospect of another night on the streets or another day without food could constrain a person to accept an offer of shelter and payment, just as such conditions could constrain a person to accept a job cleaning up hazardous chemicals or sewers that the person would otherwise not accept. The psychological effect on persons forced to choose may be similar, and a person can appropriately say in both cases, "I had no choice; it was unthinkable to refuse the offer."

PAYMENT, UNDUE INFLUENCE, AND UNDUE PROFIT

In constraining situations, monetary payments and related offers such as shelter or food give rise to questions of *undue influence* on the one hand and *undue profit* on the other. The "Common Rule" in the United States requires investigators to "minimize the possibility of" coercion and undue inducement, but it does not define, analyze, or explain these notions.[16] Issues of exploitation, undue inducement, and undue profit are inadequately handled in the bioethics literature as well.

Monetary payments seem unproblematic if the payments are welcome offers that persons do not want to refuse and the risks are at the level of everyday activities. Becoming a research subject, under these conditions, seems no different than accepting a job offer or agreeing to a contract that, without payment, one would not accept. Indeed, the offer of research involvement *is* an offer of a job or contract in which mutual benefit can and should occur (setting aside questions of sanitary conditions, impartial committee review and approval, and the like).[17] However, inducements become increasingly problematic (1) as risks are increased, (2) as more attractive inducements are offered, and (3) as the subject's economic disadvantage is exacerbated. These are the three principal conditions to be considered in assessing whether exploitation occurs.[18]

The heart of the problem of exploitation is that subjects are situationally disadvantaged and without viable alternatives, feel forced or compelled to accept attractive offers that they otherwise would not accept, and assume increased risk in their lives. As these conditions are mitigated, the problem of exploitation diminishes and may vanish; but as these conditions are heightened, the potential for exploitation increases.

As this formulation suggests, the condition of an irresistibly attractive offer is a necessary condition of "undue inducement," but this condition is not by itself sufficient to make an inducement *undue*. There must also be a risk of harm of sufficient seriousness that the person's welfare interest is negatively affected by assuming it, and it must be a risk the person would not ordinarily assume.[19] I will not try to pinpoint a precise threshold of risk, but it would have to be above the level of such common job risks as those of unskilled construction work. Inducements are not undue, then, unless they are both above the level of standard risk (hence "excessive" in risk) and irresistibly attractive (hence "excessive" in payment) in light of a constraining situation. Although these offers are not coercive, because no threat of excessive risk or of taking money away from the person is involved, the offer can be manipulative. Indeed, since irresistibly attractive payment is involved, these offers almost certainly should be categorized as manipulative.

Undue inducements should be distinguished from *undue profits*, which occur from a distributive injustice of too small a payment, rather than an irresistibly attractive, large payment. In the undue profit situation, the subject gets an unfair payment and the sponsor gets more than is justified. Often, I think, this is what critics of pharmaceutical research believe happens: The subjects are in a weak to nonexistent bargaining situation, are constrained by their poverty, and are given a pitifully small amount of money and unjust share of the benefits, while companies reap unseemly profits from the research. If this is the worry, the basic question is how to determine a nonexploitative, fair wage.

How, then, should these two moral problems of exploitation—undue inducement (unduly large and irresistible payments) and undue profit (unduly small and unfair payments)—be handled? One possible answer is that if this research involves exceptional, and therefore excessive, risk (i.e., risk having more than a minor increment above minimal risk), it should be prohibited categorically for healthy subjects, even if a good oversight system is in place. This answer is appealing, but we would still need to determine what constitutes excessive risk, irresistibly attractive payment, unjust underpayment, and constraining situations—all difficult problems that seem largely ignored in literature on the subject.

As if these problems are not difficult enough, there is a deeper moral dilemma than the analysis thus far suggests. To avoid undue influence, payment schedules must be kept reasonably low, approximating an unskilled labor wage—or possibly even lower. Even at this low level, payment might still be sufficiently large to constitute an undue inducement for some subjects. As payments are lowered down a continuum of wages to avoid undue influence—that is, to avoid making an excessively attractive offer—it is predictable that research subjects in some circumstances will be recruited largely or perhaps entirely from the ranks of the economically disadvantaged. Somewhere on this continuum the amount of money paid will be so little that it is exploitative by virtue of undue profits yielded by taking advantage of a person's misfortune. If the payment scales were reversed and run up the continuum—that is, increased to avoid undue profit—they would at some point become high enough to attract persons from the middle class. At or around this point, the offers would be declared exceptionally (and therefore excessively) attractive, and would for this reason be judged undue inducements for impoverished persons.[20] This problem becomes a more profound problem of potential injustice as the pool of research subjects is composed more or less exclusively of the economically disadvantaged. (See, further, the section on Background Justice later in this essay.)

The argument thus far yields the conclusion that exploitation occurs either when there is undue profit, offering too little for services, or when there is undue influence, offering too much for services. The most straightforward way to avoid such exploitation is a golden mean that strikes a balance between a rate of payment high enough that it does not exploit subjects by underpayment and one low enough that it does not exploit by undue inducement. If this is right, there is no a priori way to set a proper level of payment (e.g., at the level of unskilled labor) because that level might not satisfy the golden mean standard. Payment at the level of unskilled labor rates might itself be exploitative, either by creating an undue influence or generating an undue profit. The general objective should be that the research sponsor pay a fair wage at the golden mean for moderate-risk studies and not increase the wage in order to entice subjects to studies with a higher level of risk.[21] If this mean is unattainable, then any such research will be exploitative: There will be either an undue profit by underpayment or an undue influence by overpayment.[22]

If this analysis is correct, there may be situations in which payments that are too high (creating undue inducements) are, *at the same time*, payments that are too low (creating undue profits). To the desperate, $.25 per hour or $10 per hour might be irresistibly attractive while distributively unfair. Critics of the pharmaceutical industry often seem to suggest that something like this problem is common in the research context and that pharmaceutical companies routinely take advantage of these situations. If this is the charge, critics of the pharmaceutical industry could turn out to be right. As far as I know, such questions have never been carefully studied, and I have not tried to decide these questions. From what I know, at least some contexts of research conducted in North America do not involve either undue inducement or undue profit, but my argument here does not require such an assumption about North America or any other part of the world. My argument only tries to locate the moral problems and to consider possible paths to resolution.

A conclusion that is tempting to draw at this point is that pharmaceutical companies are morally obligated to avoid any situation in which the dilemma I have traced over payments cannot be satisfactorily resolved by recourse to the golden mean. That is, companies would be morally prohibited from sponsoring research in circumstances that make it exploitative by paying too much or too little. Critics of the industry would presumably be happy with this outcome, and prosperous pharmaceutical companies would also be happy with it, because it would tell them where not to locate their research in order to avoid criticism. They would then locate, or relocate, elsewhere.

I am not convinced, however, that this is the best outcome. Some moderate-risk research seems nonexploitative in adequately supervised circumstances even if an offer is irresistibly generous and choices are constrained—and perhaps even if the company could afford to pay the subjects more. However, supporting this conclusion would take more argument than I have provided, and I will not pursue it further. I make only one comment to frame the issue: An important reason for caution about prohibiting research and encouraging pharmaceutical companies to pull out of poor communities is that payments for studies are a vital source of needed funds for the economically disadvantaged as well as a way to build an infrastructure of jobs in these communities. One of the few readily available sources of money for some economically distressed persons are jobs such as day labor that expose them to more risk and generate less money than the payments generated by participation in phase I clinical trials.[23] To deny these persons the right to participate in clinical research on grounds of potential exploitation can be paternalistic and demeaning, as well as economically distressing.

Moreover, many pharmaceutical companies have the resources to make life better for subjects not only by paying them a decent wage but also by improving their lives in other respects. For example, in some countries research centers could afford to include in their budgets a range of health care benefits (including ancillary medical care not elsewhere available), financial planning, and personal counseling. These centers could make a tangible contribution to the education and social welfare of disadvantaged persons, not merely a contribution to their financial welfare. These programs too must be viewed as offers of benefits (and in this respect no different from monetary offers) and therefore as potentially creating problems of undue influence (also like monetary offers). At the same time, it would be unfeeling to disregard the contribution that such programs could make to the lives of the economically disadvantaged.

A maneuver that should be prohibited, as a matter of policy, is a sliding scale that would raise or lower payments based on an attempted assessment of risk of injury, pain, or discomfort. This maneuver would simply magnify concerns about exploitation. To reward taking risks by offering increased payment would too easily induce the most disadvantaged to take the highest risks; and to take the view that the higher the risk, the *less* one should pay in order to avoid the problem of undue inducement would be to discriminate by penalizing persons for their economic disadvantage. These are morally unacceptable outcomes that should be avoidable by not conducting research with increased risk in any location in which this problem might arise.

COMPROMISED CONSENT

Compromised consent presents another concern about the vulnerability of research subjects. The typical concerns about consent in pharmaceutical research center either on whether the *consent* is adequately informed or on whether subjects have the *ability* to give an informed consent to research participation. I am not concerned with the *ability* to consent, as I am discussing only subjects who do have this ability. I am concerned only with the process used in the research context to obtain consent and the ways in which consent can be compromised.[24]

The most frequently mentioned problems of consent in pharmaceutical research are undisclosed data, unknown risks, and inadequate discussion with trial participants about risks and inconveniences.[25] Some practices of obtaining consent are clearly shams, where consent is invalid even if a written consent document exists. Consider a paradigm case of this problem: On November 2, 2005, Bloomberg News reported that SFBC International, Inc., a global clinical research and drug development services company, had recruited a number of economically disadvantaged participants for drug-testing contracts by making inadequate disclosures regarding the risk of the research. SFBC was reported to have manipulated participants through increases of compensation during the course of the research and to have used illegal, non–English-speaking immigrants fearful of exportation, with some used in multiple trials. The amount of compensation was reported in some cases to be very high (an undue influence) and in other cases very low (an undue profit).[26] If these reports are even half correct, SFBC engaged in a blatant series of violations of nondisclosure, in the manipulation of consent, and possibly even in coercion. This case is without moral subtleties, and all morally sensitive persons would recognize it as an egregious wrong.

However, there are many subtle and difficult problems of consent, including ways in which information is presented initially and then throughout the trial.[27] Without appropriate monitoring of consent, even an *initially* informed and valid consent can become uninformed and invalid. The appropriate framework for obtaining and updating consent in pharmaceutical research is not a single event of oral or written consent, but a supervised, multistaged arrangement of disclosure, dialogue, and permission giving that takes place after adequate oversight of a protocol.

One stage in the informational process should occur during the interview that is scheduled when a potential subject responds to an advertisement announcing an upcoming study. Potential subjects should learn basic facts such as whether the study is an inpatient or outpatient study, the study's duration, forms of testing, disqualifying medical conditions, requirements such as age and smoking status, and how eating and drinking are controlled during the study. The goals should be to inform people of what they will experience and to prevent people from coming to the clinic or research center who will be excluded from the studies.

A second stage in the informed consent process should be composed of discussions that occur during in-house screening and laboratory testing. If laboratory values and other inclusion criteria are met, potential subjects should be scheduled for an interview and physical examination. If potential subjects come back, the nature and content of the consent form should be explained. At this stage potential subjects should be told about the drug being tested, the route of administration, diseases for which the drug is being developed, the amount of blood sampling, unusual risks, and the like. They should be asked whether they have understood why they are being screened, and there should be an established way of testing for adequate understanding.

A third stage should be a session devoted to the formalities of informed consent: disclosure, discussion to increase understanding, and the like. These sessions should be limited to individuals or small groups, with informed professionals in the room. The goal should be a comprehensible explanation of the study and the authorization form. Potential volunteers should come to know enough to elect to participate in the study or decide not to participate.

Answering questions, eliciting the concerns and interests of the subject, and establishing a climate that encourages questions are necessary conditions of the consent process, which is essential to justified human-subjects research. To fail to conform research to the conditions in the three stages mentioned in this section is to obtain what I am calling a compromised consent. Research that does not meet these conditions involves an inexcusable disregard of the rights of subjects, no matter who conducts it or where it occurs.

CONSIDERATIONS OF BACKGROUND JUSTICE

Several issues I have been considering should also be set against a richer background of concerns about social justice. Many considerations of justice suggest that society should take a greater interest in the economically disadvantaged than it often does—not because they have become or might become research subjects, but because of their status as exploitable members of society who are poorly served by social services.

One problem of pharmaceutical research is the potential injustice that occurs when a benefit is generated for the well-off through a contribution to research made largely by disadvantaged members of society. Research, as currently conducted, places a minority of persons at risk in order that others, or sometimes only the well-off, benefit. However, how the burdens of research involvement (if they are *burdens*, which is an underanalyzed idea) should be distributed in a population has never been established in any authoritative code, document, policy, or moral theory. The notion of "equity," commonly used in current discussions, is often poorly analyzed and poorly implemented. Today, it remains unclear, and controversial, when a research endeavor becomes a morally objectionable or marginal form of co-opting the economically disadvantaged for the benefit of the privileged.

Suppose, however, that a pharmaceutical company were to *target* the economically disadvantaged in its recruitment of subjects and were to use *exclusively* these subjects in its research. This activity raises some seldom discussed questions about disproportionate uses of the economically disadvantaged. It may be appropriate to have selection criteria that demand that the research enterprise not specifically target the economically disadvantaged and that the percentages of economically disadvantaged subjects in research protocols be restricted, while ensuring that research subjects are drawn from suitably diverse populations. This standard does not imply that it is always unfair to recruit (even heavily) from an economically disadvantaged population, only that recruitment introduces problems of

distributive justice not covered by the issues considered previously. If this judgment is right, then pharmaceutical companies should have policies requiring that
they carefully monitor the numbers and percentages of economically disadvantaged persons.

One issue is whether there is an upper level or quota of acceptable participation
by members of the economically disadvantaged in a protocol or research center.
Setting a quota would disqualify some potential subjects, which has the potential
of being unfair to them. If no categorical problem exists over the involvement of
economically disadvantaged adults as subjects, as I suggested earlier, then why
should we worry about numbers, quotas, or percentages? The relevant conditions
would seem to be that each individual in a trial, whether economically disadvantaged or not, is physically qualified, does not have a disqualifying condition, gives
an informed consent, and the like. If a given individual qualifies, there seems no
reason to set a numerical limit on the number of studies in which he or she can
participate.

This approach should be taken seriously, but it does not adequately address the
background considerations of justice that should be attended to. Requiring
diversity in a subject pool potentially protects against several conditions that
might otherwise too easily be tolerated in the research process—for example,
that drug studies would be conducted in dreary and depersonalizing environments, that the same subjects would be used repeatedly in studies, and that a
dependency on money would set in, making subjects dependent on drug studies
for their livelihood. Related problems concern whether it is problematic for
individuals to be involved by volunteering for multiple studies, a problem that
would be exacerbated as financial inducements are increased.[28]

CONCLUSION

Everyone agrees with the abstract rule that we should not exploit the economically
disadvantaged in a pharmaceutical research project. I have argued, however, that
it is not easy to determine what counts as exploitation, the conditions under
which it occurs, who is vulnerable to exploitation, how to avoid it, and whether
certain trade-offs or compromises are acceptable. The recommendations I have
made about the conduct of studies involving the economically disadvantaged
have centered on vulnerabilities and exploitation. I have argued that while
pharmaceutical research need not be exploitative or unjustified when conducted
with the economically disadvantaged, these problems are more nuanced and
difficult than they have generally been treated in literature on the subject. We
also know relatively little about the conditions under which inducements are
accepted and about whether those who accept those inducements view them as

unwelcome exploitations or as welcome opportunities.[29] We need to get clearer—conceptually, morally, and empirically—about the populations involved in research and about the difference between the unethical and the mutually beneficial when inducements are offered to those in these populations. We confront a considerable task.

Notes

1. Marcia Angell, *The Truth About the Drug Companies: How They Deceive Us and What to Do About It* (New York: Random House, 2005); House of Commons Health Committee, *The Influence of the Pharmaceutical Industry*, Fourth Report of Session 2004-05 (London: Stationery Office, 22 March 2005), esp. 43ff; T. S. Faunce and G. F. Tomossy, "The UK House of Commons Report on the Influence of the Pharmaceutical Industry: Lessons for Equitable Access to Medicines in Australia," *Monash Bioethics Review* 23, No. 4: 38–42; Department of Health and Human Services, Office of the Inspector General, *Prescription Drug Promotion Involving Payments and Gifts: Physicians' Perspectives* OEI-01-90-00481 (Washington, DC: DHHS, 1991) and also DHHS, "Pharmaceutical Company Gifts and Payments to Providers," in *Work Plan for Fiscal Plan 2002* (Washington, DC: DHHS, 2001); Jerome P. Kassirer, *On the Take: How Medicine's Complicity with Big Business Can Endanger Your Health* (Oxford/New York: Oxford University Press, 2005); Dana Katz, Arthur L. Caplan, and Jon F. Merz, "All Gifts Large and Small," *American Journal of Bioethics* 3 (2003): 39–46; Merrill Goozner, *The $800 Million Pill: The Truth Behind the Cost of New Drugs* (Berkeley: University of California Press, 2004); Jerry Avorn, *Powerful Medicines: The Benefits, Risks, and Costs of Prescription Drugs* (New York: Vintage Books, 2005); Jerry Avorn, M. Chen, and R. Hartley, "Scientific versus Commercial Sources of Influence on the Prescribing Behavior of Physicians," *American Journal of Medicine* 73 (1982): 4–8; Fran Hawthorne, *Inside the FDA: The Business and Politics Behind the Drugs We Take and the Food We Eat* (Hoboken, NJ: John Wiley & Sons, 2005); Jacky Law, *Big Pharma: How Modern Medicine is Damaging Your Health and What You Can Do About It* (New York: Carroll & Graf, 2006); Jennifer Washburn, *University Inc.: The Corporate Corruption of Higher Education* (New York: Basic Books, 2005); A. Wazana, "Physicians and the Pharmaceutical Industry: Is a Gift Ever Just a Gift?" *Journal of the American Medical Association* 283 (2000): 373–380; Arnold S. Relman, "Separating Continuing Medical Education from Pharmaceutical Marketing," *Journal of the American Medical Association* 285 (2001): 2009–2012.

2. Ezekiel Emanuel, "Ending Concerns about Undue Inducement," *Journal of Law, Medicine, & Ethics* 32 (2004): 100–105.

3. Carl Tishler and Suzanne Bartholomae, "The Recruitment of Normal Healthy Volunteers," *Journal of Clinical Pharmacology* 42 (2002): 365–375.

4. Tom L. Beauchamp, Bruce Jennings, Eleanor Kinney, and Robert Levine, "Pharmaceutical Research Involving the Homeless," *Journal of Medicine and Philosophy* (2002), 547–564; M. H. Kottow, "The Vulnerable and the Susceptible," *Bioethics* 17 (2003): 460–471; Toby L. Schonfeld, Joseph S. Brown, Meaghann Weniger, and Bruce Gordon,

"Research Involving the Homeless," *IRB* 25 (Sept./Oct. 2003): 17–20; C. E. van Gelderen, T. J. Savelkoul, W. van Dokkum, J. Meulenbelt, "Motives and Perceptions of Healthy Volunteers Who Participate in Experiments," *European Journal of Clinical Pharmacology* 45 (1993): 15–21.

5. Glenn McGee, "Subject to Payment?" *Journal of the American Medical Association* 278 (July 16, 1997): 199–200; Leonardo D. de Castro, "Exploitation in the Use of Human Subjects for Medical Experimentation: A Re-Examination of Basic Issues," *Bioethics* 9 (1995): 259–268; Laurie Cohen, "To Screen New Drugs For Safety, Lilly Pays Homeless Alcoholics," *Wall Street Journal*, Nov. 14, 1996, A1, A10.

6. Scott Halpern, Jason Karlawish, David Casarett, Jesse Berlin, and David A. Asch, "Empirical Assessment of Whether Moderate Payments Are Undue or Unjust Inducements for Participation in Clinical Trials," *Archives of Internal Medicine* 164 (2004): 801–803.

7. These problems, including the vast range of groups and populations declared to be vulnerable in the bioethics and public policy literature, are assembled and discussed in Carol Levine, Ruth Faden, Christine Grady, Dale Hammerschmidt, Lisa Eckenwiler, Jeremy Sugarman (for the Consortium to Examine Clinical Research Ethics), "The Limitations of 'Vulnerability' as a Protection for Human Research Participants," *American Journal of Bioethics* 4 (2004): 44–49; Debra A. DeBruin, "Reflections on Vulnerability," *Bioethics Examiner* 5 (2001): 1, 4, 7. For examples of treatments of these issues that assume broadly stated—and numerous classes—of vulnerable groups, see Council for International Organization of Medical Sciences, *International Ethical Guidelines for Biomedical Research Involving Human Subjects*, http://www.cioms.ch/frame_guidelines; Ruth Macklin, "Bioethics, Vulnerability, and Protection," *Bioethics* 17 (2003): 472–486; and Laura B. Sutton, et al., "Recruiting Vulnerable Populations for Research: Revisiting the Ethical Issues," *Journal of Professional Nursing* 19 (2003): 106–112.

8. See Ruth Macklin, "'Due'and 'Undue' Inducements: On Paying Money to Research Subjects," *IRB* 3 (1981): 1–6; Tishler and Bartholomae, "The Recruitment of Normal Healthy Volunteers."

9. See Debra A. DeBruin, "Looking Beyond the Limitations of 'Vulnerability': Reforming Safeguards in Research," *The American Journal of Bioethics* 4 (2004): 76–78; National Bioethics Advisory Commission, *Ethical and Policy Issues in Research Involving Human Participants*, vol. 1 (Bethesda, MD: Government Printing Office, 2001); Kenneth Kipnis, "Vulnerability in Research Subjects: A Bioethical Taxonomy," National Bioethics Advisory Commission, *Ethical and Policy Issues in Research Involving Human Participants*, vol. 2 (Bethesda, MD: Government Printing Office, 2002), G1–13

10. Gail E. Henderson, Arlene M. Davis, and Nancy M. P. King, "Vulnerability to Influence: A Two-Way Street," *American Journal of Bioethics* 4 (2004): 50–53

11. Joel Feinberg, *Harm to Others*, vol. 1 of *The Moral Limits of the Criminal Law* (New York: Oxford University Press, 1984), 32–36.

12. Cf. Anita Silvers, "Historical Vulnerability and Special Scrutiny: Precautions against Discrimination in Medical Research," *American Journal of Bioethics* 4 (2004): 56–57.

13. Ruth R. Faden and Tom L. Beauchamp, *A History and Theory of Informed Consent* (New York: Oxford University Press, 1986), Chapter 10; R. B. Cialdini, *Influence:*

The Psychology of Persuasion (New York: Quill William Morrow, 1993); Patricia Greenspan, "The Problem with Manipulation," *American Philosophical Quarterly* 40 (2003): 155–164.

14. See Robert Nozick, "Coercion," in *Philosophy, Science and Method: Essays in Honor of Ernest Nagel*, ed. Sidney Morgenbesser, Patrick Suppes, and Morton White (New York: St. Martin's Press, 1969), 440–472; and Bernard Gert, "Coercion and Freedom," in *Coercion: Nomos XIV*, ed. J. Roland Pennock and John W. Chapman (Chicago: Aldine, Atherton Inc. 1972), 36–37.

15. See Sarah E. Hewlett, "Is Consent to Participate in Research Voluntary?" *Arthritis Care and Research* 9 (1996): 400–404; Hewlett, "Consent to Clinical Research—Adequately Voluntary or Substantially Influenced?" *Journal of Medical Ethics* 22 (1996): 232–236; Robert M. Nelson and Jon F. Merz, "Voluntariness of Consent for Research: An Empirical and Conceptual Review," *Medical Care* 40 (2002) Suppl., V69–80; and Nancy E. Kass, et al., "Trust: The Fragile Foundation of Contemporary Biomedical Research," *Hastings Center Report* 25 (September–October 1996): 25–29.

16. Common Rule for the Protection of Human Subjects, U.S. Code of Federal Regulations, 45 CFR 46.116 (as revised Oct. 1, 2003); and Emanuel, "Ending Concerns about Undue Inducement," 101.

17. The justification of monetary inducement in terms of mutual benefit is defended by Martin Wilkinson and Andrew Moore, "Inducement in Research," *Bioethics* 11 (1997): 373–389; and Wilkinson and Moore, "Inducements Revisited," *Bioethics* 13 (1999): 114–130. See also Christine Grady, "Money for Research Participation: Does It Jeopardize Informed Consent?" *American Journal of Bioethics* 1 (2001): 40–44.

18. In some cases, the offers may blind prospective subjects to risks and inconveniences, but such blindness is a concern about adequately informed consent.

19. Procedures performed in the conduct of research protocols do present real risks of injury, and a threshold level of appropriate or acceptable risk must be established. Some have suggested a threshold standard of "minimal risk," which is defined in federal regulations: "Minimal risk means that the probability and magnitude of harm or discomfort anticipated in the research are not greater in and of themselves, than those ordinarily encountered in daily life or during the performance of routine physical or psychological examinations or tests." 45 CFR 46.102i (as revised Oct. 1, 2005). For many adult populations, a more realistic threshold standard is a "minor increase above minimal risk." Published evidence and commentary indicate that most phase I and phase IV studies of drugs present such minor increases over minimal risk. For studies of risks and safety in pharmaceutical research, see: M. Sibille et al., "Adverse Events in Phase one Studies: A Study in 430 Healthy Volunteers," *European Journal of Clinical Pharmacology* 42 (1992): 389–393; P. L. Morselli, "Are Phase I Studies without Drug Level Determination Acceptable?" *Fundamental and Clinical Pharmacology* 4 Suppl. 2 (1990): 125s–133s; M. Orme, et al., "Healthy Volunteer Studies in Great Britain: The Results of a Survey into 12 Months Activity in this Field," *British Journal of Clinical Pharmacology* 27 (February 1989): 125–133; H. Boström, "On the Compensation for Injured Research Subjects in Sweden," in President's Commission for the Study of Ethical Problems in Medicine and Biomedical and Behavioral Research, *Compensating for Research Injuries: The Ethical and*

Legal Implications of Programs to Redress Injured Subjects, Appendix, 309–322 (Washington, DC: U.S. Government Printing Office, Stock No. 040-000-00455-6, 1982; the Appendix to this Report is Stock No. 040-000-00456-4); P. V. Cardon, F. W. Dommel, and R. R. Trumble, "Injuries to Research Subjects: A Survey of Investigators," *New England Journal of Medicine* 295 (1976): 650–654; C. J. D. Zarafonetis, P. A. Riley, Jr., P. W. Willis, III, L. H. Power, J. Werbelow, L. Farhat, W. Beckwith, and B. H. Marks, "Clinically Significant Adverse Effects in a Phase I Testing Program," *Clinical Pharmacology and Therapeutics* 24 (1978): 127–132; J. D. Arnold, "Incidence of Injury During Clinical Pharmacology Research and Indemnification of Injured Research Subjects at the Quincy Research Center," in President's Commission for the Study of Ethical Problems in Medicine and Biomedical and Behavioral Research, *Compensating for Research Injuries: The Ethical and Legal Implications of Programs to Redress Injured Subjects*, Appendix, 275–302 (Washington, DC: U.S. Government Printing Office, Stock No. 040-000-00455-6, 1982; the Appendix to this Report is Stock No. 040-000-00456-4).

20. See Neal Dickert and Christine Grady, "What's the Price of a Research Subject?: Approaches to Payment for Research Participation," *New England Journal of Medicine* 341 (1999): 198–203; David Resnick, "Research Participation and Financial Inducements," *American Journal of Bioethics* 1 (2001): 54–56; Wilkinson and Moore, "Inducement in Research," 373–389; Macklin, "'Due' and 'Undue' Inducements: On Paying Money to Research Subjects," 1–6; Lisa H. Newton, "Inducement, Due and Otherwise," *IRB: A Review of Human Subjects Research* 4 (March 1982): 4–6; Ruth Macklin, "Response: Beyond Paternalism," *IRB: A Review of Human Subjects Research* 4 (March 1982): 6–7.

21. Compare the rather different conditions proposed by de Castro, "Exploitation in the Use of Human Subject for Medical Experimentation: A Re-Examination of Basic Issues," 264, and by Beauchamp, Jennings, Kinney, and Levine, "Pharmaceutical Research Involving the Homeless." See also Schonfeld, Brown, Weniger, Gordon, "Research Involving the Homeless: Arguments against Payment-in-Kind," 17–20.

22. One issue that will constantly have to be monitored is how to keep the offer from being irresistible. This elicits the question "irresistible by what standard?" An offer that is irresistible to one person may be resistible to another, or what one greets as a welcome offer, the other may greet as unwelcome; and this is so even if the offers are identical. How an offer is perceived and whether it will be accepted depend on the subjective responses of the persons who receive the offer. On this analysis, *undue influence* in the acceptance of increased risk occurs only if the person receiving the offer finds it irresistible.

23. See Nik Theodore, Edwin Melendez, and Ana Luz Gonzalez, "On the Corner: Day Labor in the United States," http://www.sscnet.ucla.edu/issr/csup/uploaded_files/Natl_DayLabor-On_the_Corner1.pdf.

24. I am also not concerned with situations in which there is a signed and adequately informed consent and yet the consent is invalid. For example, the protocol may be scientifically inadequate, there may have been an unjust selection of subjects, risks and inconveniences may not warrant the research, etc. I am not concerned with such invalidating conditions. I am also not here concerned with problems of consent deriving from the problems of undue inducement (controlling influences and constraining situations)

examined previously. Constraining situations may compromise the voluntariness of consent, but we need not revisit that problem here.

25. House of Commons Health Committee, *The Influence of the Pharmaceutical Industry*, 49ff.

26. Kerry Dooley Young and David Evans, with reporting by Michael Smith in Rio De Janeiro, "SFBC's Top Two Officials Quit Amid U.S. Senate Probe," *Bloomberg News*, Jan. 3, 2006. The original report of problems was by the same reporters, *Bloomberg News*, Nov. 2, 2005, "Poor Latin Immigrants Say Miami Test Center 'Is Like a Jail'." Bloomberg has issued numerous later reports in the case.

27. See Christopher K. Daugherty, Donald M. Banik, Linda Janish, and Mark J. Ratain, "Quantitative Analysis of Ethical Issues in Phase I Trials," *IRB* 22 (May–June 2000): 6–14, esp. 12–13.

28. Paul McNeill, "Paying People to Participate in Research: Why Not?" *Bioethics* 11 (1997): 390–396; Beauchamp, Jennings, Levine, and McKinney, "Pharmaceutical Research Involving the Homeless"; Michael A. Grodin and Leonard H. Glantz, eds. *Children as Research Subjects: Science, Ethics, and Law* (New York: Oxford University Press; 1994), 193–214; National Commission for the Protection of Human Subjects of Biomedical and Behavioral Research, *The Belmont Report: Ethical Guidelines for the Protection of Human Subjects* (Washington, DC: DHEW Publication (OS) 78-0012, 1978).

29. See David Casarett, Jason Karlawish, and David A. Asch, "Paying Hypertension Research Subjects: Fair Compensation or Undue Inducement," *Journal of General Internal Medicine* 17 (2002): 651–653; and Scott Halpern, Jason Karlawish, David Casarett, Jesse Berlin, and David A. Asch, "Empirical Assessment of Whether Moderate Payments Are Undue or Unjust Inducements for Participation in Clinical Trials," 801–803.

Part III

THEORY AND METHOD

9

PRINCIPLES AND OTHER EMERGING
PARADIGMS IN BIOETHICS

If a history of recent biomedical ethics were to be written, it would encompass several disciplines, including the health professions, law, biology, the social and behavioral sciences, theology, and philosophy. Principles that could be understood with relative ease by the members of these disciplines figured prominently in the development of biomedical ethics during the 1970s and early 1980s. Principles were used primarily to present frameworks of evaluative assumptions or general premises underlying positions and conclusions.[1] However, beginning in the mid-1980s, the paradigm of a system of principles was aggressively challenged. Several alternatives have since been proposed, including revivals of casuistry and virtue theory. These developments should be welcomed in bioethics, because they have improved the range, precision, and quality of thought in the field. However, the various proposed alternative approaches do not replace principles. The leading alternatives are thoroughly compatible with a paradigm of principles. Indeed, these seemingly different frameworks of norms are mutually supportive.

I will begin my argument to this conclusion by outlining the nature of a principle-based approach to ethics, concentrating on the book James Childress and I wrote in the mid-1970s entitled *Principles of Biomedical Ethics* (4th edition, 1994). After sketching our ethical framework, I will point to some limitations of the model and indicate how those limitations should be handled in the first section, Principles as a Starting Point. I will consider the nature and limits of three proposed alternatives to a principle-based approach in the second section, Alternative Paradigms.

PRINCIPLES AS A STARTING POINT

Principle-based ethical theories emphasize impartial moral obligations, but "principles" should not be *defined* in terms of obligations. Moral principles are simply relatively general norms of conduct that describe obligations, permissible actions, and ideals of action. A principle is a regulative guideline stating conditions of the permissibility, obligatoriness, rightness, or aspirational quality of an action falling within the scope of the principle. If principles are adequately expressed, more particular or specific moral rules and judgments are supported by, though not deduced from, the principles. For example, principles of justice provide support for particular rules and judgments regarding equal treatment, fair taxation, and just compensation.

A Principle-Based Paradigm

The paradigm that Childress and I defend is that various principles worthy of acceptance in bioethics can be grouped under four general categories: (*1*) respect for autonomy (a principle of respect for the decision-making capacities of autonomous persons), (*2*) nonmaleficence (a principle of avoiding the causation of harm to others), (*3*) beneficence (a group of principles for providing benefits and balancing benefits against risks and costs), and (*4*) justice (a group of principles for distributing benefits, risks, and costs fairly).

We do not sharply distinguish between rules and principles in our analyses. Both are general action guides. In addition to *substantive rules* of truth telling, confidentiality, privacy, fidelity, and the like, there are *authority rules* regarding who may and should perform actions, including rules of surrogate authority, rules of professional authority, and rules of distributional authority that determine who should make decisions about the allocation of scarce medical resources. *Procedural rules* are also important in bioethics, because they establish procedures to be followed, such as procedures for determining eligibility for scarce medical resources.

Principles, being more abstract than rules, leave considerable room for judgment about individual cases and policies. However, principles should be conceived neither as so weak that they are mere rules of thumb nor as so strong that they assert absolute requirements. Insofar as they assert obligations (but not insofar as they are used to frame ideals), principles are firm obligations that can be set aside only if they come into conflict with and do not override another obligation. In cases of a conflict of obligations, one obligation then has the potential to release the person from the other obligation. Often some balance between two or more norms must be found that requires some part of each obligation to be discharged, but in many cases one simply overrides the other.

This overriding of one obligation by another may seem precariously flexible, as if moral guidelines in the end lack backbone and can be magically waived away as not *real* obligations. But in ethics, as in all disciplines that confront principled conflicts, such as law, there is no escape from the exercise of judgment in resolving the conflicts. One function of principles is to keep judgments *principled* without removing agent *discretion*. As long as an agent does not stray beyond the demands of principles, it cannot be said that judgments are arbitrary or unprincipled, even if one principle overrides another.

I do not say that every judgment intended to resolve a principled conflict must itself be resolved by the principles that are in conflict, a manifestly false thesis. Skillful use of principles requires judgment, which in turn depends on character, moral insight, and a sense of personal responsibility and integrity; and these properties of persons are neither principles nor merely a way of conforming to principle. Sensitive, prudent, or judicious decisions are often made without being "principled" in the pertinent sense. Nonetheless, the resolution of principled conflicts will frequently appeal to (1) one or more external principles, (2) a procedure, (3) a form of authority, (4) a balancing of principles, or (5) a specification of the principles in conflict. If a procedure or an authority is the best resource for conflict resolution, this in itself will be determined by principles (or rules) that designate the procedure or authority. Principles will therefore be integrally involved in each of these five forms of appeal.

In situations of moral conflict we often need latitude to assess the various moral demands, leaving room for negotiation and compromise, but such negotiation and compromise can follow the path of (1) through (5), and so need not be unprincipled. For example, in some circumstances two or more morally acceptable alternatives are unavoidably in conflict, because both alternatives present good reasons for action. Both present good but not decisive or solely sufficient reasons. Here the best course is often to further specify the precise commitments of principles, as will be explained later.

Sources of Principles

The four categories of principles are all drawn from the common morality. By "the common morality" I mean the morality that all reasonable persons share and acknowledge—common-sense ethics, as it is sometimes called. A substantial social consensus exists about general principles and rules in the common morality, far more consensus than exists about general norms in philosophical ethical theories. From this perspective, a paradigm of philosophical theory or method should be resisted if it cannot be made coherent with preexistent common-morality understandings of what John Rawls calls our *considered judgments*—that is, those moral convictions in which we have the highest confidence and believe to have the lowest level of bias, such as principles that prohibit racial discrimination, religious intolerance, and political favoritism.

Traditional health care contexts often supply more specific moral content than principles, typically through traditions of role responsibilities. These traditions supply an understanding of obligations and virtues as they have been adapted over the centuries for professional practice. The health professional's obligations, rights, and virtues have been framed primarily as professional commitments to shield patients from harm and provide medical care—fundamental obligations of nonmaleficence and beneficence. Professional dedication to these norms has been part of the self-understanding of physicians. For example, physicians have traditionally taken the view that disclosing certain forms of information drawn from patient records can cause harm to patients under their care and that medical ethics obligates them to maintain confidentiality.

The principle of nonmaleficence provides perhaps the best example. This principle has long been associated in medicine with the injunction *primum non nocere*: "Above all [or first], do no harm," a maxim often mistakenly attributed to the Hippocratic tradition.[2] It has an equally prestigious position in the history of moral philosophy. John Stuart Mill, for example, praised the moral rules of nonmaleficence as "that which alone preserves peace among human beings."[3] British physician Thomas Percival furnished the first developed account of health care ethics, in which he maintained that principles of nonmaleficence and beneficence fix the physician's primary obligations and triumph even over the patient's autonomy rights in a circumstance of potential harm to patients:

> To a patient . . . who makes inquiries which, if faithfully answered, might prove fatal to him, it would be a gross and unfeeling wrong to reveal the truth. His right to it is suspended, and even annihilated; because, its beneficial nature being reversed, it would be deeply injurious to himself, to his family, and to the public. And he has the strongest claim, from the trust reposed in his physician, as well as from the common principles of humanity, to be guarded against whatever would be detrimental to him.[4]

Like the Hippocratics, Percival accepted as the first principle of medical ethics that the patient's best medical interest determines the physician's obligations, and he conceived the central virtues of the physician through models of benevolence and sympathetic tenderness, as they serve to promote the patient's welfare.

Recently the idea has flourished in biomedical ethics that the physician's moral responsibility should be understood less in terms of traditional ideals of medical benefit and more in terms of the patients' rights of self-determination, including rights to truthful disclosure, confidentiality, privacy, disclosure, and consent, as well as welfare rights rooted in claims of justice. These proposals have moved medical ethics from its traditional preoccupation with a patient-welfare model toward an autonomy model of the care of patient, while also confronting the field with a wider set of social concerns, such as the right to health care. For this reason, principles of autonomy and justice have increased in importance in bioethics.

The justification for choosing the particular four groups of principles that Childress and I defend is therefore partially rooted historically in medical traditions of health care ethics and partially rooted in contemporary contexts in which principles of autonomy and justice point to an important aspect of morality that was traditionally neglected in health care ethics. However, the common morality is itself the ultimate source of these basic principles.

The Need for Additional Specification of Principles

To say that principles find support in traditions of health care is not to say that their appearance in an ethical theory or in a developed paradigm of biomedical ethics is identical to their appearance in the traditions from which they spring. Even the common morality falls far short of a well-articulated and specified paradigm. Conceptual clarification and attempts to increase coherence give shape and substance to principles, much as judges in their opinions express and develop the commitments of legal precedents and principles of law to suit the cases before them.

Both ethical theories and the common morality contain regions of indeterminacy that need reduction through further development of norms in the system, augmenting them with a more specific moral content. In light of the indeterminacy found in principles and all general norms, I follow Henry Richardson in arguing that the specification of norms involves filling in details in order to overcome moral conflicts and the incompleteness of principles and rules.[5] Specification is the progressive and substantive delineation of principles and rules that gives them a more specific and practical content. Because principles are at a lofty level of abstraction, little practical content can be drawn directly from them. More precision through specification is therefore essential for regulative and decision-making contexts.

Principles are not *applied* but rather are *explicated and made suitable* for specific tasks, often by developing policies. Judgment and decision making are essential for this interpretive process. For this reason philosophers such as John Mackie rightly argue that ethics is "invented." Mackie does not mean that individuals create either the common morality or personal moral policies, but that what he calls "intersubjective standards" are creatively built up over time through communal agreements and decision making. What is morally demanded, enforced, and condemned is less a matter of what is already present in basic principles and more a matter of what we decide by reference to and in development of those principles.

As a simple example of specification and invention in this sense, consider conflicts of obligation that emerge from the dual roles of research scientist and clinical practitioner. As an investigator, the physician has an obligation to generate scientific knowledge that will benefit future patients. As a clinical practitioner, the physician has obligations of care that require acting in the best interests of present patients. The notion of a physician-as-scientist suggests two roles that pull in different directions, each role having its own specifiable set of obligations.[6] How, then, do we make these various obligations more precise, specific, and coherent when they come into conflict?

One possibility is to segregate the roles so that they cannot conflict—for example, specifying that physicians with clinical responsibilities cannot use their own patients when discharging research responsibilities. This formulation is an "invention" specifying that a physician's obligations of beneficence to patients must not be confounded or compromised by research obligations. This specification will solve some problems about the dual role, but will leave others unresolved and in need of additional inventiveness and specification. For example, it might be in everyone's best interest in some circumstances for a set of physicians to assume both roles, although we know that conflicts of interest are present for these physicians. We might then specify that "Physicians can simultaneously accept clinical and research obligations for the same patients only if a full disclosure is made to the patients of the dual role and of any conflicts of interest present in the dual role." This specification attempts to make the obligations jointly acceptable by adding obligations of disclosure that did not previously exist.

Such specifications will at times involve a balancing of principles, at times an appending of additional obligations, and at other times a development of one or more principles by making them more precise for purposes of policy. In these ways we become more specific and practical and maintain fidelity to our original principle(s). This strategy has the advantage of allowing us to unpack our evaluative commitments and to expand them as well, presumably achieving a more workable and a more coherent body of contextually relevant norms. Of course, many already specified norms will need further specification as new or unanticipated circumstances arise. All moral norms are potentially subject to this process of inventive specification, and progressive specification will increasingly reduce types of conflict and insufficiency of content.[7]

There are tangled problems about the best method to use in order to achieve specification and about how we can justify a proposed specification, but it seems clear that specification is needed, not merely a bare appeal to principles and rules. The model of analysis for reaching specification and justification in health care ethics that Childress and I have used is that of a dialectical balancing of principles against other moral considerations, in an attempt to achieve general coherence and a mutual support among the accepted norms. A now widely accepted method of this general description that can be used to help in the process of the specification of principles is "reflective equilibrium." This method was formulated by John Rawls for use in the construction of a general ethical theory. It views the acceptance of principles as properly beginning with considered judgments, and then requires a matching, pruning, and developing of considered judgments and principles in an attempt to make them coherent. We start with paradigms of what is morally proper or morally improper, and we then search for specifications of principles that are consistent with these paradigms and consistent with each other.[8]

A specified principle, then, is acceptable in a system of norms if it heightens the mutual support of other norms in the system that have themselves survived in reflective equilibrium. This understanding of the principles paradigm assumes that no canonical content exists for bioethics beyond the common morality. There is no scripture, no authoritative interpretation of anything analogous to scripture, and no authoritative interpretation of that large mass of judgments, rules, standards of virtue, and the like that we often collectively sum up by use of words such as "bioethics." A principle-based account likewise disavows models of a single ultimate principle of ethics and of absolute rules. The principles approach supports a method of inventive content expansion into more specific norms, not a system layered by priorities among rules or among categories of ethics. From this perspective, principles grounded in the common morality are the background framework, but also the point at which the real work of policy development and moral judgment begin.

ALTERNATIVE PARADIGMS

Several alternative paradigms have arisen in recent years, some of whose proponents have been sharply critical of principles. I will consider three such alternatives. Although my aim is chiefly to place criticisms of principles in a proper perspective, I have a secondary aim. Critics have often appropriately pointed to *limits* in the principles paradigm, specifically limits of scope, practicability, and justificatory power. Much can be learned from this commentary about the points at which even carefully specified principles are inadequate to provide a comprehensive account of the moral life. Alternative paradigms usually exhibit their primary strength at these points. In my assessments to follow, I will maintain that these alternatives are congenial to, and not rivals of, a principle-based account.

Casuistry as an Alternative Paradigm

The term *casuistry*, derived from the Latin *casus* for "case," is today used primarily to refer to a method of using cases to analyze and propose solutions for moral problems. Clinical bioethics is essentially casuistical, but "casuistry" usually refers to a specific *method* of analyzing and generalizing from cases. The casuistical method is to start with paradigm cases whose conclusions are settled, and then to compare and contrast the central features in these settled cases with the features of cases to be decided. Maxims drawn from past cases and specific analogies are used to support recommendations for new cases. To use an analogy to case law and the doctrine of precedent, when judicial decisions become authoritative, these decisions have the potential to become authoritative for other judges confronting similar cases in similar circumstances and with similar facts. Precedents also bind by restraining the judgments that may be made in new cases.

In casuistical ethics, moral authority proceeds from the settled paradigm cases and maxims, but there are no rigid rules or principles, because particular circumstances and their features alter the way cases are handled and decided. Just as case law (legal rules) develops incrementally from cases, so the moral law (a set of moral rules) develops incrementally in casuistry.[9] However, moral rules only pick out the salient features of cases and must be used with caution and discernment. In clinical medical ethics, for example, prior precedent cases allow us to focus by analogical reasoning on practical decision making in new cases, but very different conclusions may be reached in the new cases, depending on their novel features. Characteristic features of contemporary casuistry include this premium on case interpretation together with a strong preference for analogical reasoning over theory.[10]

A Rejection of Principles and Theory

Some contemporary casuists are dissatisfied with principle-based theories, especially in clinical contexts. They view clinical medical ethics as a discipline arising from clinical practice, rather than from an application of general ethical principles to cases.[11] However, it is not clear why some contemporary casuists react as negatively to principles as they often do. In the great Latin traditions of casuistry emanating from Cicero, students were taught how to use both principles *and* analogies from prior cases to propose resolutions in a new case. Both Rabbinical and Roman common-law traditions of casuistry continued this practice.

Although the sources of contemporary hostility to principles and theory are difficult to pinpoint, I can briefly treat some mainstream objections. A first type of objection derives from the close connection some casuists see between principles and theory, particularly when theory is depicted by its proponents as a unified theory with impartial and universal principles. The underlying aspiration of such theories seems, according to these casuists, an emulation of the natural sciences, by locating what is most general and universal in ethics, expressed in precise principles that enjoy the high measure of confidence found in scientific principles or laws. Casuists hold instead that ethics is neither a science nor a theory fashioned along the lines of traditional ethical theories such as utilitarianism and Kantianism. Rather, ethics is based on seasoned practices rooted in experience.[12] Consider an analogy to the way a physician thinks when making a diagnosis and then a recommendation to a patient. Many individual factors, including the patient's medical history, the physician's successes with similar patients, and paradigms of expected outcomes, will play a role in formulating a judgment and recommendation to a patient, which may be very different from the recommendation that will be made to the next patient with the same malady.

A second reason for hostility to principles is that moral philosophers have often regarded cases as merely a set of facts that can be used to help understand moral principles and problems, but lacking in the means to resolve the moral problems presented by new cases. Casuists maintain that when reasoning through cases, we may legitimately find that we need not appeal to principles, rules, rights, or virtues. For example, when principles, rules, or rights conflict, and appeals to higher principles, rules, or rights have been exhausted, we still need to make reasoned moral judgments. Here the casuist holds that moral reasoning invokes not principles, but narratives, paradigm cases, analogies, models, classification schemes, and even immediate intuition and discerning insight.[13]

Third, when principles are interpreted inflexibly, irrespective of the nuances of cases, some casuists find the principles "tyrannical," on grounds that they block compromise and the resolution of moral problems by generating a gridlock of conflicting principled stands; moral debate then becomes intemperate. This impasse can often only be avoided, from the casuists' perspective, by focusing on points of shared agreement about cases, not on abstract principles.[14]

Fourth, casuists maintain that principles and rules are typically too indeterminate to yield specific moral judgments (for reasons already discussed). It is therefore impossible that there be a unidirectional movement of thought from principles to cases. Indeed, *specified* principles will assume an adequately determinate form only *after* reflection on particular cases. The determinate content in practical principles will therefore, at least in part, be fixed by the authority of the cases.

Fifth, casuists argue that even carefully specified principles must still be weighed and balanced in accordance with the demands and nuances of particular circumstances. An interpreting, weighing, and balancing of principles is essential whenever the particular features of cases cannot have been fully anticipated by a prior process of specification. For example, a physician's judgment about the decisions a particular patient should be encouraged to make or discouraged from making are often influenced by how responsible the physician thinks the patient is, and every case presents a person at a different level of responsibility. Again, a principle is less an applied instrument than a part of a wider process of deliberation.

It does not follow from these five critical appraisals that casuists need be hostile to principles, but only that principles must be interpreted to be coherent with the casuists' paradigm of moral reasoning. Reasonable casuists find the gradual movement from paradigm cases to other cases to be an endeavor that eventuates in principles, which in turn can be helpful in spotting the morally relevant features in new cases. Cases can be ordered under a principle through a paradigm and then extended by analogy to new cases. As abstract generalizations, they help express the received learning derived from the struggle with cases and capture the connections between cases. However, from the casuists' perspective, principles, so understood, are merely *summaries of our experience in reflecting on cases*, not norms that are independent of cases.

Some Problems with Casuistry

Although much in these casuistical arguments is acceptable, proponents have sometimes overstated the promise and power of their account while understating their reliance on theory and principles. Casuists often write as if cases lead to moral paradigms, analogies, or judgments by their facts alone. But this claim is dubious, as the great classical casuists readily acknowledged. The properties that we observe to be of moral importance in cases are picked out by the values (and perhaps the theories) that we have already accepted as being morally important. Consider the following fact, which we might discover in a case: "Person M cannot survive without person S's bone marrow." What shall we conclude morally? Nothing, a casuist might say, until we know the full range of facts in the case. But no matter how many facts are stacked one on top of the other, we will still need some sort of *value* premise—for example, "Everyone ought to help others survive through bone marrow transplant donations" in order to reach a conclusion such as, "S ought to donate his bone marrow." The value premise, which is a principle or rule, bridges the gap between factual premises and the evaluative conclusion. Prior to adding this premise, it is not possible to reach the conclusion. The casuist will face this same problem in every case.

Appeals to "paradigm cases" may mask this fact. Paradigm cases become paradigms because of prior commitments to central values (and perhaps theories) that are preserved from one case to the next case, and principles typically play a legitimate role in determining the acceptability of what is transferred from case to case. For the casuist to move constructively from case to case, a norm of moral relevance must connect the cases. Rules of relevant features across cases will not themselves be merely a part of the case, but a way of interpreting and linking cases. Even to recognize a case as a paradigm case is to accept whatever principles or rules allow the paradigms to be extended to other cases.

Jonsen treats this problem by distinguishing descriptive elements in a case from moral maxims that inform judgment about the case: "These maxims provide the 'morals' of the story. For most cases of interest, there are several morals, because several maxims seem to conflict. The work of casuistry is to determine *which maxim* should *rule the case* and to what extent."[15] So understood, casuistry *presupposes* principles (maxims or rules) and takes them to be essential elements in moral reasoning. The principles are present prior to the decision, and then selected and weighed in the circumstances. This account agrees with the main claims in the principles paradigm, not a rival paradigm.

Jonsen notes that he does not dismiss principles even though he diminishes their importance: "When maxims such as 'Do no harm,' or 'Informed consent is obligatory,' are invoked, they represent, as it were, cut-down versions of the major principles relevant to the topic, such as beneficence and autonomy, cut down to fit the nature of the topic and the kinds of circumstances that pertain to it."[16] Jonsen goes on to point out that casuistry is "complementary to principles" in a manner that still needs to be worked out in moral philosophy. In my view, this language of "cut-down versions" of principles can be interpreted as meaning "built-up," because there is a directed specification of content, not a pruning. Jonsen points in the same direction that Childress and I do when we use the language of "specification," "support," and the like. Like us, Jonsen sees an intimate connection between principles and what we call progressive specification to rules (his maxims) in order to meet the demands of particular contexts. His main fear, which we share, is that principles will be interpreted inflexibly.

Moral reasoning can again be made analogous to legal reasoning in courts: If a legal principle commits a judge to an unacceptable judgment, the judge needs to modify or supplement the principle in a way that renders the judge's beliefs about the law as coherent as possible. If a well-founded principle demands a change in a particular judgment, the overriding claims of consistency with precedent may require that the judgment be adjusted, rather than the principle.[17] Sometimes both judgments and principles need revision. Either way, principles play a central role.

Casuists also have a problem with moral conflict. Cases are typically amenable to competing judgments, and it is inadequate to be told that cases extend beyond themselves and evolve into appropriate paradigms. Cases could evolve in disastrous ways because they were improperly treated from the outset by a perilous analogy. Casuists have no methodological resource (by appeal to case alone) to prevent a biased development of cases and a neglect of relevant features of cases. This problem caused the decline of casuistry after 1650, when it became increasingly evident that opposite conclusions could be easily "justified" by competing

casuistical forms of argument. So-called "moral laxity" destroyed classical casuistry. The same laxity will doom contemporary casuistry unless it is fortified by
stable principles.

Finally, how does *justification* occur in casuistry? Given the many different
types of appeal that might be made in any given case (analogies, generalizations,
character judgments, etc.), several different "right" answers can be offered on any
given occasion. This problem exists for virtually all moral theories, and so is not a
problem unique to casuistry. However, without a stable framework of norms,
casuists leave too much room for judgment and have too few resources to prevent
prejudiced or poorly formulated judgments and social conventions.

In the end, casuists seem ambivalent about, but not opposed to, principles. On
the one hand, a limited role is acknowledged. Jonsen says, "This casuistic analysis
does not deny the relevance of principle and theory."[18] On the other hand, casuists
denounce firm and firmly held principles as tyrannical, and criticize certain kinds
of appeals to principles as "moralistic" and "not a serious ethical analysis."[19]
Proponents of casuistry seem most deeply worried not about a reasonable use of
reasonable principles, but *excessive* forms of reliance in recent philosophy on
universal principles. It is, then, incorrect to make an account based on principles a
rival of casuistry. Casuists rightly point to the gap that exists between principles
and good decision making, but their account will fall victim to the same charge if
it leaves a similar gap between cases and good decision making.

Virtue Theory as an Alternative Paradigm

Recent ethical theory has returned to another prominent classical paradigm:
character and *virtue*. This paradigm has been used to pose a challenge to principle-based theories, which typically attend to actions and obligations rather than
agents and their virtues. The language of principles and obligations, some virtue
theorists claim, descends from assessments of virtue, character, and motives.[20]
Major writers in the virtue tradition have held that, to cite an observation of
Hume's, "If a man have a lively sense of honour and virtue, with moderate
passions, his conduct will always be conformable to the rules of morality; or if
he depart from them, his return will be easy and expeditious."[21] Various writers in
biomedical ethics have adopted this perspective, while arguing that the attempt in
an obligation-oriented account to make principles, rules, codes, or procedures
paradigmatic will result in worse rather than better decisions and actions, because
the only reliable protection against unacceptable ethical behavior is virtuous
character.[22] From this perspective, character is more important both in institutions and in personal encounters than is conformity to principles.

This line of argument has merit, but needs to be buttressed by a more careful statement of the nature of the virtues and their connection to principles. A moral virtue is a trait of character valued for moral reasons. Virtue requires properly motivated dispositions and desires when performing actions, and therefore is not reducible to acting in accordance with or for the sake of principles of obligation. We care morally about a person's motivation, and we care especially about *characteristic* forms of motivation. Persons motivated by compassion and personal affection meet our approbation when others who act the same way but from different motives would not. For example, imagine a physician who meets all of his moral obligations but whose underlying motives and desires are morally inappropriate. This physician cares not at all about being of service to people or creating a better environment in his office. He only wants to make money and avoid malpractice suits. Although this man meets his moral obligations, his character is deeply defective. The admirable compassion guiding the lives of many dedicated health professionals is absent in this person, who merely engages in following the socially required principles and rules of behavior.

Properly motivated persons do not merely follow principles and rules; they have a morally appropriate desire to act as they do. One can be disposed by habit to do what is right in accordance with the demands of principles yet be inappropriately motivated. To speak of a good or virtuous action done from principle is usually elliptical for an evaluation of the motive or desire underlying the action.[23] For example, if a person's act of benefiting another person is to elicit moral praise, the person's motive must be to benefit; it cannot be a motive such as the desire to be rewarded for supplying the benefit. Right motive is essential for virtue, and a virtuous character is constituted by an appropriate motive or motivational structure. Persons who characteristically perform morally right actions from principles without a right set of motives and desires are not morally virtuous, even if they always perform the right action from the right principle.

This paradigm of the moral person succeeds in addressing the *moral worth* of persons more adequately than does a principle-based theory of right action. The paradigm appropriately indicates that virtue cannot be reduced to right action in accordance with principles or rules. Kindness, for example, cannot be reduced to a rule-structured action or precept, as if kindness were a matter of following a recipe. Kindness is a disposition to treat people in certain ways from specific motives and desires. We are often more concerned about these motives and desires in persons than about the conformity of their acts to rules. For example, when a physician takes care of us, we expect his or her actions to be motivated from a sense of principled obligation to us, but we expect more as well. We expect the physician to have a desire to take care of us and to want to maintain our hope and keep us from despair. The physician or nurse who acts exclusively from principles may lack the virtue of caring that is implied by the term *medical care*.

Absent this virtue, the physician or nurse is morally deficient. Accordingly, to look at principled actions without also looking at virtues is to miss a large segment of the moral life.

These arguments in defense of virtue ethics are entirely compelling, but giving the virtues a central place in the moral life does not indicate that a virtue-based paradigm should bump or be granted priority over a principle-based paradigm. The two approaches have different emphases, but they can easily be mutually reinforcing if one takes the view that ethical theory is richer and more complete if the virtues are included. The strength of the virtue paradigm is in the central role played by the motivational structure of a virtuous person, which often is as serviceable in guiding *actions* as are rules and principles.[24] But the actions of persons with a virtuous character are not morally acceptable merely because they are performed by a person of good character. People of good character can perform improper actions because they have incorrect information about consequences, make incorrect judgments, or fail to grasp what should be done. We sometimes cannot evaluate a motive, a moral emotion, or a form of expression as appropriate or inappropriate unless we have some basis for the judgment that actions are obligatory, prohibited, or permissible. It is, therefore, doubtful that virtue ethics can adequately *explain* and *justify* many assertions of the rightness or wrongness of actions without resort to principles and rules.

If we rely, as we should, on traits of character such as sympathy and benevolence to motivate us morally, we should also be prepared for our motives to be partial and to need correction by impartial moral principles. For example, we are likely to judge persons more favorably as they are close to us in intimate relationships. Yet on some occasions those who are distant from us *deserve* to be judged more favorably than we are disposed to judge them. Virtues, then, do not preclude impartial principles and rules, and they often work together seamlessly. In addition, virtues such as wisdom and discernment involve understanding both that and how principles and rules are relevant in a variety of circumstances. Principles and virtues are in this respect congenial. Both require attention and sensitivity attuned to the demands of a particular context. Respect for autonomy and beneficence will be as varied in different contexts as compassion and discernment, and the ways in which health professionals manifest these principles and virtues in the care of patients will be as different as the ways in which devoted parents care for their children.

Many virtues dispose persons to act in accordance with principles and rules, and a person's virtuous character is often found in a practical understanding of how to employ a principle in a particular case through a creative response in meeting responsibilities. The ability to understand what needs to be done for patients, as well as how to do it, and then acting with sensitive and caring responses are moral qualities of character, not merely forms of practical intelligence and judgment.

These forms of caring sometimes open up discerning insights into what is at stake, what counts the most, and what needs to be done. At the same time, even a virtue such as moral integrity, which accommodates a wide variety of moral beliefs, is often a matter primarily of living in fidelity to one's moral norms and judgments. Moral integrity in science, medicine, and health care should be understood predominately in terms of fidelity to principles and rules that can be identified in the common morality and in the traditions of health care. Many other virtues, such as conscientiousness, could be similarly treated in terms of a serious commitment to follow principles and rules.

Finally, it deserves notice that some areas of the moral life are not readily frameable or interpretable in the language of virtue theory. Committee reviews in hospitals and research centers provide a typical case in contemporary bioethics. When strangers meet in professional settings, character judgments will often play a less significant role than norms that express rights and appropriate procedures. The same is true in the enforcement of institutional rules and in framing public policy. Dispensing with specified principles and rules of obligation in these settings would be an unwarranted loss in the moral life.

In his work on virtue ethics, Edmund Pellegrino has observed that "Today's challenge is not how to demonstrate the superiority of one normative theory over the other, but rather how to relate each to the other in a matrix that does justice to each and assigns each its proper normative force."[25] I quite agree. I have tried only to show that principles can provide a defensible normative framework that fits comfortably in bioethics with the virtue theory tradition.

Dartmouth Descriptivism and the Critique of Principlism

Not everyone who accepts norms of obligation and moral ideals agrees that *principles* provide the best framework for health care ethics. At the head of this line of critics are the self-described Dartmouth descriptivists—K. Danner Clouser, Bernard Gert, and Ronald Green. At the base of this account is a theory of "morality," a term that references the entire "moral system" of rules, moral ideals, and procedures for determining when it is justified to override or violate a moral rule. Paradoxically, Clouser and Gert are probably as close to Childress and me in their conception of the content of morality and philosophical method as they are to any other writers in biomedical ethics. The problem is that, although they accept general rules of obligation, they do not believe that general principles provide a reliable framework. They look to more specific rules, ideals, and procedures arranged in a structured system as the proper surrogate.

They refer to the account that Childress and I have developed as "principlism."[26] Clouser and Gert bring the following accusations against systems of general principles: (1) principles are little more than checklists or headings for values and have no deep moral substance that can guide practice in the way moral rules do; (2) analyses of principles fail to provide a theory of justification or a theory that ties the principles together, with the consequence that principles are ad hoc constructions lacking systematic order; and (3) prima facie principles often compete in difficult circumstances, yet the underlying philosophical theory is too weak both to decide how to adjudicate the conflict in particular cases and to deal theoretically with the problem of a conflict of principles.

These problems are worthy of careful and sustained reflection in moral theory. However, I doubt that Dartmouth descriptivists themselves have surmounted the problems they lay at the door of principle-based approaches. The primary difference between what Childress and I call *principles* and what they call *rules* is that their rules tend in their abstract formulation to have a more directive and specific content than our principles, thereby at first glance giving more guidance in the moral life. But we have pointed out this same fact since our first edition (in 1979). We have always insisted that turning general principles into specific rules is essential for health care ethics. Mere unspecified principles will not take us very far in bioethics.

There is also not more and not less normative content in their rules and ours, and neither more nor less direction in the moral life. It is true that principles function to order and classify as much as to give prescriptive guidance, and therefore principles do serve a labeling and organizing function. However, this feature only indicates again that principles are abstract starting points in need of additional specification. Clouser and Gert misleadingly suggest that principles only sort and classify without giving significant normative guidance. Logically, the function of principles is to guide conduct, and in pure cases free of conflicting obligations, principles often provide the needed guidance without additional rules. But principles are not stateable with an eye to eliminating the many possible conflicts among principles, because no system of guidelines (principles or rules) could reasonably anticipate the full range of conflicts.

Moreover, a set of rules almost identical to the Clouser-Gert rules is already included in the account of principles and rules that Childress and I propose. We have maintained that principles lend support to more specific moral rules, including those accepted by Clouser and Gert, and that more than one principle—respect for autonomy and nonmaleficence, say—may support a single rule (e.g., a rule of medical confidentiality). The following is a comparison between a sample of the rules we defend under the heading of the principle of nonmaleficence and a directly related sample of basic moral rules defended by Gert and Clouser:

Beauchamp & Childress	*Gert & Clouser*
4 Rules Based on Nonmaleficence	4 of the 10 Basic Rules
1. Do not kill.	1. Don't kill.
2. Do not cause pain.	2. Don't cause pain.
3. Do not incapacitate.	3. Don't disable.
4. Do not deprive of goods.	4. Don't deprive of pleasure.

No substantive moral difference distinguishes these sets of rules. The method of deriving and supporting the rules is different in our accounts, but at present I am claiming only that their rules either do not or need not differ in content from ours and that their rules are no more specific and directive than ours.

Second, Gert and Clouser are critical of us for making both nonmaleficence and beneficence principles of obligation. They maintain that there are no moral rules of beneficence that state obligations. Our only obligations in the moral life, apart from duties encountered in roles and other stations of duty, they regard as captured by moral rules of nonmaleficence, which prohibit causing harm or evil. Their reason is that the goal of morality is the minimization of evil, not the promotion of good. Rational persons can act impartially at all times in regard to all persons with the aim of not causing evil, but they cannot impartially promote the good for all persons at all times. As Clouser states the view, the moral rules all admonish us to avoid harming and are all prohibitions, but, by contrast, moral ideals are only to be encouraged. Since beneficence can only be encouraged and not required, it is a moral ideal only.[27]

This thesis is neither morally correct nor supported within the account of moral obligations presented by Gert and Clouser. The implication of this claim is that one is never morally required (i.e., obligated by moral rules) to prevent or remove harm or evil, but only to avoid causing it. There is no requirement to do anything, only to avoid causing harmful events. Childress and I believe this thesis misreads common morality. The following cases of what one is not obligated to do in the official Clouser-Gert account of obligations of beneficence point to why their view is doubtful:

1. Mr. X's life is in great peril, but if I warn him through a phone call of the peril, he will be fine. I am not obligated to make the phone call.
2. A young toddler has wandered onto a busy street, having become separated from his mother. I can save his life simply by picking him up. It would be nice of me to do so, but I am not obligated to do so. After all, there are no obligations, ever, to prevent harm, apart from roles that fix obligations for us. A policeman would be obligated to lift the child from the street, but not I.

3. A blind man on the street has obviously lost his way, and he asks me for directions. I am not obligated to provide the directions.
4. I am the only witness to a serious automobile accident that has left the drivers unconscious. I am not obligated to stop or to pick up my car telephone and call an ambulance as I speed on my way.

These examples suggest that there are moral obligations of beneficence and that they should be included in any system whose goal is to capture the nature and scope of morality. If Clouser and Gert believe that we are never under such obligations and that a morality of obligations does not contain at least as much beneficence as these four examples suggest, then we deeply disagree about the content of morality. However, as Gert points out in his book, *Morality: A New Justification of the Moral Rules,* which Clouser acknowledges to be "the basis" of his understanding of method and content in ethics, Gert does believe that one is morally obligated to act in circumstances precisely like those in my four examples. His reason is his acceptance of the general rule "Do your duty," which he gives an interpretation broad enough to incorporate the principle of beneficence. He explains his system and its commitments as follows:

> Although duties, in general, go with offices, jobs, roles, etc., there are some duties that seem more general.... A person has a duty... because of some special circumstances, for example, his job or his relationships.... In any civilized society, if a child collapses in your arms, you have a duty to seek help. You cannot simply lay him out on the ground and walk away. In most civilized societies one has a duty to help when (1) one is in physical proximity to someone in need of help to avoid a serious evil, usually death or serious injury, (2) one is in a unique or close to unique position to provide that help and (3) it would be relatively cost-free for one to provide that help.[28]

Although Gert insists that these requirements are all supported by the moral rule "Do your duty," they are effectively identical to those obligations that follow from what Childress and I call—following moral tradition in the eighteenth, nineteenth, and twentieth centuries—beneficence. It therefore cannot be the case that in Gert's system there are no obligations of beneficence in our sense of beneficence. Gert and Clouser cannot be criticizing our views about rules of beneficence (though they could object to how we ground and justify such rules), because we are in effect in agreement on all the substantive issues about what is morally required. Often when Clouser and Gert critique our views it appears that they want to categorize all obligations of beneficence as moral ideals, but it would be inconsistent to take this line about our account of beneficence, given the latent (but deep) commitments to beneficence in Gert's moral theory.

To generalize, much in principlism that Clouser and Gert appear to reject can be situated in their account under Gert's final rule, "Do your job" (or "Don't avoid doing your job"). If this interpretation is correct, our theories are far more compatible than they allow, though it is always worth bearing in mind that Childress and I are defending only a professional ethics, not a general moral theory, as Gert is. Still, it is difficult to see how the impartial rule theory of Clouser and Gert provides a real alternative to our substantive claims about the nature and scope of obligations. I have not here discussed methodology, but our methods are also, in many respects, compatible. Gert and Clouser therefore seem more like congenial partners than hostile rivals.

The major difference between our theory and theirs has nothing to do with whether principles or rules are primary or secondary normative guides in a theory, but rather with several aspects of their theory that I would reject. First, they assume that there is, or at least can be, what they call a "well-developed unified theory" that removes conflicting principles and consistently expresses the grounds of correct judgment—in effect, a canon of rules and theory that expresses the "unity and universality of morality." They fault us heavily for believing that more than one kind of ethical theory can justify a moral belief and insist that we must do the theoretical work of showing the *basis* of principles. They insist that to avoid relativism there can only be "a single unified ethical theory" and that there cannot be "several sources of final justification."[29] I reject each of these claims, but at the same time I recognize them as reasonable philosophical requests for further argument.

In the end, I think my general conception of morality and its primary elements is notably similar to Gert's moral system. We both accept the view that morality is an informal public system of norms with authority to guide the actions of all persons capable of moral agency in their behavior that affects others, and we agree that the goal of morality is to prevent or limit problems of harm, conflict, hostility, and the like through the most suitable moral norms for doing so.

CONCLUSION

I have argued that the moral universe should not be divided into rival and incompatible theories that are principle-based, virtue-based, rights-based, case-based, rule-based, and the like. Impartial rule theory, casuistry, and virtue ethics can all be interpreted as consistent with rather than rivals of a principle-based account.

In the moral life we often coherently fuse appeals to principles, rules, virtues, analogies, precedents, and parables. To assign priority to one paradigm of biomedical ethics is a suspicious project, and I have not argued that the principles paradigm is somehow more serious or more worthy than other paradigms. Even theories with a single ultimate principle, such as utilitarianism and Kantianism, deserve careful attention for what they can teach us about moral reasoning and moral theory. The more general (principles, rules, theories, etc.) and the more particular (feelings, perceptions, case judgments, practices, parables, etc.) should be coherently united in the moral life and in moral philosophy, not ripped from their natural habitat and segregated into distinct and rival species.

A careful analysis and specification of principles is consistent with a wide variety of types of ethical theory, including virtue theory and some accounts that came to prominence only recently, such as communitarian theories, casuistical theories, and the ethics of care. Many authors in biomedical ethics continue to make a mistake by addressing the field as if a principle-based approach is a one-sided and exclusionary approach to bioethics. At the same time, the principles paradigm must address the fact that principles are initially attractive because they offer an impartial instrument to resolve our moral dilemmas, but in concrete circumstances conflicts among the principles often generate dilemmas rather than resolving them. A defender of principles will therefore be grateful for help from any resource that can blunt or reduce intractable dilemmas or disagreements. Every reasonable, insightful, and useful strategy is one we can ill afford to reject if we are to successfully handle the diverse set of issues needing treatment in contemporary bioethics.

Notes

1. For example, the National Commission for the Protection of Human Subjects struggled with principles from 1974 to 1978 because of a mandate from the U.S. Congress requiring that the National Commission investigate the ethics of research and explore the "basic ethical principles" of research ethics. The National Commission ultimately developed an abstract schema of basic principles related to the subject areas of research ethics to which they primarily apply: Respect for persons applies to informed consent; beneficence applies to risk–benefit assessment; and justice applies to selection of subjects. In light of this schema, a general strategy was devised for handling problems of research ethics. See National Commission for the Protection of Human Subjects of Biomedical and Behavioral Research, *The Belmont Report* (Washington, DC: DHEW Publication No. OS 78-0012, 1978).

2. Albert R. Jonsen, "Do No Harm: Axiom of Medical Ethics," in *Philosophical and Medical Ethics: Its Nature and Significance*, ed. Stuart F. Spicker and H. Tristram Engelhardt, Jr. (Dordrecht: D. Reidel, 1977), 27–41.

3. John Stuart Mill, *Utilitarianism*, in vol. 10 of the *Collected Works of John Stuart Mill* (Toronto: University of Toronto Press, 1969), ch. 5.

4. Thomas Percival, *Medical Ethics; or a Code of Institutes and Precepts, Adapted to the Professional Conduct of Physicians and Surgeons* (Manchester, England: S. Russell, 1803), 165–166. Percival's work served as the pattern for the American Medical Association's (AMA) first code of ethics in 1847.

5. Henry S. Richardson, "Specifying Norms as a Way to Resolve Concrete Ethical Problems," *Philosophy and Public Affairs* 19 (Fall 1990): 279–310.

6. See Benjamin Freedman, "Equipoise and the Ethics of Clinical Research," *New England Journal of Medicine* 317 (July 16, 1987): 141–145.

7. See Richardson, "Specifying Norms," 294.

8. Rawls, *A Theory of Justice* (Cambridge, MA: Harvard University Press, 1971), 20ff, 46–49, 195–201, 577ff.

9. John D. Arras, "Getting Down to Cases: The Revival of Casuistry in Bioethics," *Journal of Medicine and Philosophy* 16 (1991): 31–33; Albert Jonsen and Stephen Toulmin, *The Abuse of Casuistry* (Berkeley: University of California Press, 1988), 16–19, 66–67; Jonsen, "Casuistry and Clinical Ethics," *Theoretical Medicine* 7 (1986): 67, 71; and "Casuistry as Methodology in Clinical Ethics," *Theoretical Medicine* 12 (December 1991): 298.

10. Cf. John D. Arras, "Getting Down to Cases," and "Common Law Morality," *Hastings Center Report* 20 (July/August 1990): 35–37. Arras makes the following constructive recommendations after criticizing casuistry: Use real and lengthy cases, present complex sequences of cases in which they build on one another, and be cautious regarding the limits of casuistical methods.

11. Cf. David C. Thomasma, "Why Philosophers Should Offer Ethics Consultations," *Theoretical Medicine* 12 (1991): 129–140.

12. Although some casuists are critical of theory, others encourage principles and theory construction. See Baruch Brody, *Life and Death Decision Making* (New York: Oxford University Press, 1988), 13. For a very different view, see Albert R. Jonsen, "Practice Versus Theory," *Hastings Center Report* 20 (July/August 1990): 32–34. Brody defends theory construction; Jonsen challenges the presumption that "theory is an inseparable companion to practice" and contrasts theory construction and the art of practice found in casuistry.

13. Jonsen and Toulmin, *Abuse of Casuistry*, 11–19, 66–67, 251–254, 296–299; Jonsen, "Casuistry as Methodology in Clinical Ethics," 299–302; Brody, *Life and Death Decision Making*, 12–13, 15n; Arras, "Getting Down to Cases," 31–33; Jonsen, "Casuistry and Clinical Ethics," *Theoretical Medicine* 7 (1986), 67, 71.

14. Toulmin, "The Tyranny of Principles," *Hastings Center Report* 11 (December 1981): 31–39.

15. Jonsen, "Casuistry as Methodology in Clinical Ethics," 298.

16. Albert R. Jonsen, "Casuistry: An Alternative or Complement to Principles?" *Kennedy Institute of Ethics Journal* 5 (1995): 246–247.

17. Cf. Joel Feinberg, *Social Philosophy* (Englewood Cliffs, NJ: Prentice-Hall, 1973), 34.

18. Jonsen, "Case Analysis in Clinical Ethics," *The Journal of Clinical Ethics* 1 (1990): 65. See *Abuse of Casuistry*, 10.

19. Jonsen, "American Moralism and the Origin of Bioethics in the United States," esp. 117, 125–128.

20. See Philippa Foot, *Virtues and Vices* (Oxford: Basil Blackwell, 1978), and Gregory Trianosky, "Supererogation, Wrong-doing, and Vice," *Journal of Philosophy* 83 (1986): 26–40.

21. David Hume, "The Sceptic," in his *Essays, Moral, Political, and Literary*, ed. Eugene Miller (Indianapolis: LibertyClassics/Liberty Fund, 1985), 169 (par. 29 in the essay).

22. A classic treatment is H. K. Beecher, "Ethics and Clinical Research," *New England Journal of Medicine* 274 (1966): 1354–1360. See also Gregory Pence, *Ethical Options in Medicine* (Oradell, NJ: Medical Economics Co., 1980), 177.

23. This formulation is indebted to David Hume, *A Treatise of Human Nature,* 2nd edition, ed. L. A. Selby-Bigge and P. H. Nidditch (Oxford: Clarendon Press, 1978), 478; and John Mackie, *Hume's Moral Theory* (London: Routledge and Kegan Paul, 1980), 79–80.

24. See David Solomon, "Internal Objections to Virtue Ethics," *Midwest Studies in Philosophy* 13 (1988): 439.

25. Edmund Pellegrino, "Toward a Virtue-Based Normative Ethics for the Health Professions," *Kennedy Institute of Ethics Journal* 5 (1995): 253–277, esp. 273. See, for more extensive treatment, Pellegrino's book (coauthored with David Thomasma), *The Virtues in Medical Practice* (New York: Oxford University Press, 1993).

26. See Clouser and Gert, "A Critique of Principlism," *The Journal of Medicine and Philosophy* 15 (April 1990): 219–236; and Ronald M. Green, Gert, and Clouser, "The Method of Public Morality versus the Method of Principlism," *The Journal of Medicine and Philosophy* 18 (1993). A diverse, but less focused, set of criticisms is found in Ron P. Hamel, Edwin R. DuBose, and Laurence J. O'Connell, *Beyond Principlism* (Chicago: Trinity Press International, 1993).

27. K. Danner Clouser, "Common Morality as an Alternative to Principlism," *Kennedy Institute of Ethics Journal* 5 (1995): 219–236, esp. 225–226, 231.

28. Bernard Gert, *Morality: A New Justification of the Moral Rules* (New York: Oxford University Press, 1988), 154–155.

29. Clouser and Gert, "A Critique of Principlism," 231–232; Green, "Method in Bioethics: A Troubled Assessment," *The Journal of Medicine and Philosophy* 15 (1990): 179–197.

10

A DEFENSE OF THE COMMON MORALITY

Phenomena of moral conflict and disagreement have led writers in ethics to two antithetical conclusions. Some writers maintain that there are objective, universal moral standards. Others reject all objectivity and universality. To maintain, as do most writers in bioethics, that there are valid moral distinctions between just and unjust actions, merciful and unmerciful actions, and humane and inhumane actions is either to claim that these conclusions hold universally or that they hold relative to a particular and contingent moral framework. If judgments are entirely relative to a local framework, then they cannot be applied with universal validity.

I maintain that we can consistently deny universality to some justified moral norms while claiming universality for others. I argue for this conclusion by locating universality in the common morality and nonuniversality in other parts of the moral life, which I call *particular moralities*. I defend the thesis that there are universal moral standards through (1) a theory of the objectives of morality, (2) an account of the norms that achieve those objectives, and (3) an account of normative justification (both pragmatic and coherentist). I discuss how the common morality is progressively made specific and the sense in which moral change occurs.

Several instructive articles have recently been critical of my previously published views on the common morality. I will respond here to articles by David DeGrazia and Leigh Turner, both of whom take "common morality" to refer to a broader and quite different body of norms than I do.

THE NATURE AND OBJECTIVES OF THE COMMON MORALITY

I understand the *common morality* as the set of norms shared by all persons committed to the objectives of morality. The objectives of morality, I will argue, are those of promoting human flourishing by counteracting conditions that cause the quality of people's lives to worsen.

The Nature of the Common Morality

The common morality is not merely *a* morality that differs from *other* moralities.[1] It is applicable to all persons in all places, and all human conduct is to be judged by its standards. Virtually all people in all cultures grow up with an understanding of the basic demands that morality makes upon everyone. They know not to lie, steal, break promises, and the like. The following are examples of *standards of action* (rules of obligation) in the common morality: (*1*) Don't kill, (*2*) Don't cause pain or suffering to others, (*3*) Prevent evil or harm from occurring, (*4*) Rescue persons in danger, (*5*) Tell the truth, (*6*) Nurture the young and dependent, (*7*) Keep your promises, (*8*) Don't steal, (*9*) Don't punish the innocent, and (*10*) Treat all persons with equal moral consideration.

The common morality contains standards other than principles of obligation. Here are 10 examples of *moral character traits* (virtues) recognized in the common morality: (*1*) nonmalevolence, (*2*) honesty, (*3*) integrity, (*4*) conscientiousness, (*5*) trustworthiness, (*6*) fidelity, (*7*) gratitude, (*8*) truthfulness, (*9*) lovingness, and (*10*) kindness. My claim with respect to these virtues is that they are universally admired traits of character, that a person is universally recognized as deficient in moral character if he or she lacks such traits, and that those negative traits that are the opposite of these virtues and that we call *vices* (malevolence, dishonesty, lack of integrity, cruelty, etc.) are substantial moral defects, universally so recognized. I will hereafter say no more about the virtues and vices. This area of the moral life is not my concern in this paper; instead, I focus on norms of action.

The Objectives of Morality

Centuries of experience have demonstrated that the human condition tends to deteriorate into inconvenience, misery, violence, and distrust unless norms of the sort I listed earlier—the norms of the common morality—are observed. When complied with, these norms lessen human misery and preventable death. The object of morality is to prevent or limit problems of indifference, conflict, hostility, scarce resources, limited information, and the like.

It is an overstatement to maintain that all of the norms that I listed previously are necessary for the *survival* of a society (as diverse philosophers and social scientists have maintained[2]), but it is not too much to claim that these norms are necessary to *ameliorate or counteract the tendency for the quality of people's lives to worsen or for social relationships to disintegrate.*[3] In every well-functioning society norms are in place to prohibit lying, breaking promises, causing bodily harm, stealing, fraud, the taking of life, the neglect of children, and failures to keep contracts. These norms occupy a central place in the moral life because they have proven that they successfully achieve the objectives of morality. This success in the service of human flourishing accounts for their moral authority.

PARTICULAR MORALITIES AS NONUNIVERSAL

I shift now to analysis of *particular moralities.* Turner states that I do not allow for pluralism or for the local character of "moral worlds." However, he misconstrues my view. Many moral norms are particular to cultures, groups, and even individuals. Whereas the common morality contains only general moral standards that are conspicuously abstract, universal, and content-thin, particular moralities often present concrete, nonuniversal, and content-rich norms. These moralities implement the responsibilities, aspirations, ideals, attitudes, and sensitivities that spring from cultural traditions, religious traditions, professional practice, institutional rules, and the like. In some cases, explication of the values in these moralities requires a special knowledge and may involve refinement by experts or scholars—as, for example, in the body of Jewish moral norms in the Talmudic tradition. There may also be full-bodied moral systems set up to adjudicate conflicts and provide methods for the treatment of borderline cases—for example, the norms and methods in Roman Catholic casuistry.

Professional moralities, including moral codes and traditions of practice, are one type of particular morality. These moralities may legitimately vary in the way in which they handle conflict of interest, protocol review, advance directives, and many other subjects. *Moral ideals* provide another instructive example of particular moralities. Following ideals is not morally obligatory, but ideals are universally admired aspirations.[4] Actions done from these ideals are morally good and praiseworthy, and those who fulfill their ideals can be praised and admired, but they cannot be blamed or disdained by others if they fail to fulfill aspirational ideals. Ideals are particularized in local moralities.

Turner states that I defend an ahistorical and an a priori account of morality. It should be clear from my comments on particular moralities that I do not defend this view. Particular moralities develop historically. I am also a historicist and conventionalist in regard to the common morality. However, a defense of this position, which is Hobbesian and Humean in inspiration, would require a more extended discussion than can be undertaken here. Two clarifications must suffice: First, Turner opines that pluralists form a "third theoretical camp" that is sharply distinguished from relativists and universalists. I reject this conclusion. A pluralist who repudiates universal norms is simply one form of relativist. Turner appears to be a pluralist and a relativist, though I am unsure whether his type of relativism is normative or nonnormative. He has no means to rebut the thesis that all communally initiated systems of norms are on an equally satisfactory moral footing, regardless of the principles that underlie them, the reasons for adopting them, or the consequences of their adoption. Second, Turner maintains that there are, at local levels (by contrast to the universal level), "shared, historically emergent understandings and common accounts of moral practices." This apparently empirical thesis has both wide and narrow applications. If there can be such commonly accepted practices *locally* (in cultures, tribes, religious traditions, professional organizations, and the like), then there can be commonly accepted practices *universally*. Turner and I ought not to disagree about this. Any difference between us should have to do with how to test empirically for common acceptance. I turn, then, to the problem of empirical assumptions and evidence.

THE PROBLEM OF EMPIRICAL JUSTIFICATION

Turner is tenaciously critical of what he sees as the empirical assumptions that I and my coauthor James Childress make in discussing the common morality. He says that scant anthropological or historical evidence supports the thesis that a universal common morality exists. Part of the problem is that Turner includes under "morality" many more norms—for example, norms that structure social hierarchies, stations, and gender roles—that I do not include. As best I can tell, Turner altogether ignores and perhaps rejects the distinction that I make between *common morality* and *particular moralities*.[5]

In principle, scientific research could prove me—or Turner—wrong. However, before such research is undertaken, we need to be clear about the concept, or hypothesis, being tested. For purposes of empirical investigation, my claim is that all persons committed to morality, and all well-functioning societies, adhere to the general standards of action enumerated previously. My claim is not, as Turner seems to believe, that all of the moral norms of all societies are indistinguishable. What we now know or could know empirically, and whether the propositions that I have advanced are falsifiable by scientific investigation, are nuanced questions that are not as straightforward as Turner proposes. It would be difficult to design empirical studies without either missing the target (i.e., all and only those who are committed to the objectives of morality) or begging the question. The question could be begged either by (1) designing the study so that the only persons tested are those who already have the commitments and beliefs the investigator is testing for or (2) designing the study so that all persons are tested whether or not they are committed to the objectives of morality. The first design risks biasing the study in favor of my hypothesis; the second design risks biasing the study against my hypothesis.

I have defined the *common morality* in terms of "the set of norms shared by all persons committed to the objectives of morality." Since persons not committed[6] to the objectives of morality are not within the scope of my argument, they could not appropriately be included as subjects in an empirical study. Their beliefs are not useful for testing my empirical hypothesis. Some, including Turner, will conclude that I have constructed a circular and self-justifying position; that is, they will say that I am defining the common morality in terms of a certain type of commitment and then allowing only those who accept the kinds of norms that I have identified to qualify as persons committed to the objectives of morality. In publications referenced by Turner, I have claimed that amoral people, immoral people, and people driven by ideologies that override moral obligations are not pursuing the objectives of morality, whatever else they may be pursuing.

I appreciate that this position risks stipulating the meaning and content of "morality." Nonetheless, I think the position I defend is the correct one. A full defense of this position would require a justification of all of the elements of my account—in particular, the object of morality, considered judgments, the role of coherence, pragmatic justification, and specification. Here I can do no more than note three reasons why Turner's appeals to empirical evidence are unconvincing.

First, no empirical studies known to me show that only some cultural moralities accept, whereas others reject, the several examples of standards of action that I earlier submitted as rules of obligation in the common morality. Empirical investigations of morality concentrate on differences in the way such rules are embedded in different cultures. These studies assume rather than question the most general ethical standards. Their results show differences in the *interpretation* and *specification* of shared standards; they do not show that cultures *reject* basic common-morality norms. For example, empirical studies do not test whether a cultural morality includes or rejects rules against theft, promise breaking, or killing. Instead, investigators study when theft, promise breaking, and killing are deemed in these cultures to occur, how cultures handle exceptive cases, different conceptions of killing, and the like. Empirical data show variation in what I refer to as particular moralities and in specification of the rules of the common morality. These data do not provide evidence that a common morality does not exist.

Second, the conclusions that I reach can be tested empirically, but as yet appropriate hypotheses have not been tested. Investigation would center on persons who had already been screened to ensure that they are committed to the *objectives* of morality, but not screened to determine which *particular norms* they believe to be the best means to the achievement of those objectives. That is, persons not committed to the objectives of morality would be excluded from the study, and the purpose of the study would be to determine whether cultural or individual differences emerge over the (most general) norms believed to best achieve the objectives of morality. Should it turn out that those studied do not share the norms that I hypothesize to comprise the common morality, then there is no common morality of the sort I claim, and my hypothesis has been falsified. If norms other than the ones I have specified were demonstrated to be shared across cultures, this finding would constitute evidence of a common morality, albeit one different from the account I have proposed. Only if no moral norms were found in common across cultures would the general hypothesis that a common morality exists be rejected. Of course, whatever is established about the existence of a common body of norms, nothing follows about whether those norms are justifiable, adequate, in need of change, and the like. I will later consider how this normative question is distinct from all empirical problems.

Third, and paradoxically, Turner's notion of "shared, historically emergent understandings" and "widely shared understandings of moral practices and policies" errs in the direction of presuming *more shared agreement* than actually exists. I agree with the leading thesis in Turner's paper—"We can find both zones of consensus and zones of conflict"—but even within local regions of consensus, there is sure to be dissent and controversy. Consider Turner's statement that "Moral frameworks concerning research on human subjects currently seem to constitute one region where there exist widely shared understandings of moral practices and policies." On the one hand, this statement is accurate. On the other hand, a bounty of literature in bioethics, empirical and normative, calls this judgment into question, depending on which parts of these moral frameworks are under consideration. There currently exists international agreement on major generalizations such as on most of the vague principles in the Declaration of Helsinki, but there also exists a plurality of viewpoints on virtually every major topic in research on human subjects, including such pillars of the system as the nature of the obligation to obtain informed consent and the proper way to conduct review of research by committee review.[7]

THE PROBLEM OF NORMATIVE JUSTIFICATION

DeGrazia asserts that Childress and I "reduce normative ethics to descriptive ethics" and that we attempt to justify common morality "in terms of consensus." I acknowledge that there were at one time flawed sentences regarding the role of consensus in *Principles of Biomedical Ethics*, but Childress and I are clear now that we advance both "normative and nonnormative claims" in defense of the common morality.[8] I will here clarify my own views about the distinction between the descriptive (nonnormative) and the normative.

First, descriptive ethics and consensus reports are factual; normative ethics and methods of justification are not. Descriptions are not justifications. Claims about the *existence* of the common morality need *empirical justification*, whereas claims about the *justifiability and adequacy* of the common morality require *normative justification*.

Second, I am *not* assuming that all persons in all societies do in fact accept the norms of the common morality. Unanimity of this sort is not the issue. As noted previously, many amoral, immoral, and selectively moral persons do not embrace various demands of the common morality. Some persons are morally weak, others morally depraved. Morality can be misunderstood, rejected, or overridden by other values.

Third, it is preposterous to hold that a *customary* set of norms or a *consensus* set of norms is justified by the fact of custom or consensus. More unsatisfactory still is the idea that norms qualify for inclusion in the common morality merely because they are rooted in custom or consensus. The proposition that moral justification derives from custom or consensus is a moral travesty. Any given society's customary or consensus position may be a distorted outlook that functions to block awareness of universally valid requirements. Some societies are in the grip of leaders who promote religious zealotries or political ideologies that depart from common-morality standards. Such persons may be deeply committed to their particular outlook—for example, they may be intent on converting others to their favored political ideology—but they should not be said to be *morally* committed merely because they are committed to a supremely valued point of view.[9] Fanatics in control of the Taliban in Afghanistan and Pakistan commit horrendous moral offenses. Their enthusiasm is about something other than the common morality, which to them gives no reason why they should constrain their particular zealotry.

Fourth, universal agreement about norms that are suitable for the moral life *explains* why there is a common morality, but does not *justify* the norms.[10] What justifies the norms of the common morality, in the pragmatic theory I have proposed, is that they are the norms best suited to achieve the objectives of morality. Fundamental moral norms require for their justification that we state the objective of the institution of morality. Once the objective has been identified, a set of standards is justified if and only if it is better for reaching the objective than any other set of standards. This pragmatic approach to justification is my own preferred strategy for the justification of general moral norms, but I appreciate that others may prefer a different justification (e.g., a contractarian one). In the penultimate section of this essay I will supplement this account of pragmatic justification of common-morality principles with a coherence theory of justification for particular moralities.

Fifth, DeGrazia distinguishes between *common morality 1* (widely shared moral beliefs) and *common morality 2* (moral beliefs that would be widely shared if morally committed persons reached reflective equilibrium). I find this distinction, as presented, puzzling and unsatisfactory. Common morality 2 will generate different sets of norms that constitute particular moralities, not the common morality. "Common morality 2" seems to be a general heading for the way in which particular moralities develop, or perhaps should develop, from the common morality. Despite these misgivings, this distinction between *common morality 1* and *common morality 2* can be salvaged and reconstructed as follows: *Common morality 1* is the set of universally shared moral beliefs as it now exists (a descriptive claim), whereas *common morality 2* is the set of moral beliefs that ought to be embraced in the common morality (a normative claim). I will return to this distinction between what is and what ought to be in the common morality in the final section of this essay.[11]

SPECIFICATION: MAKING GENERAL NORMS PRACTICAL

The reason why norms in particular moralities often differ is that the abstract starting points in the common morality can be coherently developed in a variety of ways to create practical guidelines and procedures. DeGrazia and I agree that Henry Richardson's account of specification presents an important way in which general norms are made suitably practical. Specification is not a process of producing general norms such as those in the common morality; it assumes that valid general norms are available. Specifying the norms with which one starts, whether those in the common morality or norms previously specified, is accomplished by *narrowing the scope* of the norms, not by explaining what the general norms *mean*. The scope is narrowed, as Richardson puts it, by "spelling out where, when, why, how, by what means, to whom, or by whom the action is to be done or avoided."[12]

For example, the norm that we must "respect the autonomy of competent persons" cannot, unless specified, handle complicated problems of what to say or demand in clinical medicine and research involving human subjects. A definition of "respect for autonomy" (as, say, "allowing competent persons to exercise their liberty rights") might clarify one's meaning in using the norm, but would not narrow the general norm or render it more specific and contextually appropriate. Specification is a different kind of spelling out than analysis of meaning. It adds content. For example, one specification of "respect the autonomy of competent persons" could be "respect the autonomy of competent patients when they become incompetent by following their advance directives." This specification will work well in some medical contexts, but will confront limits in others, thus necessitating further additional specification. Progressive specification can continue indefinitely, but to qualify as a specification, a transparent connection must be maintained to the initial norm that gives moral authority to the resulting string of norms.

I come now to a critical matter about the way in which particular moralities are developed through specification. There is always the possibility of developing more than one line of specification when confronting practical problems and moral disagreements. Different persons and groups will offer conflicting specifications of the same norm. In any given problematic or dilemmatic case, several competing specifications may be offered by reasonable and fair-minded parties, all of whom are committed to the common morality. We should not hold persons to a higher standard than that of making judgments conscientiously in light of the relevant basic and specified norms while attending to appropriate factual evidence. It is to be expected that conscientious and reasonable moral agents will disagree with other conscientious persons over moral weights and priorities in circumstances that involve a contingent conflict of norms, and it may be that multiple particular moralities will be developed.

JUSTIFYING SPECIFICATIONS USING THE METHOD OF COHERENCE

I earlier suggested that it is reasonable to hold that the norms of the common morality are justified pragmatically. In addition to this form of justification, I accept a coherentist justification that helps determine when the specified norms that comprise particular moralities are justified.

A specification is justified if and only if there is good reason to believe that it will maximize the coherence of the overall set of relevant beliefs. DeGrazia and I share this view. These beliefs could include empirically justified beliefs, justified basic moral beliefs, and previously justified specifications. This is a version of so-called wide reflective equilibrium.[13] No matter how wide the pool of beliefs, there is no reason to expect that the process of rendering norms coherent through the process of specification will come to an end or be perfected. Particular moralities are continuous works in progress—a process rather than a finished product. There is no reason to think that morality can be rendered coherent in only one system through the process of specification. Many particular moralities are coherent ways to specify the common morality. Normatively, we can demand no more than that agents faithfully specify the norms of the common morality with an attentive eye to overall coherence.

The moral life will always be plagued by forms of conflict and incoherence that need reduction. Our goal should be a method that *helps* in a circumstance of conflict and disagreement, not a *panacea*. Although DeGrazia conjectures that Childress and I have an "excessive aversion to disagreement," his thesis must confront the accusation commonly brought against us that we allow for *too much conflict and disagreement*. My view is that we countenance disagreement (in moral theory and in moral practice) more readily than many writers in bioethics. Indeed, it appears that we tolerate disagreement more readily than DeGrazia himself, judging from his comments regarding "standing up for what's right." Standing up for what a person believes to be right is often admirable, but without more explanation than DeGrazia offers, such resolve can descend into little more than an insistent inflexibility that refuses to recognize legitimate disagreement.

DeGrazia speculates that our "excessive aversion to disagreement" leads us to an "excessive accommodation of existing moral beliefs and/or competing constituencies," resulting in "reduced coherence and justification." He offers three examples. I will consider only his third example, which he seems to find the most flagrant example because "compromise apparently leads to contradiction." This example centers on our support for physician-assisted suicide—thereby, he says, accommodating "liberal commentators"—and the way we take seriously slippery-slope arguments in opposition to physician-assisted suicide—thus, he says, accommodating "conservative participants in this debate." DeGrazia greets with skeptical disbelief our assertion that these two points of view can be reconciled.

He offers no argument for his conclusion that our position is incoherent and contradictory, and he does not reconstruct the arguments that Childress and I present in our book. To see how the two views can be coherently reconciled, we need before us the distinction that Childress and I use between the justification of *policies* and the justification of *acts*. Public rules or laws sometimes justifiably prohibit conduct that is morally justified in individual cases. Two moral questions about physician-assisted suicide need to be distinguished: (1) Are physicians ever morally justified in complying with first-party requests that they assist patients in acts of suicide? (2) Is there an adequate moral basis to justify the legalization of physician-assisted suicide? Childress and I argue that there are justified *acts* of assisting patients in committing suicide. However, once public considerations external to the private relationship between a physician and a patient are brought into the picture—such as the implications of legalized physician-assisted suicide for medical education and medical practice in hospitals and nursing homes—these considerations may provide good and sufficient moral reasons for disallowing physicians from engaging in such actions as a matter of public law. We argue that some policies that legalize physician hastening of death would, under at least some circumstances, be morally problematic. It may turn out that the worries about legalization advanced in some slippery-slope arguments have force, but it may also turn out they have little or no force. There is no incoherence in this position on the multiple sides to the controversy over physician-assisted suicide.

DeGrazia also maintains that Childress and I have had relatively little to say about the question, What is coherence? He suggests that coherence is simply "the holistic embodiment of theoretical virtues, the characteristics we expect of any good theory." Coherence seems to reduce for him to conformity to the criteria of good theories. This issue is too involved to be addressed here, but, as DeGrazia specifically notes, Childress and I have a defensible set of criteria of good theories, and therefore, by his account, we have an acceptable core notion of coherence. Nevertheless, he would find it an underdeveloped notion, and I would agree.

CHANGE AND STABILITY IN THE COMMON MORALITY

I turn, finally, to issues about whether morality changes over time. Moral change entails that what was not previously morally required (or prohibited) is now morally required (or prohibited). Particular moralities, customary practices, and so-called consensus moralities can and do change; they may even change by reversal of a position. For example, a code of research ethics might at one time endorse placebo-controlled trials only to reverse itself and condemn such trials at a later time. When relevant circumstances change or new insight is achieved, such revisions are warranted.

Change in *particular moralities* is not, however, at issue. The issue is whether *the common morality* can and does change. Is it possible in principle or in practice for this morality to change? Could it come to be the case that we no longer have to keep our promises, that we can lie and deceive, or that a vice can become a virtue? To the extent that we can envisage circumstances in which human society is better served by substantively changing or abandoning a norm in the common morality (i.e., we can envision that some alternative norm would better serve to counteract the tendency for the quality of life to worsen or disintegrate in social relationships), change in the common morality could occur and could be justified. For example, it is possible, however unlikely, that the obligation to tell the truth could become severely dangerous to the well-being of our friends and acquaintances, and we might therefore abandon the rule altogether.

Justification of a change in the common morality either would require that one or more moral *norms* remain unchanged in the moral system or would require that the *objectives* of morality not change. Without some stability of this sort in the system, moral change is incomprehensible and would lack justification. The point is that justification of the new norm will require recourse to some unchanged norms or goals.[14]

In principle, all moral norms in the common morality could change over time, but such change is extraordinarily unlikely in practice. It is difficult to construct actual or even plausible hypothetical examples of a moral principle in the common morality that has been valid only for a limited duration. Moreover, I do not believe that we do or will in the future handle problems of profound social change by altering norms in the common morality. Instead, we will do what we have always done: As circumstances change, we will find moral reasons for saying that there is either a valid *exception* to a particular obligation or a need to specify it in a somewhat different way. For example, "Do not kill" is a basic moral rule, but we have never allowed prohibitions against killing to prevail in all circumstances. Particular moralities have carefully constructed exceptions in cases of war, self-defense, criminal punishment, martyrdom, misadventure, and the like. We also will continue to handle social change through the structure of one or more norms in the common morality overriding one or more different norms.

However, moral change in the common morality may occur in at least one important respect. Even if the abstract principles of the common morality do not change, the scope of individuals to whom the principles are deemed to apply has changed—a problem of moral status. Consider the norm that we should "Treat all persons with equal moral consideration." Imagine that we are able to teach both language and the norms of the common morality to the great apes. It is possible under these conditions that we would collectively come to the conclusion that the great apes, not just human apes, should be included in the category of "persons," or some comparable category of moral status, and therefore are owed equal moral consideration. This would be a momentous change in the scope of individuals covered by the protections of the common morality. It seems unlikely to occur, as do other changes of this magnitude, but we can conceive of conditions under which such change could occur.

It can be argued that the common morality has already been refined in a conspicuously similar manner by changes in the way slaves, women, people of color, and persons from many other groups have come to be acknowledged as owed a deeper level of moral consideration than had been previously recognized. This sort of change constitutes a major—and an actual rather than a hypothetical—modification in the scope of moral rules. But are the changes that have taken place in recent centuries truly changes *in the common morality*? Changes in the way slaves, women, and people of various ethnicities are regarded seem to be changes in particular moralities or ethical theories rather than in the common morality.

The most defensible view, I suggest, is that the common morality does not now, and has never in fact, included a provision of equal moral consideration for all individuals. However, this norm *could become* part of the common morality, which would constitute a substantive modification. I am confident, however, that empirical investigation of rules determining who should receive equal consideration would show considerable disagreement across individuals and societies, even among people who could reasonably be said to be committed to the objectives of morality. This finding is consistent with the normative thesis that the common morality should include rules of equal moral consideration for slaves, women, people of color, and other relevant parties now excluded.

Descriptive ethics analyzes where we are (which rules we do accept); normative ethics ventures into the waters of where we should be (which rules we ought to accept). Where we are in the common morality is not necessarily where we should be according to a normative theory. By appeal to what I have called the objectives of morality, we can (arguably) justify the claim that rules of equal moral consideration ought to be applied to all persons—not merely to limited groups of persons. I will not attempt to justify this normative thesis, but I wish to mark its importance. Among the most momentous changes to occur in the history of moral practice have been those regarding the scope of persons to whom moral norms are applied. A theory of the common morality that deprives it of the capacity to criticize and evaluate existing groups or communities whose viewpoints are morally deficient would be an ineffectual theory. A profoundly important feature of the common morality is its provision of cross-cultural standards of evaluation. To the extent that the common morality itself stands in need of improvement, we can hope to make those improvements by revising the normative guidelines necessary to achieve the fundamental objectives of morality. We need to think not merely in terms of what universally is the case, but also in terms of where we might be in the future.

Notes

1. Although there is only one universal common morality, there is more than one theory of the common morality. For a diverse set of theories of the common morality, see Alan Donagan, *The Theory of Morality* (Chicago: University of Chicago Press, 1977); Bernard Gert, Charles M. Culver, and K. Danner Clouser, *Bioethics: A Return to Fundamentals* (New York: Oxford University Press, 1997); and W. D. Ross, *The Foundations of Ethics* (Oxford: Oxford University Press, 1939).

2. See Sissela Bok, *Common Values* (Columbia, MO: University of Missouri Press, 1995), 13–23, 50–59 (citing several influential writers on the subject).

3. Compare the arguments in G. J. Warnock, *The Object of Morality* (London: Methuen & Co., 1971), esp. 15–26; John Mackie, *Ethics: Inventing Right and Wrong* (London: Penguin, 1977), 107ff. I have been deeply influenced on this subject by Warnock and Mackie, and no less by Thomas Hobbes and David Hume.

4. See Richard B. Brandt, "Morality and Its Critics," in his *Morality, Utilitarianism, and Rights* (Cambridge: Cambridge University Press, 1992), chap. 5.

5. I concur that virtually all of the norms mentioned by Turner are not in the common morality and that we can differentiate societies by the different norms that each society accepts.

6. When I say that some persons are not committed to morality, I do not mean that they are not dedicated to a way of life that they consider a moral way of life. Religious fanatics

and political zealots clearly have this self-conception even as they act against or are neglectful of the demands of morality.

7. For an overview of persistent problems and controversies, see Committee on Assessing the System for Protecting Human Research Participants, Institute of Medicine, *Responsible Research: A Systems Approach to Protecting Research Participants* (Washington, DC: The National Academies Press, 2002).

8. Tom L. Beauchamp and James F. Childress, *Principles of Biomedical Ethics*. 5th edn. (New York: Oxford University Press, 2001), 4.

9. For a once influential literature suggesting that moral norms are those that a person or, alternatively, a society accepts as supreme, final, or overriding, see *The Definition of Morality*, ed. G. Wallace and A. D. M. Walker (London: Methuen, 1970), and William K. Frankena, *Perspectives on Morality*, ed. K. E. Goodpaster (Notre Dame, IN: University of Notre Dame Press, 1976), chaps. 10, 15. A criterion of supremacy would permit almost anything to count as moral if a person or a society is committed to its overriding pursuit.

10. Cf. Mackie, *Ethics: Inventing Right and Wrong*, 22–23.

11. I agree with DeGrazia that there are many forms of "moral prejudice" and that "moral judgment can be distorted in many ways." However, I disagree with him that these distorted judgments "reflect common morality 1." These judgments do not reflect common morality as I use the term.

12. Henry Richardson, "Specifying, Balancing, and Interpreting Bioethical Principles," *Journal of Medicine and Philosophy* 25 (2000): 285–307, quote on p. 289. See also Richardson, "Specifying Norms as a Way to Resolve Concrete Ethical Problems," *Philosophy and Public Affairs* 19 (1990): 279–310; David DeGrazia, "Moving Forward in Bioethical Theory: Theories, Cases, and Specified Principlism," *Journal of Medicine and Philosophy* 17 (1992): 511–539; DeGrazia and Beauchamp, "Philosophical Foundations and Philosophical Methods," in Daniel Sulmasy and Jeremy Sugarman, eds. *Methods in Medical Ethics* (Washington, DC: Georgetown University Press, 2001), 31–46.

13. Norman Daniels, "Wide Reflective Equilibrium and Theory Acceptance in Ethics," *Journal of Philosophy* 76 (1979): 256–282; Daniels, "Wide Reflective Equilibrium in Practice," in L. W. Sumner and J. Boyle, eds., *Philosophical Perspectives on Bioethics* (Toronto: University of Toronto Press, 1996).

14. See the argument to this conclusion in Joseph Raz, "Moral Change and Social Relativism," in Ellen Paul, Fred Miller, and Jeffrey Paul, eds., *Cultural Pluralism and Moral Knowledge* (Cambridge: Cambridge University Press, 1994), 139–158.

11

FROM MORALITY TO COMMON MORALITY

For some 19 years, Bernard Gert has feasted on my views about moral philosophy and the principles of biomedical ethics. Between 1990 and 1994, Gert and his coauthors published a group of articles[1] critical of my work with James Childress.[2] These articles were widely read in biomedical ethics, and Gert has since continued to engage my work. Rather than answering his criticisms, I here consider a single problem at the heart of Gert's moral philosophy: the justification of claims about the common morality. My goal is to identify and provide a limited defense of three forms of justification of claims about the common morality.

Despite Gert's many efforts, and my own, the common morality is little studied in contemporary philosophy and rarely embraced as foundational in a moral theory. In much of the literature on the subject, Gert and I, together with our coauthors, are treated as the *only* defenders of common morality theory. This assessment may be correct. Clearly many philosophers are skeptical of appeals to a common morality. My graduate students, my colleagues, and the critics[3] Gert and I share in common have frequently recommended that I abandon common morality theory. Their advice is that I rely exclusively on considered moral judgments and reflective equilibrium, following the path charted by John Rawls, Norman Daniels, and others.[4] However, both Gert and I have rejected this advice.[5]

A HISTORY OF THE GERT CORPUS: HOW COMMON MORALITY BECAME DOMINANT

I start with a brief history of Gert's movement from morality to the common morality. His first published book was entitled *The Moral Rules: A New Rational Foundation for Morality.*[6] This title draws attention to three notions: "the moral rules," "morality," and "rational foundation." Gert was at the time centering his theory on rules, rationality, and morality. Eighteen years later, in a 1988 revision, the term *rational* was removed from the subtitle and the revised book was issued as *Morality: A New Justification of the Moral Rules.*[7] This "new justification" in 1988 was fundamentally identical to the justification in the 1970 book. Another revised edition in 1998 removed the word *new* from the subtitle.[8] As this history of titles indicates, over a period of 35 years of publication (now 40 years ago) only one word—*morality*—has remained constant in the titles of Gert's theoretical masterwork.

In 2004, Gert published his *Common Morality: Deciding What to Do.*[9] This title suggests that the term *morality* may be on the way to replacement by the term *common morality*. The first appearance of the term *common morality* in the publications of the Gert group[10] (or the "Dartmouth descriptivists," as they once described themselves) known to me was published in 1995 by Gert's friend and longtime coauthor, Dan Clouser, in an article he published specifically as a criticism of my work with Childress.[11] In the same year Sissela Bok published her underappreciated book *Common Values.*[12] Childress and I had begun to use the term *common morality* in our edition published in 1994, under the influence of a 1977 book by Alan Donagan that used the language of "common morality."[13] Something seems to have been in the air around 1994 that led to the wider use of the term "common morality."[14]

THE NATURE OF THE COMMON MORALITY

Gert and I both understand the common morality as universal morality.[15] It is not relative to cultures or individuals and is to be distinguished from norms that bind only members of special groups such as cultures, religions, or professional associations. All persons committed to morality accept its core moral norms. They know not to lie, not to steal others' property, not to kill or incapacitate innocent persons, to keep promises, to respect the rights and liberties of others, and the like.

Gert views the nature and number of the rules in the common morality as precisely determinable,[16] whereas I regard these matters as less than precisely determinable. I will not address this issue, but I note that it is of the highest importance in the interpretation of Gert's writings that we not concentrate excessively on the moral rules. "Morality" references the entire "moral system" for him. His full system includes moral rules, moral ideals, and a two-step procedure for determining when a violation is justified. An undue emphasis on rules can cause neglect of the full system, which in turn can cause us to misunderstand how Gert views the common morality and to interpret him as having an unduly narrow moral theory. When he says that the "phrase 'moral system' . . . has the same meaning as 'morality,'"[17] he means that "morality" includes the full spread of shared moral norms, whether or not they are norms of moral obligation.

THE JUSTIFICATION OF CLAIMS ABOUT THE COMMON MORALITY

I come now to my main question: Which types of justification of the common morality may be offered, and for which types of claims about the common morality are they suitable?

I distinguish three types, or strategies, of justification: (1) normative theoretical justification of the sort found in ethical theories; (2) normative conceptual justification that rests on conceptual analysis; and (3) empirical justification reached through empirical research. I do not claim that each each of these strategies of justification justifies the same conclusion or set of conclusions about the common morality, nor do I claim to produce here a justification that uses any of the three strategies. Rather, my limited aim is to identify three available types of justification. In bringing empirical justification into this picture, I obviously must distinguish justification of norms of the common morality (Gert's principal project) from justification of claims that there is a universally shared common morality (which is, as yet, of little or no interest to Gert).[18]

NORMATIVE THEORETICAL JUSTIFICATION

Gert has argued convincingly that the norms of the common morality can be justified by a moral theory. This is not to say that he has convinced me of the rightness of his moral theory in particular. I mean that he has shown that an ethical theory can be put to the work of justifying the norms of the common morality. In his theory common morality is justified on the basis of rationality. To justify morality, one must show that it is a public system that all rational persons would accept as universally valid. Gert regards it as clear to all rational persons that we should not act irrationally because irrational actions are those that should not be performed:

Rational persons want to avoid death, pain, disability, loss of freedom, and loss of pleasure, and they know not only that they are fallible and vulnerable but that they can be deceived and harmed by other people. They know that if people do not act morally with regard to them, they will be at significantly increased risk of suffering some harm. If they use only rationally required beliefs, it would be irrational not to endorse common morality as the system to be adopted to govern the behavior of all moral agents.[19]

Acting irrationally has a close relationship to acting in ways that will increase the likelihood of certain basic harms, and Gert argues that moral rules have the goal of prohibiting the causing of these harms or contributing to conditions that may cause them.[20]

Ethical theories other than Gert's could be employed to justify the common morality. Gert himself often suggests that Hobbes and Kant more or less had this strategy in mind,[21] and he has commented that, "Like Mill, most moral philosophers begin by trying to see what support, if any, can be given to common morality."[22] I have previously used a form of pragmatism to illustrate a type of theory that is particularly suited to serve this purpose; this theory also has similarities to Gert's conception of the goals of morality.[23] Pragmatic justification holds that moral norms are justified by their effectiveness in achieving the object of morality. In its most general formulation, pragmatic justification can be used to justify a wide array of types of norms, not merely *moral* norms: Once an operative purpose or objective of an institution or system of thought has been identified, a set of standards is considered most suitable, and therefore is vindicated, if it can be shown to be better for reaching the identified objectives than any alternative set of standards.[24] I am not altogether endorsing pragmatic justification. I am maintaining that pragmatic justification is positioned to provide a theoretical justification of the common morality that has similarities to Gert's recent statements about justification.

Notably close to Gert's formulation of the goal of morality is the pragmatist starting point that I call, using G. J. Warnock's term, "the object of morality." Gert likely would regard such pragmatic justification as threatening the secure status of the privileged norms of common morality and as introducing too much contingency into the system of basic norms and ideals of morality. He would be concerned that the theory would justify a set of norms other than those of the common morality, much as utilitarianism does. Nonetheless, Gert's description of the goal of morality is conspicuously similar to the starting point that I am proposing for pragmatic justification. Gert has consistently argued that morality's goal is the lessening of evil or harm and has insisted that this goal is a major characteristic of morality.[25] While only slightly modifying this account of the goal of morality, a pragmatist can conceive the goal as that of promoting human flourishing by counteracting conditions that cause the quality of people's lives to worsen. The goal is to prevent or limit problems of indifference, conflict, suffering, hostility, scarce resources, limited information, and the like. We have learned from centuries of experience that the human condition tends to deteriorate into misery, confusion, violence, and distrust unless norms of the common morality are enforced through what Gert calls an informal public system—that is, a public normative system which, by not having authoritative judges and formal decision procedures, is structured informally.[26] When complied with, these norms lessen human misery, foster cooperation, and promote human flourishing. Such norms may not be necessary for the *survival* of a society, as some have maintained,[27] but it is reasonable to claim that they are necessary to ameliorate the tendencies for the quality of people's lives to worsen and for the disintegration of social relationships. This formulation of the object of morality bears a closer resemblance to Warnock's theory than to Gert's,[28] but Gert's formulations are similar to my formulations, and we are both indebted to elements of Hobbes's theory, especially his accounts of human nature and the human condition.

In the pragmatist theory as I conceive it, the norms of morality are those the evidence indicates best serve the object of morality. That is, once the object of morality has been identified, a set of standards is pragmatically justified if and only if it is the best means to the end identified when all factors—including human limitations, shortcomings, and vulnerabilities—are taken into consideration. If one set of norms will better serve the object of morality than a set currently in place, then the former should displace the latter. It is here that Gert will see pragmatic justification as giving only contingent support to moral rules. I will not now pursue this problem, but later I will discuss the contingency of moral norms in general and whether it is plausible to believe that there are good candidates to displace what Gert and I consider to be the norms of the common morality.

In other publications I have supported the method of reflective equilibrium as a valid form of justification. It might seem inconsistent that I do not call on it in the present discussion of justification in ethics. However, reflective equilibrium theory is not a candidate for justifying the common morality. Reflective equilibrium needs the common morality to get off the ground, and so is in no position to offer a justification of it. It would obviously be circular to use the norms of the common morality to justify the norms of the common morality. Rawls says that reflective equilibrium begins with considered judgments, none of which is foundational and all of which are provisionally fixed points, subject to emendation or even elimination. Rawls uses this term to refer to "judgments in which our moral capacities are most likely to be displayed without distortion."[29] My view is that the norms of the common morality *are* considered judgments and are most unlikely to be subject to alteration by reflective equilibrium.[30]

Another problem of circularity also deserves a brief comment. It might be argued that ethical theories cannot provide a noncircular justification of the common morality because they presuppose the same norms the theory is presumed to justify, just as reflective equilibrium does. Here the question is, "How can a theory of morality proceed without presuming morality?" However, this objection is not relevant to what Gert and I have proposed. Gert's theory of rational justification does not presuppose particular norms of the common morality, nor does the pragmatic justification that I have sketched. In pragmatic justification, many norms could qualify as justified norms of morality, and it could turn out that there is no single justified morality. That is, there might be no common morality at all.

NORMATIVE CONCEPTUAL JUSTIFICATION

Now I come to a thornier issue: Can the norms of the common morality be justified by analysis of the *concept* of morality? The problem originates in the looseness of the ordinary-language use of the term *morality* and a lack of clarity in the way philosophers commonly employ the term. To shed light on the meaning of "morality," Gert provides an instructive distinction, which I will here adopt. He distinguishes between the *descriptive* and the *normative* senses of the term. The descriptive sense has no implications for how persons *should* behave, whereas the normative sense determines that some behaviors are immoral and others morally required.[31]

Morality in the Descriptive Sense

In the descriptive sense, "morality" refers to a group's code of conduct, or perhaps to important beliefs and attitudes of individuals. In this sense moralities can differ extensively in the content of beliefs and in practice standards. One society might emphasize the liberty of individuals, while another emphasizes the sanctity of human and animal life. Rituals may be established in one society, but disavowed in another. What is immoral in one society may be condoned, or even deemed morally required, in another.

"Morality" in the descriptive sense needs no further examination here, because it will not help us in identifying types of justification of the norms of the common morality. However, I will return in my final section to ways in which social scientists interested in descriptive morality can constructively investigate whether a common morality exists and can provide empirical justification of their findings.

Morality in the Normative Sense

Gert writes that, "'Natural law' theories of morality . . . claim that morality applies to all . . . persons, not only those now living, but also those who lived in the past. These are *not empirical* claims about morality; they are claims about *what is essential* to morality, or about *what is meant* by 'morality' when it is used normatively."[32] These claims are conceptual. Gert seeks the substantive norms that constitute the common morality and are essential to the concept of morality. He sometimes presents the questions as definitional, rather than conceptual and justificatory, but I will not address these distinctions.

Moral pluralists claim that there are multiple concepts of morality in the normative sense, but moral pluralism is a group-relative notion best interpreted as a version of descriptive morality. It would be incoherent to formulate the normative meaning of the term *morality* as composed of the norms of multiple moralities, because contradictory advice would be given. One could deny that the term is univocal and then formulate two or more normative senses (ns_1, ns_2, etc.), each with a different set of substantive norms, just as we can distinguish descriptive and normative senses. However, this maneuver is again the functional equivalent of analyzing morality descriptively rather than normatively. Accordingly, I will not further pursue conceptual pluralism.

Gert's natural law approach enables him to connect his views, as he should, to traditional theories that take a universal normative approach. His personal inspiration is Hobbes, but other philosophers serve just as well. For example, Locke seems a perfect fit for Gert when he writes that "the law of nature [is] plain and intelligible to all rational creatures, yet men [when] biassed by their interest, as well as ignorant for want of studying it, are not apt to allow of it as a law binding to them in . . . their particular cases."[33]

Extensive discussion of Gert's views about the essential normative content of morality is beyond the scope of this paper, but a brief observation will serve to situate his account as conceptual in nature. In the 2005 revised edition of his masterwork, Gert has brought part-and-chapter divisions to his book for the first time in 35 years. Part I, which contains six chapters, is titled "Conceptual Foundations." This part, when joined with his *Stanford Encyclopedia* article, shows that he conceives his work as conceptual: The project is a conceptual analysis of "morality" in the normative sense. Part II, "The Moral System and Its Justification," provides Gert's justification of the common morality and is an example of what I earlier discussed as normative theoretical justification. It might seem that Gert here presents a moral justification of his normative theory, but this is not his stated goal. He says that he offers a justification of a public system of morality that applies to all moral agents.[34]

Gert's work in the early chapters is a wide-ranging conceptual analysis of morality in the normative sense, but his work can be misunderstood because of its movement between the language of the *conceptual analysis* of morality and that of the *nature* of morality. There also may be unclarity as the language shifts between "morality," the "concept of morality," and a "theory of morality." However, I will here be satisfied to agree with Gert that there is a concept of "morality" in the normative sense and that its analysis requires the provision of specific normative content in the form of rules and ideals.

Nonetheless, I worry that what Gert claims to discover in the concept of morality reduces it, more than he acknowledges, to the normative content of his ethical theory and to certain presumptions he makes about the nature of the common morality. He denies it, however, and adds the following perceptive observation:

> The differences in content among those philosophers who use "morality" to refer to a universal guide that all rational persons would put forward for governing the behavior of all moral agents are less significant than their similarities. For all of these philosophers, such as Kurt Baier, Philippa Foot, and Geoffrey Warnock, morality prohibits actions such as killing, causing pain, deceiving, and breaking promises. . . . As Hobbes said in both *Leviathan* and *De Cive* morality is concerned with promoting people living together in peace and harmony, not causing harm to others, and helping them. . . . The differences among those philosophers who hold that there is a universal morality are primarily about the foundation of morality, not about its content.[35]

This passage correctly acknowledges that many philosophers with different conceptions of the theoretical justification of universal morality largely agree on the general norms that comprise morality in the normative sense, even though they may disagree on justified exceptions to those norms. Put another way, philosophers converge on the principles, rights, and responsibilities that are essential to morality, and in doing so converge on essential conditions of the concept of morality.[36] They also agree on paradigm cases such as the judgment that rules legitimizing the slave trade are unacceptable independent of any cultural framing of ethics and independent of any framework of law, whether past or present, national or international. Slavery is inconsistent with morality, and rights against being treated as a slave are cross-culturally valid. As Locke's comment implies, it is plain to any reasonable person who turns attention to the notion of morals that slavery is morally wrong and inconsistent with "morality" in the normative sense. I understand Gert to stand in this tradition of moral philosophy, and I locate myself there as well.

The Definition of Morality

How, then, shall we define the term *morality* in the normative sense? Gert proposes the following definition: "Morality is an informal public system applying to all rational persons, governing behavior that affects others, and has the lessening of evil or harm as its goal."[37] This definition is acceptable for the most part, but I prefer to modify it slightly. Instead of "all rational persons," I prefer "all persons capable of moral agency" (a formulation Gert himself sometimes uses[38]); and instead of "lessening of," I prefer to be specific about whether "lessening of" is restricted to "not causing" harm or is a broader notion. Gert acknowledges that his notion of "lessening" (which is not the term he always uses to express his views on this subject[39]) is controversial: "The final characteristic of morality—that it has the lessening of evil or harm as its goal—is also somewhat controversial.... [But] even those precepts that require or encourage positive action, such as helping the needy, are almost always related to *preventing or relieving* harms."[40]

This formulation in terms of preventing or relieving is an important clarification of his views, as is the previously quoted description Gert offers when mentioning Hobbes ("morality is concerned with promoting people living together in peace and harmony, not causing harm to others, *and helping them*"). Gert seems to have eased up on his nonmaleficence-oriented conception of the moral rules at the heart of the content of "morality" in the normative sense, though his theory has never been narrowly nonmaleficence-oriented in the content of the moral ideals. In his article on the "Definition of Morality" and in recent book revisions, he implies, however guardedly, that we can set aside disputes about whether nonmaleficence shades into beneficence.[41] Gert is, in my judgment, now well positioned to work out any looming inconsistency or narrowness in his earlier work by using his distinction between the moral ideals and the moral rules.

Gert and I are agreed that the concept of morality will not be analyzed appropriately unless there is a delineation of the particular set of substantive norms that are essential to morality. Philosophers who attempt to analyze the concept of morality exhaustively in terms of formal or nonsubstantive conditions will miss what is most important. Examples are theories that analyze morality in terms of (1) norms that are regarded as supremely authoritative and of overriding social importance; (2) norms that are prescriptive in form (i.e., action-guiding imperatives that do not describe states of affairs); or (3) norms that harmonize pro and con interests.[42] These once popular approaches to the definition of morality— possibly the received approach in moral philosophy—are ways of investigating how conceptually, we can identify something as a morality. They are appropriate and useful in the context of the study of morality in the descriptive sense; but, by design, these accounts do not address whether there is a specific normative content that is privileged and constitutive of morality.

My work, and Gert's, would probably be improved by making it clear that the conceptually privileged content of morality in the normative sense entails that certain moral norms that are discovered through work in descriptive ethics are conceptual errors and are necessarily false (which is not to say they are absolute rather than prima facie). For example, it is a conceptual mistake, when using morality in the normative sense, to assert that morality allows persons to trade in slaves. The proposition that the slave trade is permissible might be true of the morality of certain groups when "morality" is used in the descriptive sense, but it is conceptually incorrect when speaking of morality in the normative sense. Similarly, the proposition that "lying is morally permissible" is necessarily false; it contradicts the norm "lying is not morally permissible," which is a conceptually privileged norm in "morality" in the normative sense. "Lying is morally permissible" is not necessarily false when using "morality" in the descriptive sense, but it is necessarily false in the normative sense.

Similarly, it is inconceivable that a person who rejects the principle of nonmaleficence, or who makes vices into virtues and virtues into vices, has coherent moral beliefs in the normative sense of morality, even if he or she has a self-perception of embracing morality. Morality in the normative sense has here been stretched beyond its conceptual boundaries. Similarly, its boundaries are exceeded if one asserts that a good mariner is necessarily a morally good person or that all judgments about good tennis are moral judgments. Some sort of conceptual confusion is at work. However, I will not further address ideas about the methods of analysis that might be used to investigate the concept of morality.

I conclude this section by returning to the definition of morality in the normative sense. As noted earlier, Gert states, as a definition, that "Morality is an informal public system applying to all rational persons, governing behavior that affects others, and has the lessening of evil or harm as its goal." I have proposed modifications, and, accordingly, recommend the following formulation, which follows Gert's wording as far as my own analysis allows: Morality in the normative sense is a single informal public system of norms with authority to guide the actions of all persons capable of moral agency in their behavior that affects others; its goal is to prevent or limit problems of indifference, conflict, hostility, vulnerability, scarce resources, and the like. This definition is reasonably consistent with Gert's recent formulations and explanations using the language of lessening.[43]

This definition does not provide a full conceptual analysis of morality in the normative sense. I have not provided such an analysis, whereas Gert has attempted to do so. Whether he has done so successfully will depend on a close assessment of his work in Part I of *Morality: Its Nature and Justification*.

Conceptual Change

My suggestions so far leave unresolved whether it is possible for conceptually privileged norms of morality to change, in which case it could not be claimed that there is a conceptually essential body of norms constituting morality in the normative sense. If norms are not fixed, then they could evolve into different norms, thereby altering the concept of morality in the normative sense. In Gert's theory, change cannot occur in the norms of morality because the basic moral rules are essential and not time bound: "A *general* moral rule concerns actions open to all rational persons in all societies at all times. . . . A general moral rule is unchanging and unchangeable; discovered rather than invented. . . . Since general moral rules apply to all rational persons at all times, obviously they cannot be invented, or changed, or subject to the will of anyone."[44] But is Gert correct in this assessment?

To the extent that we can envisage circumstances in which human society is better served by substantively modifying or abandoning a norm in the common morality, change could in principle occur and could be justified under the account of pragmatic justification that I earlier sketched. It is conceivable, for example, that the rule that we are obligated to tell the truth could become sufficiently dangerous that we would abandon the rule of truth telling altogether. However unlikely, the possibility of such change might be taken to weaken the claim that there is a *common* morality with essential conditions and that holds a timeless normative authority for all moral agents.

It is easy to see that morality in the descriptive sense has changed and continues to change, but it is not clear whether such change actually might occur in morality in the normative sense. It would be dogmatic to assert without argument that the privileged norms of "morality" in the normative sense cannot change, but it is difficult to construct a historical example of a basic moral norm that has been valid for a limited duration and was dropped because some good moral reason was found for its displacement. No evidence known to me suggests that societies have handled moral problems by either rejecting or altering basic norms in the common morality. As circumstances change, we find moral reasons for saying that there are valid *exceptions* to a norm or new *specifications* of it, but we do not discard basic norms.

Nonetheless, I do not conclude, as Gert does, that morality in the normative sense is a web of norms so fixed that those norms *cannot* be altered, no matter the circumstances. It is not difficult to envision a situation in which a rule might be *added* to the common morality, by contrast to rules being abandoned or swapped out. For example, the common morality could be expanded to include a basic rule of equal moral consideration (or nondiscrimination), and inclusion of such a rule could constitute a substantial change in the common morality.[45] I am assuming that a rule of equal moral consideration is not a basic rule in the common morality. There lurks here the problem that rules of nondiscrimination are similar to antislavery rules: Historically neither has been socially sanctioned in most societies for everyone in those societies. Slavery, like other forms of discrimination, and in every society in which slavery abounds, has always involved scope questions about which group is protected by the rules of morality. I do not believe that the common morality has ever addressed the question of precisely who is protected. However, this issue about scope questions would distract from the current argument and I put it aside here.[46]

My ideas about the pragmatic justification of moral norms clearly suggest that, were human nature or human social conditions to be altered sufficiently, a change of moral rules to accommodate these changes might be justified. Gert rejects this possibility, but perhaps without a full consideration of the range of possible changes that might occur. It should be apparent by now that I find Gert's thesis that the norms of morality are atemporally fixed to be an overly demanding conceptual condition of morality in the normative sense. A less demanding condition, and one I think more plausible, is that there is a body of basic moral norms that distinguish universal morality, or the common morality, from particular moralities. Particular moralities certainly change, but even universal morality allows for the possibility of conceptual change. At the same time, it is empirically unlikely that there will be shifts in universal morality, and for this reason it is unlikely that the normative concept of morality will undergo change.

Any philosopher's position on these questions is sure to be influenced by his or her more general theoretical commitments. My defense of the possibility of moral change is facilitated by the fact that I appeal to pragmatic justification: If contexts shift sufficiently, new norms may be required to improve protections from harm. Gert is not committed to pragmatic justification or to social contingencies as important considerations, and his commitments take him down a different path. From this perspective I cannot be said to have shown that his views are not correct, and such an argument is more than I will undertake here.

EMPIRICAL JUSTIFICATION

I move on now to the third type, or strategy, of justification. Some have opined that, as Gert and I conceive it, "common morality theory is empirical in nature."[47] But are questions about the common morality empirical matters? And what might it mean to say that there could be an empirical justification of the claim that a common morality exists?

As far as I can determine, no empirical studies throw into question whether some cultural moralities accept, whereas others reject, what Gert and I describe as the norms of the common morality. Existing empirical data are, of course, from studies of moralities in the descriptive sense. These empirical investigations have studied differences in the way rules of the common morality have become embedded and applied in cultures and organizations, but they more assume than investigate what Gert and I have in mind when we speak of the common morality. Empirical studies succeed in showing cultural differences in the interpretation and specification of moral norms, but they do not show whether cultures accept, ignore, abandon, or reject the standards of the common morality. For example, empirical studies have not tested whether certain cultural moralities reject rules against theft, promise breaking, or killing. Instead, investigators study the conditions under which these acts are judged to occur in cultures, how cultures handle exceptive cases, and the like.

Nonetheless, facts about moralities in cultures and the morality held (or not held) in common are important for philosophers interested in the common morality, and they are more important for Gert's claims about the common morality than he acknowledges. He says that "Every person subject to moral judgment knows what kinds of actions morality prohibits, requires, discourages, encourages, and allows."[48] Gert also writes that the common morality exists independent of a moral theory,[49] that "the existence of a common morality is supported by widespread agreement on most moral matters by all moral agents,"[50] and that "I regard morality or the moral system as the system people use, often unconsciously, when they are trying to make a morally acceptable choice."[51] He argues that although societies regard morality as concerned primarily with practices that prevent or minimize harms, it is "doubtful that any actual society has a morality that contains only this feature.... Nonetheless, this feature of morality . . . is included in everything that is regarded as morality in all societies."[52] And to all of this Gert adds, "There are many religions but only one morality."[53]

These claims are empirical, not meta-ethical or normative. Gert seems to claim (1) that all rational persons know the same things about basic moral conduct, (2) that all societies have a morality oriented around the feature of avoiding and minimizing harm, and (3) that it is doubtful whether avoiding and minimizing harm are included in the full scope of what is regarded as morality in any society. Empirical investigation is needed to support these statements.[54] Otherwise, they are merely speculative generalizations drawn from anecdote, limited experience, and philosophical theories of human nature.

Despite his own apparent reliance on empirical claims, Gert has been unfriendly to the idea that important claims about the common morality rest on factual assumptions that merit empirical study. His view seems to be one of a distanced disregard of the relevance of empirical evidence. His work presumably relies exclusively on normative theoretical content and normative conceptual analysis, as informed by a theory of human nature. He seems to think that no additional form of inquiry bears on either his claims or his assumptions. Gert says:

> It is very tempting to think that I am simply starting with an account of human nature, including an account of human rationality, fallibility, and

vulnerability, and simply generating a code of conduct that all rational persons would favor adopting to guide everyone's behavior. But I am not doing this, because it would not count as *justifying morality* unless the code of conduct being justified was virtually identical to the moral system that is now implicitly used in deciding how to act morally and in making moral judgments. . . . The starting point has to be common morality.[55]

I do not disagree with this statement, but I would add to it that we are certain to encounter different conceptions of how to formulate the precise content of the common morality, including the content of what Gert calls the starting point. This formulation is not a purely philosophical matter, and I believe that empirical work could be conducted that would add additional support to a general program defending the claim that there exists a common morality of a certain sort, by contrast to the claim that there is an adequate justification of the common morality. Such empirical work has the potential to help clarify claims of the actual moral content in the common morality. Scientific studies sometimes confirm our beliefs, but at other times they upset or correct our beliefs. As things now stand, we can only create hypotheses about the proper starting point.

Oliver Rauprich has argued, I think appropriately, that common morality theory, if it is to be credible, must more carefully address empirical claims about the status of a shared morality. He proposes that studies should be designed to capture the moral beliefs that prevail in societies and that are shared by a vast majority of people. He recommends that investigators study the *extent* to which there is shared agreement. For example, he thinks we need to find out whether "shared beliefs" means that, say, "95 or even 99% of the people" share the norms.[56]

A frequent criticism of common morality theory is that anthropological and historical evidence already speak against the empirical hypothesis that a universal morality exists.[57] I earlier suggested that this thesis misconstrues the findings of historians and anthropologists. I add now that these critics of common morality theories, unlike Rauprich, seem to me unappreciative of the nuances that would surround the design of empirical research on the common morality. In principle, scientific research could either confirm or falsify the hypothesis that there exists a universal common morality containing the norms that Gert and I envisage, but, as with all empirical research, it must be stated which hypotheses are to be tested, how the inclusion/exclusion criteria for study subjects are to be formulated, and why these hypotheses and criteria were selected. To date, critics who appeal to available empirical studies as falsifying common morality claims have not attended to the specific concerns that must be addressed in the scientific investigation of hypotheses about the common morality.

What are these concerns? I have elsewhere emphasized the importance of an inclusion criterion for study subjects that would allow only persons who are committed to morality.[58] Persons not committed to morality, such as criminals and sociopaths, should be excluded because their inclusion introduces a fatal bias. When I say that some persons are not committed to morality, I do not mean that they are not dedicated to a way of life that they consider a moral way of life. However, this commitment may be no more than a set of intolerant and narrow-minded beliefs—a commitment of little interest in confirming or falsifying hypotheses about the common morality.

It would be devious of me to deny that many millions of people from many societies likely would be excluded by this criterion, which leads to its own nest of theoretical and practical problems. Here I think both philosophers and social scientists have to bite the bullet and assert that massive swaths of some societies are indeed inappropriate subjects because of their beliefs. It should not matter whether the number of persons excluded is large or small: The issue is whether inadequate impartiality or concern for others renders persons inadequate as test subjects, and I think that the answer is yes. Even if these individuals are committed religious persons of emulable moral integrity within the framework of their beliefs—for example, certain Christian, Jewish, or Muslim fundamentalists—they may not have a proper impartiality and concern for the welfare of others beyond their affiliations.

The main hypothesis that I propose be empirically tested is this: All persons *committed to morality and to impartial moral judgment in their moral assessments* adhere to the norms in what Gert and I have called the common morality. The persons to be included in the study, with other potential subjects excluded, are (1) persons who pass a rigorous test of whether their beliefs conform to some critical component feature of the normative sense of morality (with this feature to be designated in the study design); and (2) persons who qualify as having the ability to take an impartial moral point of view.

It would be difficult, but not impossible, to design this study without either missing the target—namely, the beliefs of all and only those who are committed to both *morality* and *impartiality*—or begging the question by insisting on studying only persons known to accept what Gert and I call morality in the normative sense. The question could be begged either by (1) designing the study so that the only persons who are included as subjects are those who already have precisely the commitments and beliefs the investigator is testing for or (2) designing the study so that all persons are tested whether or not they are committed to morality and impartiality. The first design biases the study in favor of the hypothesis that there exists a common morality. The second design biases the study against the hypothesis.

These problems of potential bias and circularity can be controlled through proper research design. It is reasonable to require, for example, that study subjects believe in impartial application of a general principle of nonmaleficence. Acceptance of this principle would serve as an inclusion criterion, and nonacceptance an exclusion criterion. It is unimaginable that a morally committed person would not take this principle seriously. This choice of a single general moral norm does not bias the study by preselecting study subjects for the norms Gert and I judge to constitute the common morality. Study subjects would not be screened for any norms other than nonmaleficence and impartiality. The purpose of the study is to determine the extent to which cultural or individual differences emerge, or do not emerge, in study subjects over a wide range of basic norms other than nonmaleficence and impartiality, such as respect for autonomy, keeping promises, helping disabled persons, and not punishing the innocent. The design of the study is not biased because these norms are not entailed by, or an intrinsic part of, the principle of nonmaleficence or a requirement of impartiality.

Should it turn out that the persons studied do not share one or more of the norms that Gert or I hypothesize to comprise the common morality, this result would show that study subjects have different conceptions about either the content of morality or the concept of morality in the normative sense than those that Gert or I have hypothesized. The study might even show that there is no common morality or no concept of morality of the sort we claim. More optimistically, if the norms that Gert and I hypothesize to constitute morality in the normative sense were found to be shared by study subjects selected from a broad array of cultures, this finding would constitute good initial evidence of the existence of the common morality, though the study would undoubtedly need to be replicated.

No matter how careful in design, a single study is not likely to give us a complete picture. Moreover, the results will likely not come packaged in the distilled form a philosopher might prefer. It should be no surprise if an empirical study of fundamental moral norms does not turn up exactly the same norms and conclusions found in a conceptual analysis of fundamental moral norms in philosophy. Conceptual analysis does not have to confront the complicated web of moral beliefs found in social moralities, not to mention differences in individual beliefs. Conceptual analysis and empirical investigation are such different tools that they are likely to identify or discover somewhat different features in the landscape of morals.

I have not claimed in this final section that *empirical confirmation* of the hypothesis that there exists a common morality would constitute a *normative justification* of the norms of the common morality, and I leave open whether, if the common morality were found to exist, investigators would thereby be able to establish its normative content. A well-designed empirical study has the potential to justify or falsify the claim that some form of common morality exists, but it would probably not discover every feature of the common morality. Still, empirical study stands to inform us in the work of philosophical ethics, and we ignore it at our peril.

CONCLUSION

In this essay I have tried to show that three types or strategies of justification of claims about the common morality can be identified. My goal has been to classify and provide a limited defense of the three methods. I have not offered a justification of the common morality that satisfies the conditions of any of the three forms, nor have I shown that Gert's work is fatally flawed. Indeed, I have warmly supported his view that the common morality merits the most careful attention by philosophers, an attention it has rarely received, and never better than by Gert himself.

References

Ainslee, Donald C. 2002. "Bioethics and the Problem of Pluralism." *Social Philosophy and Policy* 19, 1–28.

Arras, John. 2009. "The Hedgehog and Borg: Common Morality in Bioethics." *Theoretical Medicine and Bioethics*, as published online [unpaginated]. Available at: http://www.springerlink.com/content/95x81214715395r2/.

Beauchamp, Tom L. 2003. "A Defense of the Common Morality." *Kennedy Institute of Ethics Journal* 13, 259–274.

Beauchamp, Tom L., and James F. Childress. 1st edition 1979, currently 6th edition 2009. *Principles of Biomedical Ethics.* New York: Oxford University Press.

Bok, Sissela. 1995. *Common Values.* Columbia, MO: University of Missouri Press.

Brock, Dan W. 2001. "Gert on the Limits of Morality's Requirement." *Philosophy and Phenomenological Research* 62, 435–440.

Clouser, K. Danner. 1995. "Common Morality as an Alternative to Principlism." *Kennedy Institute of Ethics Journal* 5, 219–236.

Daniels, Norman. 1979. "Wide Reflective Equilibrium and Theory Acceptance in Ethics." *Journal of Philosophy* 76, 256–282.

_____. 1996a. "Wide Reflective Equilibrium in Practice." In L. W. Sumner and J. Boyle, eds., *Philosophical Perspectives on Bioethics.* Toronto: University of Toronto Press, 96–114.

_____. 1996b. *Justice and Justification: Reflective Equilibrium in Theory and Practice.* New York: Cambridge University Press.

_____. 2003. "Reflective Equilibrium." *Stanford Encyclopedia of Philosophy.* Online, first published, April 28, 2003; accessed August 24, 2007 at http://plato.stanford.edu/entries/reflective-equilibrium/.

DeGrazia, David. 2003. "Common Morality, Coherence, and the Principles of Biomedical Ethics." *Kennedy Institute of Ethics Journal* 13, 219–230.

Donagan, Alan. 1977. *The Theory of Morality.* Chicago: University of Chicago Press.

Engelhardt, H. Tristram, Jr. 1996. *The Foundations of Bioethics.* New York: Oxford University Press.

Feigl, Herbert, 1950. "De Principiis Non Disputandum . . . ?" In Max Black, ed., *Philosophical Analysis*. Ithaca, NY: Cornell University Press, 119–156.

Frankena, William K., 1980. "What is Morality?" In his *Thinking about Morality*. Ann Arbor: University of Michigan Press, Chapter 1.

Gert, Bernard. 1970. *The Moral Rules: A New Rational Foundation for Morality*. New York: Harper and Row.

_____. 1988. *Morality: A New Justification of the Moral Rules*. New York: Oxford University Press, 1988.

_____. 1998. *Morality: Its Nature and Justification*. New York: Oxford University Press.

_____. 2001. "Reply to Dan Brock." *Philosophy and Phenomenological Research* 62, 466–470.

_____. 2004. *Common Morality: Deciding What to Do*. New York: Oxford University Press, paperback edition 2007.

_____. 2005. *Morality: Its Nature and Justification*. New York: Oxford University Press.

_____. 2008. "The Definition of Morality." *The Stanford Encyclopedia of Philosophy*. First published Wed. April 17, 2002; here using the substantive revision of Mon. Feb. 11, 2008. Pages in this article are determined by a file downloaded from the Stanford site, as accessed March 15, 2009: http://plato.stanford.edu/entries/morality-definition/.

Gert, Bernard, and K. Danner Clouser. 1990. "A Critique of Principlism." *Journal of Medicine and Philosophy* 15, 219–36.

_____. 1994. "Morality vs. Principlism." In *Principles of Health Care Ethics*, ed. Raanan Gillon and Ann Lloyd. London: John Wylie & Sons, 251–266.

_____. 1999. "Concerning Principlism and Its Defenders: Reply to Beauchamp and Veatch." In *Building Bioethics: Conversations with Clouser and Friends on Medical Ethics*, ed. Loretta Kopelman. Boston: Kluwer Academic, esp. 191–193.

Gert, Bernard, Charles M. Culver, and K. Danner Clouser. 1997. *Bioethics: A Return to Fundamentals*. New York: Oxford University Press.

_____. 1997. *Bioethics: A Systematic Approach*. New York: Oxford University Press, 2006.

_____. 2000. "Common Morality versus Specified Principlism: Reply to Richardson." *Journal of Medicine and Philosophy* 25, 308–322.

Gert, Bernard, Ronald M. Green, and K. Danner Clouser. 1993. "The Method of Public Morality versus the Method of Principlism." *Journal of Medicine and Philosophy* 18, 179–197.

Hartland-Swann, John. 1960. *An Analysis of Morals*. London: George Allen & Unwin.

Herissone-Kelly, Peter. 2003. "The Principlist Approach to Bioethics, and its Stormy Journey Overseas." In *Scratching the Surface of Bioethics*, ed. Matti Hayry and Tuija Takala. Amsterdam: Rodopi, 65–77.

Holm, Søren. 1994. "Not Just Autonomy—The Principles of American Biomedical Ethics." *Journal of Medical Ethics* 21, 332–338.

Lindsay, Ronald A. 2005. "Slaves, Embryos, and Nonhuman Animals: Moral Status and the Limitations of Common Morality Theory." *Kennedy Institute of Ethics Journal* 15, 323–346.

_____. 2009. "Bioethics Policies and the Compass of Common Morality." *Theoretical Medicine and Bioethics*, as published online [unpaginated] at http://www.springerlink.com/content/jhol7t2034x72744/.

Locke, John. 2006. *A Treatise Concerning the True Original Extent and End of Civil Government*, Second Treatise, Chap. 9. In *The Longman Standard History of Modern Philosophy*, ed. Daniel Kolak and Garrett Thomson. New York: Pearson Longman, 276.

Mackie, John. 1977. *Ethics: Inventing Right and Wrong*. London: Penguin.

Rauprich, Oliver. 2008. "Common Morality: Comment on Beauchamp and Childress." *Theoretical Medicine and Bioethics* 29, 43–71.

Rawls, John. 1971. *A Theory of Justice*. Cambridge, MA: Harvard University Press; revised edition, 1999.

———. 1996. *Political Liberalism*. New York: Columbia University Press.

Richardson, Henry S. 1990. "Specifying Norms as a Way to Resolve Concrete Ethical Problems," *Philosophy and Public Affairs* 19, 279–310.

Ross, W. D. 1939. *The Foundations of Ethics*. Oxford: Oxford University Press.

Salmon, Wesley. 1966. *The Foundations of Scientific Inference*. Pittsburgh, PA: University of Pittsburgh Press.

Strong, Carson. 2009. "Exploring Questions about Common Morality." *Theoretical Medicine and Bioethics*, as published online [unpaginated], section entitled "Objections to Common Morality." Available at http://www.springerlink.com/content/tk66rojwou061804/.

Turner, Leigh. 1998. "An Anthropological Exploration of Contemporary Bioethics: The Varieties of Common Sense." *Journal of Medical Ethics* 24, 127–133.

———. 2003. "Zones of Consensus and Zones of Conflict: Questioning the 'Common Morality' Presumption in Bioethics." *Kennedy Institute of Ethics Journal* 13, 193–218.

Wallace, Gerald, and A. D. M. Walker. 1970. *The Definition of Morality*. London: Methuen & Co., Ltd.

Wallace, K. A. 2009. "Common Morality and Moral Reform." *Theoretical Medicine and Bioethics*, published online [unpaginated], section on "Pragmatic Common Morality and Moral Reform." Available at: http://www.springerlink.com/content/h6529372046v5220/.

Warnock, G. J. 1971. *The Object of Morality*. London: Methuen & Co.

Notes

1. K. Danner Clouser and Bernard Gert (1990); Ronald M. Green, Gert, and Clouser (1993); and Clouser and Gert (1994).

2. Tom L. Beauchamp and James F. Childress (1979, as in the 6th edition 2009).

3. Good examples are John Arras (2009), Oliver Rauprich (2008), Peter Herissone-Kelly (2003), and Søren Holm (1994). Other skeptical appraisals are given by H. Tristram Engelhardt, Jr. (1996) and David DeGrazia (2003).

4. Norman Daniels (1979); Daniels (1996a); Daniels (1996b); and Daniels, *Stanford Encyclopedia* (online, first published, April 28, 2003; accessed Aug. 24, 2007).

5. Gert rejects reflective equilibrium altogether—see Gert (2005), 380–381—whereas I accept it for certain types of justification. See Beauchamp and Childress (2009), 381–387.

6. Gert (1970).

7. Gert (1988).

8. Gert (1998). Gert at last has a title not in need of revision, and the title, *Morality: Its Nature and Justification*, is retained seven years afterward in the next edition (2005).

9. Gert (2004, paperback edition 2007). Gert (2005, vii) describes this common morality book as "a short version of my theory."

10. Gert and Clouser published, with Charles M. Culver (1997), a sustained criticism of views that Childress and I had developed. This criticism is carried into the second edition of the work (2006). See also Gert, Culver, and Clouser (2000); and Gert and Clouser (1999).

11. Clouser (1995). Clouser's article was a later version of lecture delivered on March 6, 1994, at the Kennedy Institute of Ethics, Georgetown University. In this lecture he did not use the language of "common morality"—thus suggesting that the mid-1994 to early-1995 period was pivotal for the change of language used by both Clouser and Gert.

12. Sissela Bok (1995).

13. Alan Donagan (1977).

14. My views on the common morality were originally formed by reflection on Donagan's book (1977). He had a distinct view of the common morality as heavily informed by Kantian and Judeo-Christian thought—more of a western common morality theory than a universal account. In retrospect I would have profited at the time more by a careful assessment of Gert's account of morality. My views wound up considerably closer to Gert's, and I came to regard his theory as far superior to Donagan's.

15. Although there is only one universal common morality, there is more than one *theory* of the common morality. For a variety of theories, see Donagan (1977); Gert (2004, paperback edition 2007); Beauchamp and Childress (2009); and W. D. Ross (1939).

16. Gert readily acknowledges disagreement among philosophers on the point and says that there is not even "complete agreement concerning what counts as a moral rule." Gert (2005), 13.

17. Gert (2005), 3; and see 159–161, 246–247.

18. I am indebted for my own views to Gert's books and especially to his extensive article in the *Stanford Encyclopedia* on the definition of morality (2008). The 2005 revision of Gert's masterwork covers the subject of "The Definition of Morality" in a single page (13–14, but see also the preparatory work on p. 10).

19. Gert (2004, paperback 2007), 84.

20. Gert (2005), 29–33, 39–41, 181.

21. Gert (2005, 6) contains a more critical view of Hobbes, Kant, and Mill, who "provide only a schema of the moral system" (not an "adequate account").

22. Gert (2005), 18; (1998), 18.

23. Beauchamp (2003), 259–274. See also Rauprich (2008), 68; and K. A. Wallace (online 10 Feb. 2009), section on "Pragmatic Common Morality and Moral Reform."

24. This particular formulation is indebted to Herbert Feigl (1950), 119–156; and Wesley Salmon (1966).

25. Gert (2005), 13, 109, 246.

26. Gert (2005), 11–14.

27. See the sources referenced in Bok (1995), 13–23, 50–59 (citing several influential writers on the subject).

28. G. J. Warnock (1971), esp. 15–26; also John Mackie (1977). I am indebted to both.

29. John Rawls (1971), esp. 1971, 20ff, 46–50, 579–580 (revised edition, 1999, 17ff, 40–45, 508–509). See also Rawls's comments on reflective equilibrium in his later book (1996), esp. 8, 381, 384, and 399.

30. My view is that the norms are most plausibly understood as subject to what I call, following Henry Richardson, *specification*—that is, the process of reducing the indeterminate character of abstract norms and generating more specific action-guiding content. Though constrained by standards of reflective equilibrium, specification is not identical to reflective equilibrium. See Richardson (1990), 279–310.

31. Gert (2008), 2.

32. Gert (2008), 8 (italics added).

33. John Locke (2006), 276 (chap. 9.124).

34. Gert (2005), 7, 11–13, 219; Gert (1998), 160.

35. Gert (2008), 9.

36. Cf. Beauchamp and Childress (2009), 260–261, 361–363.

37. Gert (2005), 14.

38. Gert says that, "To say that moral rules apply to all moral agents means essentially the same as to say that they apply to all rational persons" (2005, 112). In his *Stanford Encyclopedia* article (2008, 11), he writes that "Since the normative sense of 'morality' refers to a universal guide to behavior that all rational persons would put forward for governing the behavior of all moral agents, it is important to provide at least a brief account of what is meant by 'rational person.' In this context, 'rational person' is synonymous with 'moral agent' and refers to those persons to whom morality applies. This includes all normal adults with sufficient knowledge and intelligence to understand what kinds of actions morality prohibits, requires, discourages, encourages, and allows, and with sufficient volitional ability to use morality as a guide for their behavior." See further Gert (2005), 23, 136–147.

39. For example, see Gert (2004, paperback 2007), 7; and Gert, Culver, and Clouser (1997), 7 ("the purpose of morality is to minimize the amount of evil or harm suffered by those protected by morality"), and see also 62–68; Gert, Culver, and Clouser (2006), 89–93; and Gert (2005), 17, 124–128.

40. Gert (2008), 13 (italics added here and in the paragraph following). In explicating the normative sense of "morality," Gert writes as follows (12): "That morality is a public system does not mean that everyone always agrees on all of their moral judgments, but only that all disagreements occur within a framework of agreement."

41. For Gert's tough line on confining moral obligation to the scope of a principle of nonmaleficence, see Gert, Culver, and Clouser (1997), 7–8; and (2006), 11–13. For some problems with Gert's views and some concession on Gert's part, see Dan W. Brock (2001), 435–440; and Gert, "Reply to Dan Brock" (2001), 466–470.

42. Such a philosophical analysis is advanced in John Hartland-Swann (1960) and pursued in various articles in Gerald Wallace and A. D. M. Walker (1970), and also William K. Frankena (1980).

43. Gert (2008), 13.

44. Gert (2005), 114–115. For more on the thesis that morality is unchanging, see Gert, Culver, and Clouser (2006), 104.

45. Compare Ronald A. Lindsay (2005), 323–346.

46. I deal with this question in Beauchamp (2003).

47. Herissone-Kelly (2003), 65–77; and similarly Lindsay (2009), first section.

48. Gert, Culver, and Clouser (2003), 310.

49. Gert, *Common Morality* (2004, paperback edition 2007), v.

50. Gert, *Common Morality* (2004, paperback edition 2007), 8.

51. Gert (2005), 3.

52. Gert (2008), 4.

53. Gert (2005), 6.

54. Arras's critique turns on Gert's failure to deal adequately with questions of empirical evidence and with whether it bears on his claims about morality. See "The Hedgehog and the Borg" (2009), in the subsection "What is Common Morality?"

55. Gert (2005), 3.

56. Rauprich (2008), 47.

57. See Leigh Turner (2003); Turner (1998); Donald C. Ainslee (2002); Carson Strong (2009), section entitled "Objections to Common Morality"; David DeGrazia (2003).

58. Beauchamp and Childress (2009), 392–394.

12

ON ELIMINATING THE DISTINCTION BETWEEN APPLIED ETHICS AND ETHICAL THEORY

"Applied ethics" has been a major growth area in North American philosophy in recent years, yet robust confidence and enthusiasm over its promise are far from universal in academic philosophy. It is considered nonphilosophical in Germany, and has largely failed to penetrate British departments of philosophy. Whether it has any intellectually or pedagogically redeeming value is still widely debated in North America, where many who have tried to teach some area of applied ethics for the first time have seen their courses grind to a halt in irresolvable quandaries, practical exigencies, or unavailable technical information. Consequently, some departments are at war over whether to hire or confer tenure on those who teach these subjects. Many also remain unconvinced that philosophical generalizations or theories can play any significant role in practical contexts. They even doubt both that applied ethics is truly philosophical ethics and that philosophy should accommodate this blossoming field in its curriculum.

Against the skeptical side of these opinions, I argue that no significant differences distinguish ethical theory and applied ethics as philosophical *activities* or *methods*. Philosophers do what they have always done since Socrates. I do not argue that there are no differences in *content*, but this basis for a distinction can be misleading because the essence of "applied ethics" is not captured by such differences. Initially I argue for eliminating the distinction between applied ethics and ethical theory. I then turn in subsequent sections to a particular method—the case method. The methodology in this method is unsettled and may be discipline specific, but it has played and will continue to play a significant pedagogical role in "applied" ethics. I argue that this method has a scholarly as well as a pedagogical value for philosophy and that the method can be used to enhance traditional reflective uses of cases and examples in ethical theory. Ethical theory, no less than applied ethics, can be enhanced by this method.

THE STRANGE IDEA OF "APPLYING" ETHICAL THEORY

I shall not here attempt a deep conceptual analysis of "applied ethics," but a basic working understanding of the term is needed. Bernard Gert has provided a standard definition: "the application of an ethical theory to some particular moral problems or set of problems." Gert maintains that applied ethics can be concerned either with particular moral situations or with general moral problems such as those found in political theory. For both the general and the particular, ethical theory determines which facts count as morally relevant and which actions can be considered morally justified or unjustified.[1]

For reasons that will become clear, I prefer not to use the term *application*, as Gert does. While his definition is mainline, it is too restricted and does not capture significant features of applied ethics. I will use "applied ethics" more broadly to refer to the use of philosophical theory and methods of analysis to treat fundamentally moral problems in the professions, technology, public policy, and the like. Biomedical ethics, political ethics, journalistic ethics, jurisprudence, and business ethics are fertile professional areas for such philosophical activity, but "applied ethics" is not synonymous with "professional ethics" and does not necessarily require an ethical theory. Staple problems such as the allocation of scarce social resources, the entrapment of public officials, research on animals, and the confidentiality of tax information are problems beyond those of professional conduct and relationships, and they may not be best addressed by a general ethical theory.

APPLICATIONS OF CONTENT AND APPLICATIONS OF METHOD

Under this broad conception, there need not be a special philosophical *method* for applied ethics even when the work is fundamentally philosophical. Traditional conceptions of the role or activity of philosophy typically undergo no major shift to accommodate a new subject matter for philosophical reflection. New methods of normative and conceptual analysis did not emerge with the development of the philosophy of economics, for example, and nothing about our new interest in the philosophy of sociobiology requires new methods for the philosophy of science.

Applied ethics, and applied philosophy more generally, are no different. "Applied philosophers" do what philosophers have always done: They analyze concepts; submit to critical scrutiny various strategies that are used to justify beliefs, policies, and actions; examine the hidden presuppositions of various moral opinions and theories; and offer criticism and constructive accounts of the moral phenomena in question. They seek a reasoned defense of a moral viewpoint, and they use guides to duty and virtue in order to distinguish justified moral claims from unjustified ones. They try to stimulate the moral imagination of their students, promote analytical skills, and prevent the substitution of purely personal attitudes or intuitions for a reasoned and justified moral position. Prejudice, emotion, false data, false authority, and the like are weeded from the premises of arguments, and moral reasons are advanced and defended by recognizably philosophical modes of argument. Inquiry into the meta-ethics of applied ethics invites a wild goose chase if one expects to find activities different from those philosophers have pursued since Socrates submitted the great issues of his day to philosophical scrutiny.

When we turn from method to *content*, we expect and find differences. Courses in business ethics or engineering ethics vary as much in content from courses in ethical theory as courses in philosophy of sociobiology and philosophy of psychology differ from those in the philosophy of science. In each case, however, it is not an easy matter to say how or why they vary, and indeed they often do *not* vary to the degree we might anticipate. Courses in philosophy of psychology commonly begin with an introductory text in the philosophy of science, and courses in business ethics typically begin with a major section on ethical theory. Yet, as the courses proceed, differences in content from the "parent" field will emerge: The concepts analyzed will be different, the topics treated will be different, the presuppositions examined will be different, and the principles employed or investigated will vary.

Rather than analyze the word *good*, or other tasks of meta-ethics, philosophers interested in applied ethics turn their efforts to the analysis of a range of concepts including confidentiality, medicine, trade secrets, environmental responsibility, euthanasia, authority, undue influence, free press, privacy, and entrapment. But in noting these differences of content, we should note the similarities as well. Some notions on this sample list play a significant role in both applied ethics *and* ethical theory, with privacy and authority being obvious examples. In journals such as *Philosophy and Public Affairs*, no sharp line of demarcation can be drawn between ethical theory and applied ethics when such notions are examined. There is not even a discernible continuum from theoretical to applied concepts or principles. While there are discernible differences in content between ethical theory and applied ethics, it is difficult to specify the respects in which they differ.

THE IDEA OF APPLYING GENERAL AND FUNDAMENTAL PRINCIPLES

A critic might object that there are more fundamental differences of content than I have acknowledged. It seems widely presumed in contemporary ethics that the "applied" part of "applied ethics" involves the application of basic principles of ethical theory to particular moral problems, as Gert suggests. This outlook promotes the thesis that ethical theory develops *general* and *fundamental* principles, virtues, rules, and the like—the "groundwork" in the German tradition—while applied ethics treats *particular* contexts through less general, *derived* principles, virtues, rules, judgments, and the like. There is no new or special ethics (of general normative principles), but only the application of existing theories and principles to specific cases and controversies. For example, principles of the confidentiality of information in medicine, journalism, and political theory derive from more general and fundamental principles of respect for persons, promise keeping, and the like.

This thesis helps explain why some believe that applied ethics is doomed to secondary importance. They think applied work fails to treat what is basic to philosophical ethics—analysis of the most general and fundamental principles, virtues, presuppositions, and theories. The conventional wisdom behind the distinctions in analytic philosophy between normative ethical theory and applied ethics, in the Catholic tradition between general ethics and special ethics, and in the German tradition between philosophical ethics and bureaucratic application seems in each case to be that a general normative ethics collects the set of principles presupposed by or needed for application to specific moral problems such as abortion, widespread hunger, and research involving human subjects. These general principles are more *fundamental* than other principles or rules because the latter can be derived from them, while the general principles are not similarly dependent on these other sources.

Presumably, the same general principles apply across many particular contexts. If so, this is further witness to their status as fundamental. For example, one might appeal to the same set of principles of justice to examine issues of taxation, delivery of health care, criminal punishment, and reverse discrimination. Similarly, general principles of veracity apply to debates about secrecy and deception in international politics, misleading advertisements in business ethics, accurate reporting in journalistic ethics, and the disclosure of the nature and extent of an illness to a patient in medical ethics. Greater clarity about the conditions in general under which truth must be told and when it may permissibly be withheld should enhance understanding of what is required in all these areas and would help us evaluate the moral actions of persons in a broad spectrum of human activities.

Consider the example of an eight-chapter text in biomedical ethics that has the following structure: The first chapter introduces morality and ethical theory, the second chapter treats types of ethical theories, and the third through sixth chapters treat the basic moral principles of respect for autonomy, nonmaleficence, beneficence, and justice. The attempt throughout is to show how moral problems in modern medicine and biology can be analyzed by appeal to these principles as they pertain to specific problems. Many case studies and empirical studies are examined, and the basic principles are used to argue for derivative rules such as those governing valid third-party consent, permissible instances of letting die, and medical paternalism.

Although the book mentioned is one I coauthored, I reject portions of this *interpretation* of both the book and the method at work in applied ethics. This interpretation neglects, for example, the role that case studies and empirical studies play in the "derivation" of rules for biomedical ethics. The rules and judgments proposed for acceptance are hammered out in this volume through an adjustment of abstract moral principles to concrete cases and factual findings. For example, rules about the disclosure of information are developed by appeal to the principle of respect for autonomy, clinical cases of medical decision making, and empirical studies of comprehension. While principles of respect for autonomy, nonmaleficence, and beneficence all play significant roles in the justification of rules and judgments about both disclosure and nondisclosure, psychological information about and clinical experience in the practical problems of the patient–physician relationship are no less important. Paradigm cases may significantly shape rules, as may empirical studies of effective communication and legal theories of liability that govern medical malpractice.

This description is typical of applied ethics contexts: Rules are shaped by (1) moral principles, (2) empirical data, (3) paradigm cases, and (4) moral reflection on how to put (1) through (3) into the most harmonious unit. I want to be clear, however, about what I accept and what I reject in this interpretation. I *accept* the view that certain broad *fundamental* moral principles give support to numerous other principles, rules, and judgments (as part of their "foundation" or justification); but support is not entailment, and the underlying ideas of generality, application, and fundamentalness (as well as derivation) in this interpretation can lead to a view that has more falsity and misleading statement than truth and insight. Moral principles are rallying points for justification. They provide vital premises, but before we render them the queen of the applied moral sciences, we had better be sure they have the power to fulfill the assigned function.

Hegel was properly critical of Kant for developing an "empty formalism" in a theory that preached duty for duty's sake, but lacked the power to develop an "immanent doctrine of duties" or any particular duties. All "content and specification" in a living code of ethics (and reflection on it) had been replaced by abstractness.[2] Although Kant is an extreme case in moral theory, Hegel's point has force for an evaluation of the abstract principles and rules in contemporary ethical theory. They are relatively empty formalisms with little power to identify or assign specific duties in almost any context in which moral *problems* are present. Principles help us see the moral dimensions of such problems and help us get started, but they are too weakened by their abstractness to give us particular duties or to assign priorities among various assignable duties. For example, if nonmaleficence is the principle that we ought not to inflict evil or harm, this principle gives us but a weak start on the moral problem of whether active euthanasia can be morally justified; and if we question whether physicians ought to be allowed to be the *agents* of active euthanasia, we compound the problems further.

The whole of the corpus of writings of Kant, Mill, and Aristotle will not take us very far in answering such questions, even if they do provide some important insights that help us supply answers. I am not denying that principles of ethical theory can be *applied*—in, for example, the way Gert suggests. Of course they can. But they are applied as premises along with a great many other considerations; moreover, the principles and their "derivative rules" are formulated, shaped, and reshaped by the moral codes and judgments of everyday life. On this point Hegel and the pragmatists have it over Kant.[3]

Much can also be learned in these discussions by the ingenuity that has been devoted in recent epistemology to showing that foundationalist or level-derivation theories misconstrue the structure and development of human knowledge. Similar arguments could be deployed to show that morality is not structured in a layered system of principles from which other items such as rules and judgments are derived. If, as I claim, moral theories should not be modeled on geometrical systems, but rather on the sciences whose principles have been, and continue to be, shaped and modified by new data, unexpected cases and situations, predictive failures, and modified hypotheses, then we need to be very careful with the notion of *fundamental* principles and its ally *general* ethical theory, because they may do more to obscure the nature of moral thinking than to illuminate it.

Consider an example from recent philosophical literature that shows how these distinctions can prove to be more confusing than helpful. Norman Daniels has devoted a major effort to addressing problems of macroallocation and health policy, in an attempt to establish a theory of the just distribution of health care resources.[4] While he calls on Rawls at various points—the opportunity principle being especially important—Daniels goes on to argue for principles specifying resource allocation priorities and physician responsibilities that are in no respect directly derived from Rawls or from anywhere else in ethical theory. Is Daniels's effort any more or less philosophical, fundamental, theoretical, or general than Rawls's? Despite what might be called his "applications" of Rawlsian arguments and assumptions, is his work intrinsically different from Rawls's own "application" of Kant in order to develop his theory of "the basic structure"? Is Rawls an applied philosopher because he adopts parts of Kant's more general ethical theory? Both Rawls and Daniels are writing about distributive justice, developing philosophical theories, and using similar methodologies and content—all of which I would prefer to call ethical theory in each instance and be done with misleading descriptions in terms of "applied ethics."

I do not, however, want to be associated with critics[5] who have claimed that Kantian and Rawlsian theories are irrelevant to and provide no helpful background for discussion of the moral problems under investigation in areas of applied ethics. Daniels, Onora O'Neill, and others have shown by their labors that this view of Rawls and Kant is mistaken.[6] But Rawls himself has commented that his is a strict compliance and ideal theory that does not provide major applications to "pressing and urgent matters" such as regulation of the liberty of conscience, restraining violence, just war, unjust regimes, and problems of compensatory justice[7]:

> [In nonideal theory] we must ascertain how the ideal conception of justice applies, if indeed it applies at all, to cases where rather than having to make adjustments to natural limitations, we are confronted with injustice. The discussion of these problems belongs to the partial compliance part of nonideal theory. It includes, among other things, the theory of punishment and compensatory justice, just war and conscientious objection, civil disobedience and militant resistance. These are among the central issues of political life, yet so far the conception of justice as fairness does not directly apply to them.[8]

What we need at present in philosophy is a realistic estimate of the limited power of theories such as Rawls's to cultivate moral wisdom, while also appreciating—as he does—how they can help nourish more rigorous work in areas now labeled "applied."

We ought to turn our eyes in the other direction as well, as Alasdair MacIntyre and Arthur Caplan have urged.[9] Traditional ethical theory has as much to learn from "applied contexts" as the other way around, as Caplan has noted:

> There are many ways currently in vogue for constructing theories in ethics.... [Rawls's and Nozick's] are not the only starting points for moral theorizing. One might want to start with a rich base of moral phenomena and, inductively, construct a moral theory that captures the richness and complexity of moral life.... Far from being *atheoretical*, medical ethics and its related enterprises in applied ethics compel attention to deep philosophical questions about optimal research strategies in ethical

theorizing.... Theoreticians are always in danger of oversimplifying, overidealizing, or underestimating the complexity of human behavior.[10]

Our greatest philosophical writings have been plagued by the latter problems, and by the difficulty that no theory adequate to serve as the *foundation* for application to concrete moral problems has ever been devised. Accordingly, the conception of a unilateral direction to the flow of ethical knowledge, together with a presumption of special professional expertise, is a posture of insularity and arrogance that practitioners of ethical theory ought never to adopt.

CLOUSER'S ANALYSIS

Danner Clouser has offered arguments that expand on the approach found in Gert's definition and that offer a challenge to the conclusions I have defended. Clouser accepts the distinction between applied ethics and ethical theory and proposes that applied ethics must not be expected to have the "depth" that ethical theory has. Bioethics and other applied areas are simply "ordinary morality applied to new areas of concern." New "derived rules" are yielded, but they are not "special principles" because they are not new "basic moral rules." Applied work need not, he argues, have a "very sophisticated level of ethical theory or foundations." Instead, worthwhile applied ethics requires a detailed "ground preparation" in "the field to which the ethics is being applied." This ground preparation includes a thorough acquaintance with the concepts, behavior, beliefs, strategies, and goals of the field. New principles do not emerge; rather, we "squeeze out all the relevant implications from the ones [ethics] already has." Clouser argues that philosophical "purists" who dismiss applied ethics as not "real ethics" miss the rigor and careful analysis that goes into the ground preparation and the squeezing procedure. They dismiss it, he suggests, because they "never looked" closely either at the field or at what is accomplished in applied ethics. A part of the problem is that the philosophical purist does not possess the adequate ground preparation and so misses the essence of the application.[11]

Clouser is right about the purist, but his pedagogical model of applied ethics causes him to miss its potential, and in some cases actual, nature and contribution. ("Perhaps it is the 'ground preparation,'" he comments, "which is the essence of applied ethics.") Consider Clouser's major example—"the issue of informed consent." Here, he says, we find that:

Endless articles say essentially the same thing; seldom is anything conceptually new accomplished—that is, in terms of moral theory; but the need for informed consent is uncovered and emphasized in new circumstances and settings. At their intellectual and conceptual best, biomedical ethics articles will interestingly explore or extend or challenge ethical theories in light of the details of biomedicine, ... so that the implications of the old and familiar morality (whatever that might be) can be more accurately "applied," or more decisively rejected.[12]

The endless stream of boring articles cannot be denied, but a more accurate characterization of the literature on informed consent is that "the old and familiar morality" ("whatever that might be") has *not* been skillfully applied in philosophy to yield compelling insights into "the issue of informed consent." "Squeezing" is a misplaced metaphor; "drilling a dry hole" would be closer. Disciplines other than philosophy have fared better in treating this moral problem. In law, the health professions, and the social sciences[13] a rich literature with multiple methodological commitments and interdisciplinary affiliations has been generated. To be sure, certain philosophical analyses of voluntariness, coercion, and related concepts have well served those who have carefully analyzed the issue of informed consent. But the most helpful among these analyses (Nozick's work on coercion and Feinberg's on voluntariness, say) have not in even a *circuitous* fashion led to a theory of informed consent or to new normative rules of informed consent.

We are currently beginning to appreciate in moral theory that the major contributions in this area have recently run from "applied" contexts to "general" theory rather than from general to applied. In examining case law and other literature on informed consent, philosophers have learned a great deal about moral problems in the disclosure of information that are requiring us to rethink and modify traditional conceptions of truth telling, disclosure, lying, withholding information, understanding, consenting, contracts, and the like. To the extent that sophisticated philosophical treatments of these notions are now emerging, they are due in many cases to the examinations and refinements occurring in applied contexts, and they are beginning to fortify rather than squeeze juice from "the old and familiar morality." The works produced by Sissela Bok, Gerald Dworkin, Bernard Gert and Charles Culver, and the President's Commission (which counted Dan Wikler, Dan Brock, and Allen Buchanan among its staff philosophers)—all forged in a heavily interdisciplinary environment—have pushed us along on issues surrounding informed consent and truth telling more than any treatise in ethical theory in decades. But we have been pushed even further along on informed consent by the *legal* analyses presented by Alan Meisel, Jay Katz, Alex Capron, and the landmark cases from *Schloendorff* to *Canterbury*. This contribution to the moral problems of informed consent came not by the application of ethical theory, but rather by a sensitive attention to the moral inadequacies of various legal approaches.

There was no model ethical theory in the pages of philosophers X, Y, and Z for the advances made by the aforementioned philosophers and legal scholars. No "sophisticated" background had been prepared from which an application could be squeezed into a moral theory of informed consent. This should not be surprising once we understand the nature and limits of philosophy's potential contribution. The obligation to obtain informed consent in research and clinical contexts is generally understood to be grounded in a principle of respect for autonomy, but many issues about the nature and limits of this principle remain unsettled. For example, what are the exact demands that the principle makes in the consent context as to disclosure requirements? There is also much debate about whether respect for autonomy demands informed consent where a relatively low level of risk is attached. These questions are too specific for general normative ethics to hope to determine answers from its repertoire of fundamental principles and virtues. More important is that a philosophical account of respect for autonomy—not merely of informed consent—is likely to be shaped by the practical realities and scholarly studies in other disciplines that engage such problems as those of informed consent.

A model system of general normative ethics is so unavailable for this work that no such application has been attempted. Even Gert's *The Moral Rules* could not be milked to provide a theory or set of foundational rules in terms of which his conceptual analyses and normative proposals for informed consent, competence, and the like could be "derived" in his *Philosophy in Medicine*.[14] As important as *The Moral Rules* is to Gert's subsequent work—and he is a model of a philosopher attempting to make the proper connections—his "applied" work is no less "ethical theory" than the treatment of moral rules. One reason applied ethics has flourished of late, along with the revival of social and political philosophy, is because these endeavors have shown more insight into the moral life than most of the previous course taken by philosophical ethics in the twentieth century. I am not arguing that "applied" work is displacing or should displace traditional ethical theory, but only that recent work by the philosophers I have named should help displace some shopworn ideas of what ethical theory *is* and can be. Until philosophy has learned that "applied" work is not a separate category from ethical theory—a double-deck conception of ethics, where one deck is the cheap bleachers—the profession will not have understood the potential in this area of investigation.

It might be maintained that I am only stipulatively defining "ethical theory" to suit my own conceptual preferences and that my argument does not exceed stipulation, but this objection mistakes my meaning. My argument is that worthy philosophical activity need not be modified or compromised by "applied ethics." I do not mean to alter the meaning of "ethical theory" or to stipulate a new meaning. The new content supplied by these applied contexts will simply revive an ethical theory troubled by an overdose of meta-ethics and the ever less exciting wars between deontological and utilitarian theories.

TRADITIONAL CASE METHODS

I earlier invoked a distinction between method and content, and I want now to return to the subject of method, in particular the case method. This method is widely used in applied contexts, but is regarded by many philosophers as having about the same degree of rigor and significance as teaching Kant's categorical imperative through audio-visual aids. I want to argue, however, that not only is the case method a sound pedagogical technique with a distinguished history, but also that it can be used to make important contributions to ethical theory. This will lend further support to my arguments favoring elimination of the distinction between ethical theory and applied ethics.

Only recently has applied ethics drawn attention in philosophy to the importance of case studies and the case method. There has been some attempt to say why the method is important and how it can be effective. For example, Daniel Callahan and Sissela Bok have suggested that "case studies are employed most effectively when they can readily be used to draw out broader ethical principles and moral rules ... [so as] to draw the attention of students to the common elements in a variety of cases, and to the implicit problems of ethical theory to which they may point."[15] This method seems well suited to certain conceptions of applied ethics—as a way to apply, draw out, and illustrate the general principles explored in theory. If anything illustrates *applications of theory*, it might be thought, this method does. It is not obvious, however, how to apply theory, draw out principles, or find common elements. I argue in this section that proper use of the case method undermines rather than supports the belief in two worlds of theory and application.

This argument requires a brief examination of the history of reflection on the use of case studies and the case method—a history to which philosophy has yet to make a notable contribution. Yet this history has much to teach us about discovering, modifying, and using ethical principles. I shall begin with two methods of case analysis that have been widely employed outside of philosophy departments in American universities for nearly a century. This procedure will have the additional advantage of distancing our investigations from philosophical preconceptions about theory and its areas of application.

THE CASE METHOD IN LAW

The most extensive body of thought on strategies for analyzing cases is found in the law, where "case law" establishes precedents of evidence and justification. The earliest developments in the history of the legal use of the case method in law schools occurred shortly after 1870, when Christopher Columbus Langdell revolutionized academic standards and teaching techniques by introducing "the case method" at the Harvard Law School.[16] Langdell's casebooks were composed of cases selected and arranged to reveal to the student the pervasive meaning of legal terms, as well as the "rules" and "principles" of law. He envisioned a dialectical or Socratic manner of argument to reveal how concepts, rules, and principles are found in the legal reasoning of the judges who wrote the opinions. The skillful teacher or legal scholar presumably could extract these fundamental principles, much as a skillful biographer might extract the principles of a person's reasoning by studying his or her considered judgments.

Langdell held that legal theory is a science, resting on an inductive method modeled on the "scientific method" of the natural sciences. Teachers and students were viewed as developing hypotheses in their dissection of cases and landing on principles, just as any good scientist does. In the law, he argued, one extracts from cases a select body of principles that frame the English common law. Even though the many particulars in cases vary and their judicial conclusions are sometimes at odds, the principles of judicial reasoning need not vary. Using this method, one could presumably study exactly how far a principle validly extends, including where it is invalidly applied.

Langdell's dream of making the law a science and making its essence a few abstract principles was eccentric by almost any standard. His vision tended to suppress such matters as the politics of legislation, particular historical circumstances, jurisdictional variations, and actual legal practice. These were dismissed as irrelevant, because historical development and political context were less important in his conception than abstract principle. Langdell's "principles" also did not prove to be as uniform across court, context, or time as had been envisioned, and incompatible and even rival theories or approaches of judges tended to be controlling in many precedent cases. Scientific legal theory proved unattainable, and the idea of abstract fundamental principles worked no better here than it has for ethical theory. Eventually, legal realism shattered Langdell's dream.

There are, however, important reasons why the case method, with appropriate modifications, ultimately prevailed in American law schools and persists as a basic model. Analysis of cases offers teachers a powerful and attractive tool for generalizing from cases. Spanning the tangled web of details in particular cases are something like what Langdell declared "the principles of law." Judges must have them in order to render opinions. Legal theory and its fundamental doctrines are arguably *found in and applied to cases*. Moreover, such training in the case method can sharpen skills of legal reasoning—both legal analysis and legal synthesis. One can tear a case apart and then construct a better way of treating similar cases. In the thrust-and-parry classroom setting, teacher and student alike have to think through a case and its rights and wrongs. The method in this way prepares the student for the practice of the law—the application to new cases—and not merely for theoretical wisdom about it.

In the end, the method's most enduring value is the way it teaches students to distinguish principles and evidence. By examining cases, students learn which courts are considered most adept at legal reasoning and where "the weight of the evidence" lies. The case method has come to stand as a way of learning how to assemble facts and judge the weight of evidence to enable the transfer of that weight to new cases. This is done by generalizing and mastering the principles that control the transfer, usually principles at work in the reasoning of judges.

THE CASE METHOD IN BUSINESS

The case method has also dominated many business schools, where it has never been hailed as a science or even as a single uniform method. Rather, the emphasis has been on deliberation and decision making—making analyses, weighing competing considerations, and reaching a decision in complex and difficult circumstances.[17] Judgment is taught rather than doctrine, principle, or fact. Cases that involve puzzles and dilemmas without any definitive solution along lines of principles or rules are therefore preferred over those that fail to present a difficult dilemma. Cases are not primarily used to illustrate principles or rules, because the latter are inadequate to achieve the goals of the enterprise. Their inadequacy is part of the problem from the perspective of business: There are no reliable rules that can be generalized and transferred. There is no parallel to "the law." The objective, then, is to develop a capacity to grasp problems and to find novel solutions that are contextually workable. To adapt Gilbert Ryle's distinction: Knowing *how* is more prized than knowing *that*.[18]

Business and law are not the only fields that employ a case-studies methodology from which philosophers can learn. Case studies in the history of science have been used by historians, social scientists, and philosophers in order to rationally reconstruct conceptions of scientific methodology and theory. The reconstruction itself can be a form of normative theory.[19] Even in a field seemingly as remote from "theory" as textual bibliography, series of case studies have been used both to develop principles for establishing authoritative critical texts for classical writings and to caution against overly rigid principles. A leading bibliographer—Philip Gaskell—has argued that rather than sticking with a set of a priori bibliographical principles, it is best to *adapt* contingently held principles for each particular case to which they are to be *applied*.[20] The history of recent bibliography has shown that attachment to a preconceived theory or set of principles in textual bibliography has produced utterly bizarre outcomes when applied to some texts.

There are, of course, dangers in transferring the case methods in law, business, and other fields to philosophical ethics if, in their examination, the cases are uninformed by ethical theory. Not much is drearier than a tedious and unrewarding exposure to the moral opinions of those who are ignorant of theoretical materials that transmit sustained philosophical reflection. However, this fact does not lead to the conclusion that studying cases must be informed by theory while theory can remain in isolation from modification by case study.

THE CASE METHOD IN PHILOSOPHY

The case method has made minor inroads in philosophy courses in recent years because cases assist in focusing and dramatizing moral problems while locating them in real-life rather than hypothetical circumstances. This development may at first glance seem novel, and perhaps even pedagogically revolutionary, but Socrates knew it well. His own case of struggling with obedience to the state, and whether or not to escape from its clutches, is a classic source of philosophical reflection emerging from a particular occasion. But this is no isolated instance of the Socratic style of reflection. While he published no ethical theory as we now frame it, everyone recognizes that he taught ethical theory by using a method that richly deserves the association with his name that it currently enjoys.

It takes little acquaintance with that method to know that Socrates served as a midwife by eliciting from the student reflection, insight, and both theoretical and practical judgment. The method starts with a profession of ignorance (*not* a parading of theory) and proceeds to pointed questions that eventuate in proposed principles or definitions. The latter are tested by hypotheses, then modified and tested further until insight into principles or definitions is achieved. Modifications specifically involve repeated appeals to cases, as in the *Meno* when Socrates is discussing whether virtue can be taught. In his discussion with Anytos and Meno, a string of cases of Sophists and fathers and sons is detailed to get at this question, and at the end of his analysis of the various cases, Socrates says that he fears that virtue cannot be taught. His cases are short, but they are constantly at work in shaping his general moral views.

Philosophy has generally neglected to adapt something like the style of case method successfully used in law and business to the philosophical method practiced no less successfully by Socrates. Philosophers have generally preferred in their writings to confine their attention to "hypothetical cases" or "paradigm cases" of a few sentences. Usually they are explicitly fashioned to *support* a theory, although the method of counterexample improves this defect by presenting "the hard cases." The best practitioners of this method do adjust the theory through the counterexamples. While I think philosophy could have been stimulated by using the more complex cases presented in business schools, I have no quarrel with or reservation about an example–counterexample method of philosophizing. I do, however, quarrel with those who associate the use of more extensive case analyses with an "applied" rather than "theoretical" orientation to ethics. They are under the false assumption that theory is not extracted from the examination of cases but only *applied to* cases. My view, by contrast, is that Socrates was on the right track in using cases to develop and modify theory, as was Hegel in his reflection on the cultural roots of moral theory. Cases provide not only data for theory but also its testing ground. Cases lead us to modify and refine embryonic theoretical claims, especially by pointing to inadequacies in or limitations of theories.

A more extensive case analysis in philosophy might be joined with other philosophical methods such as John Rawls's account of reflective equilibrium, which I shall modestly redescribe for present purposes. In developing a normative ethical theory, he argues, it is appropriate to start with the broadest possible set of our considered judgments about a subject such as justice, and to erect a provisional set of principles that reflects them. These principles can then be pruned and adjusted by bringing cases under them. If, for example, some problems in "applied ethics"— say, deceptive advertising or environmental responsibility—are under examination, widely accepted principles of right action (moral beliefs) might be taken, as Rawls puts it, "provisionally as fixed points," but also as "liable to revision."[21] Paradigm cases of what clearly are right courses of action could first be examined, and a search could then be undertaken for principles consistent with our judgments about these paradigm cases. These principles could be tested by reference to other paradigm cases and other considered judgments found in similar cases in order to see if they yield counterintuitive or conflicting results. Through this process, moral theories and principles could be made to cohere with considered judgments about particular cases. That is, general ethical principles and particular judgments can be brought into equilibrium. The principles and theory are *justified* by the process. Presumably, the more complex and difficult the cases that force revisions, the richer the resultant theory will be.

Although Rawls uses this strategy as a supplement to his Kantian moral theory, reflective equilibrium has been subjected to criticism in recent ethics on grounds that it merely brings judgments and intuitions into coherence, without thereby providing theoretical justifications. In effect, this amounts to the standard objection to coherence theories of truth. However, the account can probably be formulated to overcome these difficulties,[22] and in any event I am not arguing that all of moral theory should be derived from this form of analysis. I am arguing only that moral thinking resembles other forms of theorizing in that hypotheses must be tested, buried, or modified through relevant experiments. Principles can be justified, modified, or refuted—and new insights gained—by examination of cases that function as experimental data. Likewise, our developed principles allow us to interpret the cases and arrive at moral judgments in a reflective and accomplished manner. This is the dialectic in moral thinking that Socrates symbolizes. One promise of the case method is that philosophers could increase the quality and applicability of their ethical theories by more careful attention to complicated, real-world cases that provide opportunities for testing the scope, consistency, and adequacy of those theories.

There is no single method delineating how cases are to be used in either law or business, and we should not expect an entirely uniform conception in philosophy. I have presented a programmatic proposal about the promise of the case method for pedagogical as well as theoretical objectives. It is an undervalued tool for reflection that stands to enhance ethical theory more than philosophers presently seem to appreciate. If philosophy can learn to move easily from case studies and issues in private, professional, and public ethics to various more traditional concerns in ethical theory—while training students to reason both without fear of theoretical "irrelevancies" and without disdain for practical applications—the profession will have taken to heart the lesson that Socrates long ago taught. However, as warmly as I endorse the case method, we must not expect too much of it, just as we must not expect too much of moral philosophy generally in the way of final methods or solutions to moral problems. Philosophical ethics provides reasoned and systematic approaches to moral problems, not finality.

Notes

1. Bernard Gert, "Licensing Professions," *Business and Professional Ethics Journal* 1 (Summer 1982): 51–52.

2. G. W. F. Hegel, *Philosophy of Right*, trans. T. M. Knox (Oxford: Clarendon Press, 1942), 89–90, 106–107.

3. On the promise of pragmatism for applied ethics, see Andrew Altman, "Pragmatism and Applied Ethics," *American Philosophical Quarterly* 20 (April 1983): 227–235.

4. See, for example, Daniels's "Health Care Needs and Distributive Justice," in *Philosophy and Public Affairs* 10 (Spring 1981). Daniels's book on the subject is forthcoming from Cambridge University Press (1985).

5. Cf. Ched Noble, "Ethics and Experts," *The Hastings Center Report* 12 (June 1982): 7–10, with responses by four critics.

6. See Onora O'Neill, "The Moral Perplexities of Famine Relief," in Tom Regan, ed., *Matters of Life and Death* (New York: Random House, 1980), pp. 260–298, esp. section IV.

7. John Rawls, *A Theory of Justice* (Cambridge, MA: Harvard University Press, 1971), 8–9, 245–247.

8. Ibid., 351.

9. Alasdair MacIntyre, "What Has Ethics to Learn from Medical Ethics?" *Philosophic Exchange* 2 (Summer 1978): 37–47; Arthur L. Caplan, "Ethical Engineers Need Not Apply: The State of Applied Ethics Today," *Science, Technology, and Human Values* 6 (Fall 1980): 24–32, and reprinted in S. Gorovitz, et al., eds., *Moral Problems in Medicine*, 2nd ed. (Englewood Cliffs, NJ: Prentice-Hall, 1983).

10. Caplan, "Ethical Engineers Need Not Apply," in Gorovitz, et al., 40–41.

11. K. Danner Clouser, *Teaching Bioethics: Strategies, Problems, and Resources* (Hastings-on-Hudson, NY: The Hastings Center, 1980), 53–57; "Bioethics: Some Reflections and Exhortations," *The Monist* 60 (1977): 47–61; and "Bioethics," *Encyclopedia of Bioethics*, Vol. I, ed. Warren T. Reich (New York: Free Press, 1978).

12. Clouser, *Teaching Bioethics*, 55.

13. For the best philosophy has had to offer, see Gerald Dworkin, "Autonomy and Informed Consent," in President's Commission for the Study of Ethical Problems in Medicine and Biomedical and Behavioral Research, *Making Health Care Decisions*, Vol. 3 (Washington, DC: U.S. Government Printing Office, 1982), 63–82.

14. *Philosophy in Medicine: Conceptual and Ethical Issues in Medicine and Psychiatry* (New York: Oxford University Press, 1982) contains surprisingly little of the *moral* theory developed in *The Moral Rules* (New York: Harper Torchbooks, 1975). The application comes almost exclusively in discussions of paternalism. See *Philosophy in Medicine*, 130–163. (Chapter 2 in this book also relies on an account of rationality developed in the earlier book.) See also pp. 42–63 for discussions of informed consent and competence that rely surprisingly little on the earlier book. The best example of his attempts at *application* is Gert's "Licensing Professions," which *is* developed almost entirely within the framework of *The Moral Rules*. This essay suffers, in my judgment, from an overdose of ethical theory and a miniscule treatment of licensing professions (as Gert hints, on pp. 57 and 59). The essay serves, however, to show how difficult it is to bring a systematic moral theory to bear on such concrete problems without a total immersion in the surrounding "nonphilosophical" material.

15. Daniel Callahan and Sissela Bok, *The Teaching of Ethics in Higher Education* (Hastings-on-Hudson, NY: The Hastings Center, 1980), 69. See also Thomas Donaldson, "The Case Method," in his *Case Studies in Business Ethics* (Englewood Cliffs, NJ: Prentice-Hall, 1984), 1–12.

16. Langdell's first casebook on *Contracts* is treated in Lawrence M. Friedman, *A History of American Law* (New York: Simon and Schuster, 1973), 531f. The general account of the case method in this section is indebted to this source, and also to G. Edward White, *Tort Law in America: An Intellectual History* (New York: Oxford University Press, 1980).

17. See M. P. McNair, ed., *The Case Method at the Harvard Business School* (New York: McGraw-Hill, 1954).

18. Gilbert Ryle, "Knowing How and Knowing That," *Proceedings of the Aristotelian Society* XLVI (1945–1946): 1–16.

19. See Richard M. Burian, "More Than a Marriage of Convenience: On the Inextricability of History and Philosophy of Science," *Philosophy of Science* 44 (1977): 1–42.

20. Philip Gaskell, *From Writer to Reader* (Oxford: Oxford University Press, 1978), and *A New Introduction to Bibliography* (Oxford: Oxford University Press, 1972).

21. John Rawls, *A Theory of Justice*, 20f.

22. See Norman Daniels, "Wide Reflective Equilibrium and Theory Acceptance in Ethics," *Journal of Philosophy* 76 (1979): 256–282. See also Altman, "Pragmatism and Applied Ethics," 229–231.

13

DOES ETHICAL THEORY HAVE A FUTURE IN BIOETHICS?

The last 25 years of published literature and curriculum development in bioethics suggest that the field enjoys a successful and stable marriage to philosophical ethical theory. However, the next 25 years could be very different. I believe the marriage is troubled. Divorce is conceivable and perhaps likely. The most philosophical parts of bioethics may retreat to philosophy departments while bioethics more generally continues on its current course toward a more interdisciplinary and practical field.

I make no presumption that bioethics is integrally linked to philosophical ethical theory. Indeed, I assume that the connection is contingent and fragile. Many individuals in law, theological ethics, political theory, the social and behavioral sciences, and the health professions carefully address mainstream issues of bioethics without finding ethical theory essential or breathtakingly attractive. This is not surprising. Moral philosophers have traditionally formulated theories of the right, the good, and the virtuous in the most general terms. A practical price is paid for this theoretical generality[1]: It is often unclear whether and, if so, how theory is to be brought to bear on dilemmatic problems, public policy, moral controversies, and moral conflict—which I will here refer to as problems of practice. By "problems of practice" I mean the moral difficulties and issues presented in health policy and the health professions when decisions must be made about a proper action or policy.

Historically, no moral philosopher has developed a detailed program or method of practical ethics supported by a general ethical theory. There is no well-developed conception of practical ethics or its relation to theoretical ethics. Many philosophers—including Peter Singer and Richard Hare, as utilitarians, or Alan Donagan and Alan Gewirth, as nonutilitarians—could be presented as counterexamples, but I am skeptical of this assessment. None has offered a detailed statement of a method for moving from a general theory to the practical implications of the theory; nor has any developed a fine-grained conception of notions such as "practical ethics" and "practical method." Further, although many moral philosophers are, at present, actively involved in problems of bio-medical ethics such as clinical and corporate consulting, policy formulation, and committee review, questions are open regarding what their role as moral philosophers should be and whether they can successfully bring ethical theories and methods to bear on problems of practice.

I will use the term *ethical theory* to refer to normative philosophical theories of the moral life and philosophical accounts of the methods of ethics. Writers in bioethics such as Peter Singer, Bernard Gert, and Norman Daniels have offered or discussed ethical theories, method in ethics, and practical ethics in the relevant sense. While my definition of "ethical theory" is narrow, it should be suitable for present purposes. I do not assume that only philosophers develop normative theories or that the theories of philosophers occupy a privileged position. I simply restrict the discussion to philosophical theories. I also will not discuss the value of philosophical argument as a resource for the treatment of specific issues in bioethics. For example, I will not discuss whether philosophical ethics can be brought to bear on topical questions such as whether theories of distributive justice and methods of philosophical analysis are currently contributing to the discussion of population ethics and global inequities in health care, which is a promising but still developing area of philosophical investigation.

My concerns are principally with the types of theory and method that have been under discussion in bioethics in the last quarter-century. Three interconnected areas have been prominent: (1) general normative moral theories (from utilitarian and Kantian theories to principlism, casuistry, virtue ethics, feminist ethics, particularism, etc.); (2) moral and conceptual analyses of basic moral notions (informed consent, the killing/letting-die distinction, etc.); and (3) methodology (or how bioethics proceeds—e.g., by use of cases, narratives, specified principles, theory application, reflective equilibrium, legal methods, etc.). I leave it an open question whether (2) or (3) can be successfully addressed without addressing (1), an unresolved problem in ethics.

I will question philosophy's success in all three areas, laying emphasis on its failure to connect theory to practice. In order to survive and flourish in the interdisciplinary environment of bioethics, work will have to improve in philosophical quality and will have to directly engage problems of practice such as whether public laws need modification, whether consensus is an acceptable standard in committee review, ways in which the system for protecting human subjects needs reform, and how decision-making rights are best protected in the health care system. I believe that bioethics needs philosophical theory and stands to profit from it, but better conceptions of method and applied argument are also needed.

In assessing the contemporary literature and how it should change, I will confine attention to three areas of the intersection between bioethics and ethical theory: cultural relativity and moral universality, moral justification, and conceptual analysis. In each case I will argue that philosophers need to develop theories and methods that are more closely attuned to practice. The future of philosophical ethics in interdisciplinary bioethics may turn on whether this challenge is met.

CULTURAL RELATIVITY AND MORAL UNIVERSALITY

Prior to the early 1970s, there was little reason to conceive medical ethics or research ethics as intimately connected to philosophical ethical theory. However, the 1970s brought fears in medicine that the cement of its moral universe—the Hippocratic tradition—was woefully inadequate for clinical ethics and inappropriate for research ethics. A felt need arose for moral norms that could guide investigation of prevailing clinical and research practices. Frameworks drawn from moral philosophy suggested that bioethics could be given universal and principled moral foundations as well as practical methods of inquiry. It was reassuring that medical-moral judgments are not like leaves blowing in the shifting winds of cultural relativism, subjective feelings, institutional commitments, and political voting. Thus, there arose in the late 1970s and early 1980s the idea that universal principles drawn from moral philosophy could be made theoretically interesting and practically relevant in medical ethics.[2]

Internal Challenges to Ethical Theory

For some years thereafter this assumption went largely unchallenged in the literature of bioethics. However, approaches that invoke universal principles began to be vigorously challenged in the late 1980s. Two prominent moral philosophers, Danner Clouser and Bernard Gert, wrote an article that captured widely shared concerns about appeals to universal principles that had emerged in bioethics. At approximately the same time, Albert Jonsen and Stephen Toulmin introduced objections to all principles that were interpreted as rigid universal principles. They judged such principles unsuitable for bioethics.[3] Soon there appeared case-based approaches, rights-based approaches, virtue-based approaches, feminist approaches, and assorted attempts to show that one approach to moral thinking in bioethics is superior to others. Some approaches, though not all, seemed to incorporate an ethical relativity or subjectivity that mitigated the hope for universal norms.

After two decades of clashes of "theory," this discussion has helped clarify many matters, but there is no need to embrace only one of the frameworks that have seemed in intractable conflict. One can without inconsistency embrace principles, rules, virtues, rights, narratives, case analysis, and reflective equilibrium. Bioethics is no longer profiting from these discussions of theory conflict. Moreover, these disputes have long had little to do with clinical and research practices.

I expect this "theory" part of the landscape of bioethics to vanish soon, because it is serving no useful purpose. What is enduring, as a legacy, is how to handle the original hope for universal principles, rights, or virtues—and how to make these norms relevant to practice. Those, including me, who defend universal norms are currently under attack on grounds either that we make inadequately defended claims of universality or that we claim too much universality. This issue has implications for practice in both clinical medicine and research. If there are no transcultural, transinstitutional norms, then it appears that any set of rules may be as viable as any other set of rules and that external criticism of rules has no substantive basis.

External Challenges to Ethical Theory

Before coming to philosophical treatments of this problem, I will discuss two critics of universal norms who hail from disciplines other than philosophy. They propose that universalist ethics be replaced in bioethics by pluralism, multiculturalism, postmodernism, or a practice-based account of morals. The first critic is Nicholas A. Christakis:

> The proper approach to ethical conflict recognizes that culture shapes (1) the content of ethical precepts, (2) the form of ethical precepts, and (3) the way ethical conflict is handled. Medical ethics may be viewed in cross-cultural perspective as a form of "local knowledge." ... The hallmarks of such an approach are ethical pluralism and humility rather than either ethical relativism or universalism.[4]

Christakis commends the approach of Barry Hoffmaster and supports a "contextualist view of medical ethics." He endorses the surprisingly influential thesis of Renee Fox and Judith Swazey (a thesis advanced without evidence or argument) that mainstream ethical theory—based in "AngloAmerican analytic philosophical thought"—has led "American bioethics" into "an impoverished and skewed expression of our society's cultural tradition."[5]

The second critic is Leigh Turner, who agrees that contextualism is a worthy model. He argues that the

> presuppositions that many bioethicists seem to find persuasive fail adequately to recognize the moral conflicts that can be found in a multiethnic, multicultural, multifaith country such as the United States. As a conceptual package, [these presuppositions] lead to a style of moral reasoning that drastically overestimates the ability of bioethicists to "resolve" moral issues because they exaggerate the extent to which morality exists in a stable, orderly pattern of wide reflective equilibrium. This criticism is relevant to the work of principlists [Beauchamp and Childress], casuists [Jonsen and Toulmin], and the common morality approach of Gert, Culver, and Clouser.... My chief criticism of universalist and generally ahistorical accounts [is that they] ... have not made a persuasive argument in support of the claim that there are cross-cultural moral norms supporting a "universal" common morality.[6]

These two statements are notable for their dismissiveness, even hostility, with regard to mainstream ethical theory. Only contextualism, which is more antitheory than theory, survives unbesmirched. Cultural anthropology ("an ethnography of the practice of morality in medical contexts"[7]) is judged to be better positioned than ethical theory to address questions of cultural conflict, transcultural bioethics, and shared principle. These representations seem to rest on both misunderstandings of ethical theory and an extraordinary faith in a vague and undefended contextualism. However, my objective is not to assess the conclusions that Turner and Christakis reach about universalist ethical theory. My intention is to focus on their reservations about ethical theory to see what can be learned from them.

There is much to be learned. The problem is that the philosophical literature in bioethics on universal principles and rationally required behavior is often bereft of a compelling defense and of a clear statement of implications for practice. I will now argue that the literature fails to engage challenges presented by other disciplines or to connect theory to practice and practice to theory.

Moral Philosophers on the Threat of Relativism

Philosophers in bioethics often condemn a specific cultural practice more by assuming the wrongness of the distasteful practice than by rebutting it through a careful analysis or a general theory. But if their claims to differentiate warranted and unwarranted practices are not grounded in a defensible moral account, then relativism, pluralism, and multiculturalism become more, rather than less, attractive.

As an example, I turn to the best work thus far published in bioethics as an attempt to refute relativism and support universalism: Ruth Macklin's *Against Relativism: Cultural Diversity and the Search for Ethical Universals in Medicine.*[8] This book is motivated by her understandable dismay over literature in bioethics in which it is asserted that all norms are socially constructed and that context is everything. She is flabbergasted that this view has become fashionable. In response, Macklin endorses "fundamental principles" that "can be universally applied" and proposes valid cross-cultural judgments. She grants that many norms are relative to the moralities of particular cultures while insisting that violations of basic human rights are universally proscribed. Macklin deftly handles the thesis that acceptance of universality does not undercut acceptance of appropriate measures of particularity. She argues, rightly in my view, that we can consistently deny universality to some justified moral norms while claiming universality for others. Cultural diversity therefore does not entail moral relativism.

Macklin's book is the most thorough treatment of relativism in bioethics by a universalist. It contains compelling cases based on her experience in diverse cultures. She presents stimulating reflections on moral progress, cultural imperialism, basic human rights, cultural sensitivity, and the like. She goes out of her way to make her views accessible to an interdisciplinary audience and to avoid writing, as she says, in an "ahistorical" or "acontextual" manner. Her book displays experience with and practical wisdom about many problems in bioethics.

But is this book an example of bioethics grounded in ethical theory, Macklin's native discipline? Does she either bring a well-defended ethical theory to bear on practice or use practice as the springboard to ethical theory? And does she defend her universalism by philosophical argument? In a notably negative assessment of Macklin's book, Daniel Sulmasy rightly argues that Macklin does not attempt to defend the principles at the core of her arguments through ethical theory, does not distinguish her principles from certain exceptionless moral rules that she rejects, and sometimes relies more on moral intuitions than on universal principles:

> She never makes any arguments for where [her] principles come from or why they should be considered universal, but for her, these are clearly cross-cultural truths. Nonetheless, distinguishing between fundamental moral principles and more specific moral rules, she claims that such universal truth only exists at the abstract level of principles. She states unequivocally,

"I don't believe that exceptionless moral rules exist." Thus, there is plenty of room for moral rules to vary among cultures and individuals.... I looked forward to understanding how a more liberal author might ground an anti-relativist position. However, Macklin has provided no such ground. The book is almost devoid of philosophical argument.... Those looking for ethical justification for their positions should look elsewhere.[9]

Sulmasy provides criticisms of Macklin that—independent of the specific content and issues in her book—capture my sense of deficiencies in the use and nonuse of ethical theory in bioethics. The defects he sees in her book are problems that I find ubiquitous in bioethics: There is a failure to engage the arguments of the opposition (more dismissal than confrontation by argument)[10] and an absence of theory to support central conclusions.

At the same time, Macklin is understandably distressed by multiculturalism's current attractiveness. She finds that pluralism, relativistic multiculturalism, and contextualism are rarely supported by careful argument or grounded in an ethical theory. Everything that Sulmasy says in critical evaluation of Macklin's book could be directed at some of the leading defenses of contextualism. This debate over universalism, pluralism, and relativism—like many discussions in bioethics—needs a more careful grounding in a literature controlled by argument that seriously engages opposition cases and disagreement.[11]

No less important, I shall now argue, is the lack of a serviceable literature on moral justification. I have proposed that philosophers who proceed from a thorough understanding of practice often fail to produce or to ground their conclusions in an ethical theory. I now reverse the direction of argument and maintain that philosophical theories commonly fail to reach down to problems of practice.

MORAL JUSTIFICATION

Philosophers are, by reputation and in self-conception, experts on the theory of justification. No issue is more central to the work of a philosopher. However, one would not know this by looking at the literature of ethical theory as it has been used in bioethics. It is often doubtful whether and, if so, how philosophers in bioethics conceive of justification and how they attempt to justify their claims. It can be unclear whether the justification is normative or nonnormative, what the method of justification is, and even whether a justification is being offered. Detailed discussions of the nature and standards of justification are rare, and, when they do appear, are generally unhelpful to other philosophers and confusing to an interdisciplinary audience.

The Reflective Equilibrium Model

The best work by a figure in bioethics on the theory of justification, in my judgment, is that of Norman Daniels.[12] Using Rawls's celebrated account of "reflective equilibrium,"[13] Daniels argues that moral principles, theoretical postulates, and moral judgments about particular situations should be rendered coherent. His method requires consolidation of an array of moral-theoretical beliefs as well as principles and concepts drawn from diverse ethical theories, ethical traditions, and cultures. Here is Daniels's streamlined statement of the method:

> All of us are familiar with the process of working back and forth between our moral judgments about particular situations and our effort to provide general reasons and principles that link those judgments to ones that are relevantly similar. Sometimes we use this process, which is what Rawls calls "narrow reflective equilibrium," to justify our judgments, sometimes our principles. We can still ask about the principles that capture our considered judgments: Why should we accept them? To answer this question, we must widen the circle of justificatory beliefs. We must show why it is reasonable to hold these principles and beliefs, not just that we happen to do so. Seeking wide reflective equilibrium is thus the process of bringing to bear the broadest evidence and critical scrutiny we can, drawing on all the different moral and nonmoral beliefs and theories that arguably are relevant to our selection of principles or adherence to our moral judgments. Wide reflective equilibrium is thus a theoretical account of justification in ethics and a process that is relevant to helping us solve moral problems at various levels of theory and practice.[14]

This is sweet reason, but is it more than common knowledge ("all of us are familiar")? Is reflective equilibrium a theory that, as Daniels's last sentence implies, can be brought to bear on practice? If so, whose practice and in which ways? Even basic notions such as "evidence" and "selection of principles" are underanalyzed. The more Daniels has elaborated and deepened the theory, the less accessible it has become to those not heavily invested in ethical theory and the more the theoretical discussion has become distanced from argument about practical affairs.[15] Anyone inexperienced in ethical theory will find it difficult to follow the analysis, to grasp its methodological importance, or to see its practical importance.

To the extent that Daniels has been successful in bioethics—where his contribution to issues of distributive justice is unmistakable—his success seems to me curiously detached from his theory of justification. He asserts that throughout his bioethical writings he is appealing to and employing the method of reflective equilibrium. Perhaps he is, but it is obscure what the method requires, how one could check on whether the method has been used, and even whether Daniels follows his model of justification. I am not asserting that Daniels fails to follow his method. I am asserting that it has never been made clear how the method connects to practical problems, how one would know whether it has been followed, and how it might be used by others in bioethics.[16] Daniels states that "the best defense" of the method of reflective equilibrium is "to put it into action . . . and let it be judged by its results."[17] Fair enough, but to assess the results, one must understand what one is assessing. The theory is elegant; the bearing on practice remains more promise than achievement. It continues to be unclear whether anyone in bioethics has followed the reflective-equilibrium model (I include myself), despite its standing as the most widely mentioned model.[18]

Substantial contributions in bioethics to the theory and practice of justification are rare. One can cite examples such as Bernard Gert's able justification of the rules in his moral system,[19] but, like most of Daniels's work, it is not easy to see how this philosophical accomplishment is connected to practical problems of bioethics.

Practice Standards as the Model

Daniels aspires to a close link between theory and practice, but some moral philosophers in bioethics imply that practice has no close confederation with theory. These writers seem to recoil from the abstractness of theory and its distance from practice.

Few theoretical discussions have been more influential in recent bioethics than Alasdair MacIntyre's conception of a moral practice as a cooperative arrangement in pursuit of goods that are internal to a structured communal life.[20] Building on this conception, various philosophers have proposed that what it means to be a good practitioner in health care and research rests on internal (and sometimes evolving) standards of practice, rather than on an external moral theory. Here is a statement by Howard Brody and Frank Miller:

Physicians, by virtue of becoming socialized into the medical profession, accept allegiance to a set of moral values which define the core nature of medical practice. These values give rise to at least some of the moral duties incumbent upon physicians in their professional role and indicate the virtues proper to physicians. . . . The professional integrity of physicians is constituted by allegiance to this internal morality.[21]

Brody and Miller may seem to be illicitly grounding duties and virtues in existing practice standards without justifying those standards. However, they note that "Even the core of medical morality must be thoughtfully reevaluated and reconstructed at intervals."[22] They observe that existing standards of practice may be shallow and in need of reexamination. Their test case of standards of practice currently in need of reevaluation is medical morality's prohibition of physician-assisted suicide. Although medical tradition has insistently condemned this activity, Brody and Miller say, "today's physicians might [legitimately] still conclude that so many things have changed since the time of Hippocrates . . . [that the times] warrant a reconstruction of the internal morality so that assisted suicide in certain defined circumstances is permissible."[23]

What would "warrant a reconstruction"? Brody and Miller propose that physician-assisted death may turn out, upon careful consideration, to be justifiable in terms of the internal morality of medicine. The first line of justification, they suggest, should be to show that internal standards of professional integrity and moral duty are not violated by active assistance in dying. However, realizing that this morality may not support the entirety of needed reforms, Brody and Miller propose that external standards will sometimes be needed:

> Professional integrity does not encompass the whole of medical ethics. Moral considerations other than the norms of professional integrity may be appealed to in favor of, or against, permitting a practice of limited physician-assisted death. . . . An experimental public policy of legalizing the practice should be undertaken, subject to stringent regulatory safeguards.[24]

What sort of "moral considerations" would supply a justification? One might reasonably expect moral philosophers such as Brody and Miller to turn to moral philosophy. Having asserted that justification is a central issue and that internal justification using practice standards may come up short, they make no attempt at justification beyond a vague statement that "the reconstruction will be carried out by those who live in modern society who are inevitably influenced by societal values as they interpret the history."[25] In short, their first-line appeal is to internal standards of medical morality; their second-line appeal is to societal values; and there is no third-line appeal to ethical theory or even a hint that it might be relevant.

I am not arguing that Brody and Miller are mistaken. I am pointing out that their training in ethical theory is removed from their venture and that their approach is characteristic of much of the current literature by philosophers in bioethics. Many prefer to ground their claims in institutional standards, societal values, paradigm cases, narratives—indeed, in virtually any source other than ethical theory. When, subsequently, it appears that neither institutions nor societies provide the needed justification, few hints are provided about how to proceed. Just at the point ethical theory seems relevant, it is ignored. This neglect transparently conveys the impression that moral philosophy is ill-equipped to help us solve problems.

CONCEPTUAL ANALYSIS

I turn now to the third of the three areas I said I would investigate, conceptual analysis. This method is of the first importance in moral philosophy. Although it is rarely expected to resolve practical moral problems, it is widely thought to play an important role in such argument.

One example in bioethics of the philosophical and practical importance of conceptual analysis is work on the concept of "informed consent." Appropriate criteria must be identified if we are to define and classify an act as an informed consent. Overdemanding criteria such as "full disclosure and complete under-standing" mischaracterize informed consent, and so-called informed consents are then impossible to obtain. Conversely, underdemanding criteria such as "the patient signed the form" misconceive informed consent, and so-called informed consents then become too easy to obtain. In the literature of informed consent over the last 30 years, conceptual and moral analysis of informed consent has, beyond a reasonable doubt, been vital to advances in both clinical and research ethics. This work is ongoing and incomplete, but it has changed our under-standing as well as our practices in research and clinical settings.

The Concept of Autonomy

Though the notion of informed consent has received extensive attention in bioethics, many other concepts have not received comparable attention—or at least not with an eye to professional and policy areas. Paradoxically, the more fundamental and philosophically challenging the concept, the less it seems that moral philosophers in bioethics have attended to it or spelled out a theory's implications for practice. I will use "autonomy" as an example. In moving to this example, I start with an engaging 1988 statement by Jonathan Moreno that was intended to motivate his important research on the role of consensus in bioethics: "Unlike the concept of autonomy, consensus has not yet undergone systematic and intense scrutiny in medical ethics."[26] I agree about consensus, but still today no clear connection has been made between conceptual analysis of autonomy and practical areas of bioethics.

It is agreed in the literature that "autonomy," "respect for autonomy," and "rights of autonomy" are very different concepts. "Respect for autonomy" and "rights of autonomy" are moral notions, whereas "autonomy" and "autonomous person" are not obviously moral notions. To many writers the latter seem more metaphysical than moral, and literature in both ethical theory and bioethics generally supports this idea.[27] However, the distinction between the metaphysical concept of autonomy and the moral concept of autonomy has fostered confusing views, and uncertainty currently surrounds the meaning of autonomy, its relationship to the concept of persons, the descriptive or normative character of these concepts, and the connection of these notions to that of respect for autonomy (and respect for persons). What it is about autonomy that we are to respect remains unclear, and it remains obscure what "respect" means. Most obscure of all is how practice is affected by a theory of autonomy.

The contemporary literature in bioethics contains no theory of autonomy that spells out its nature, its moral implications, its limits, how respect for autonomy differs from respect for persons (if it does), and the like. Much of the literature relies on notions of liberty and agency. The most detailed theory of autonomy by a writer in bioethics is Gerald Dworkin's.[28] He offers a "content-free" definition of autonomy as a "second-order capacity of persons to reflect critically upon their first-order preferences, desires, wishes, and so forth and the capacity to accept or attempt to change these in the light of higher-order preferences and values."[29] For example, consider a person who has desires for low-quality foods (a first-order desire or preference). To qualify as autonomous, the person must have the capacity to reflect on his or her desires and form a desire about whether to change or retain those desires (a second-order desire or preference).

This theory has many problems. There is nothing to prevent a reflective acceptance or preference at the second level from being caused by and assured by the strength of a first-order desire. The individual's acceptance of or identification with the first-order desire would then be no more than a causal result of an already formed structure of preferences, not a new structuring of preferences. For example, if I decide that I prefer to continue eating low-quality food because I have a passion for doing so, this choice seems determined by my initial desires. At first I wanted cheeseburgers; then I discovered that I desire to desire cheeseburgers and that I want this second-order desire to be my controlling desire. This example may seem superficial, but the two-tier theory embraced by Dworkin and Frankfurt lacks adequate conditions to protect even against such a simple case. To make the theory plausible, a component, supplementary theory would have to be added that distinguished between influences or desires that rob an individual of autonomy and influences or desires consistent with autonomy.[30]

More worrisome for present purposes is that, like Daniels's account of justification, Dworkin's theory of autonomy has not been carefully assessed or used in bioethics. Its implications for practice are unclear and untested. This neglect is not surprising, as there seem to be no practical implications of the theory. Dworkin himself does not appear to use the theory in his writings on applied topics of bioethics. He devotes the second half of his book *The Theory and Practice of Autonomy* to "Practice," where he treats five issues in bioethics. He scarcely mentions the theory developed in the first half of the book and never attempts to decide an important question in bioethics by reference to the theory. In his "Epilogue" to the book, Dworkin points out that a number of conceptual issues must be worked out to develop the research program he initiated. It is two decades later, and nothing has appeared.

If I could point to a more penetrating or successful theory of autonomy in bioethics than Dworkin's, I would, but it does not exist. We await a carefully crafted philosophical theory as well as a connection between theory and practice.

The Concepts of Killing and Letting Die

Consider, as a second example of skimpy conceptual analysis, the distinction between killing and letting die. Many issues have been raised in the literature of bioethics about the conceptual conditions under which physicians do or do not kill patients, let them die, or neither. Most recently, physician-assisted suicide has been the primary concern. Various problems of moral justification are at work in these debates, but I will focus here entirely on the concepts that drive the discussion: killing and letting die.

In medical tradition killing by physicians is prohibited and letting die permitted under specified conditions. Despite a remarkable convergence of opinion in support of this traditional outlook, no one has yet produced a cogent analysis of the distinction between killing and letting die as it functions in medicine so that meaningful law and professional ethics can be developed through the distinction. Philosophical writers on the subjects of euthanasia, assisted suicide, terminal sedation, and the like are typically concerned about killing rather than letting die. However, their work does little to explicate the conditions under which killing by physicians occurs; indeed, the work is sketchy to nonexistent on whether "physician-assisted suicide" actually involves suicide by patients. I am not aware of a philosophical article or book on killing that carefully addresses what counts as killing in medical contexts and how that notion is to be distinguished from letting die.[31]

The notion of letting patients die has often been ignored in this literature, though conceptually it is no less important than killing. "Letting die" occurs in medicine under two circumstances: cessation of medical technology because it is useless and cessation of medical technology because it has been validly refused.

The latter notion applies to both first-party and proxy refusals, though I will not address this distinction here. Honoring a valid refusal of a useful treatment knowing of a fatal outcome is a letting die, not a killing. The type of action—a killing or a letting die—can depend entirely on whether a valid refusal justifies the forgoing of medical technology. This brings evaluative appraisal into the heart of the concept. (See my Essay 7 on hastened death in these *Collected Essays*.)

In the medical context, "letting die" is value laden in the sense that it is tied to *acceptable* acts, where acceptability derives either from the futility of treatment or a valid refusal. Killing, by contrast, is conceptually tied in medical contexts to *unacceptable* acts. Thus, the value neutrality of "killing" and "letting die" found in ordinary moral discourse (as when we say "the disease killed her"; "she was killed in an auto accident"; or "he killed an enemy soldier") is not present in medical morality, where letting die is prima facie justified and killing prima facie unjustified. A thorough philosophical analysis would have to work through the subtleties of these problems. This is the sort of problem that philosophers should be well equipped to address and also the sort of problem that stands to affect medical practice and contribute to bioethics.

However, philosophers generally miss these key issues. A common strategy in philosophical literature is to present two cases differing only in that one is a killing and the other a letting die (usually involving some harm or wrong), and then to investigate conceptually what the difference is and morally whether the difference is relevant to judgments of right and wrong. The hypothesis is that the conceptual or moral difference in the two cases shows that the distinction either is or is not viable or morally relevant. In treating such cases, philosophers seem to prefer to retreat from the messiness of the medical situation—that is, they distance their analyses from the real problems of practice—to achieve conceptual clarity and deal with problems of concern to fellow philosophers. They utilize cases of runaway trolleys, minuscule releases of toxic substances, persons who drown in bathtubs, rescuing drowning persons by killing someone in the path of the swimmer, and the like. These examples and accompanying analyses fail to illuminate whether doctors kill or let die, whether they act justifiably or not, and how to think about the acts of patients who refuse life-saving technologies.

In short, philosophical literature tends to evade the central context in which the distinction arises in bioethics—real encounters between doctors and patients—and, as a result, the analyses turn out to be too pure and general to illuminate that context. The fit is poor. I do not say that philosophical analysis fails to illuminate circumstances of killing or letting die beyond medical practice. I claim only that the available conceptual analyses are largely unilluminating in regard to medical practice, which is the domain of bioethics.

CONCLUSION

The controversies I have discussed largely originated in philosophy and have been perpetuated using philosophical discourse. Consequently, outsiders have had a hard time looking in. The more the issues have been philosophically refined, the less serviceable and influential ethical theory has become in bioethics. Philosophical theories today have a diminished stature in bioethics by comparison to their standing of 10 or 20 years ago. The reasons for the demotion of ethical theory are the lack of distinctive authority behind any one framework or methodology, the unappealing and formidable character of many theories, the indeterminate nature of general norms of all sorts, the turn in bioethics to more practical issues, and—most important—the stumbling and confusing manner in which philosophers have attempted to link theory to practice.

How theory can be connected to practice is a problem of greater urgency today than it was 30 years ago, when philosophers were not in touch with medical morality and virtually nothing was expected of them in this domain. In 1974 Samuel Gorovitz and I drove back and forth from Washington, D.C., to Haverford College over a six-week period to discuss with a group of philosophers whether bioethics had a future in philosophy. The word *bioethics* had just been coined, and no one understood quite what it meant or encompassed. Few philosophers had exhibited an interest in the subject. While traveling on Interstate 95, Gorovitz and I reflected on how developments in biomedicine present a treasure chest of fundamentally philosophical issues. Gorovitz was puzzled that philosophers ignored such matters. He thought these issues "a natural" for philosophers. I think he was right, and I still believe that many issues in bioethics are fundamentally problems that should be handled by the methods of moral philosophy. However, thousands of publications later, the grand promise of ethical theory for bioethics remains mostly promise.

For 15 years or so it seemed that Gorovitz would be proved right: Bioethics did seem a natural for philosophers. In limited respects he has been proven correct by the profound influence that philosophers have enjoyed in various areas of bioethics. However, the literature of an interdisciplinary bioethics has shifted in the last two decades or so toward greater levels of comfort with law, policy studies, empirical studies, standards of practice, government guidelines, and international guidelines—progressively marginalizing the role of ethical theory. Moral philosophers have not convinced the interdisciplinary audience in bioethics, or themselves, that ethical theory is foundational to the field and relevant to practice. To continue on this path will call into question whether ethical theory has a significant role in bioethics. It is a question worth considering.

Notes

1. See R. K. Fullinwider, "Against Theory, or: Applied Philosophy-A Cautionary Tale," *Metaphilosophy* 20 (1989): 222–234.

2. For works published during the period, see National Commission for the Protection of Human Subjects, *The Belmont Report: Ethical Guidelines for the Protection of Human Subjects of Research* (DHEW Publication No. (OS) 78-0012, 1978); J. V. Brady and A. R. Jonsen, "The Evolution of Regulatory Influences on Research with Human Subjects," in R. Greenwald, et al. eds., *Human Subjects Research* (New York: Plenum Press, 1982): 3–18; R. J. Levine, *Ethics and Regulation of Clinical Research*, 1st edn. (Baltimore: Urban & Schwarzenberg, 1981); E. D. Pellegrino and D. C. Thomasma, *A Philosophical Basis of Medical Practice* (New York: Oxford University Press, 1981); and F. W. O'Connor, et al. *Deviance and Decency: The Ethics of Research With Human Subjects* (London: Sage Publications 1979). For later studies or accounts of the period, see J. D. Moreno, *Deciding Together: Bioethics and Consensus* (New York: Oxford University Press, 1995); Advisory Committee on Human Radiation Experiments, *Final Report of the Advisory Committee on Human Radiation Experiments* (New York: Oxford University Press, 1996); D. DeGrazia, "Moving Forward in Bioethical Theory: Theories, Cases, and Specified Principlism," *Journal of Medicine and Philosophy* 17 (1992): 511–539; J. Arras, "Principles and Particularity: The Role of Cases in Bioethics," *Indiana Law Journal* 69 (1994): 983–1014; and R. M. Veatch, "From Nuremberg through the 1990s: The Priority of Autonomy," in H. Y. Vanderpool, ed. *The Ethics of Research Involving Human Subjects: Facing the 21st Century* (Frederick, MD: University Publishing Group 1996): 45–58.

3. K. D. Clouser and B. Gert, "A Critique of Principlism," *The Journal of Medicine and Philosophy* 15 (1990): 219–236. A. Jonsen and S. Toulmin, *The Abuse of Casuistry* (Berkeley: University of California Press, 1988).

4. N. A. Christakis, "Ethics are Local: Engaging Cross-Cultural Variation in the Ethics for Clinical Research," *Social Science and Medicine* 35 (1992): 1079–1091, quotation from 1079, 1089.

5. Ibid., 1088.

6. L. Turner, "Zones of Consensus and Zones of Conflict: Questioning the 'Common Morality' Presumption in Bioethics," *Kennedy Institute of Ethics Journal* 13 (2003): 193–218, esp. 196.

7. Christakis, supra note 4, 1088.

8. R. Macklin, *Against Relativism: Cultural Diversity and the Search for Ethical Universals in Medicine* (New York: Oxford University Press, 1999).

9. D. P. Sulmasy, "Review of Against Relativism," *The National Catholic Bioethics Quarterly* 1 (2001): 467–469, esp. 468–469. See, however, Macklin's explicit statement in her "Preface" (p. v.) regarding the way she limits her theoretical goals.

10. For an example of the sorts of arguments of the opposition in publications in bioethics that need to be addressed, see the essays in *Cross-Cultural Perspectives on the (Im)Possibility of Global Bioethics*, ed. Julia Tao Lai Po-Wah (Dordrecht: Kluwer, 2002).

11. For nuanced accounts of the use of moral philosophy to defend both relativism and antirelativism, see G. Harman and J. J. Thomson, *Moral Relativism and Moral Objectivity*

(Cambridge, MA: Blackwell Publishers, 1996). Thomson mounts a compelling philosophical defense of "objectivity." A very different and engaging approach, more concrete but not appropriately described as practical ethics, is provided by M. C. Nussbaum, *Women and Human Development: The Capabilities Approach* (Cambridge: Cambridge University Press, 2000), especially chapter 1, "In Defense of Universal Values."

12. N. Daniels, *Justice and Justification. Reflective Equilibrium in Theory and Practice* (Cambridge: Cambridge University Press, 1996); N. Daniels, "Wide Reflective Equilibrium in Practice," in L. W. Sumner and J. Boyle, eds., *Philosophical Perspectives on Bioethics* (Toronto: University of Toronto Press, 1996), 96–114; N. Daniels, "Wide Reflective Equilibrium and Theory Acceptance in Ethics," *Journal of Philosophy* 76 (1979), 256–282; and, with A. Buchanan, D. W. Brock, and D. Wikler, *From Chance to Choice: Genetics and Justice* (Cambridge: Cambridge University Press, 2000), esp. 371ff.

13. J. Rawls, *A Theory of Justice* (Cambridge, MA: Harvard University Press, 1971; revised edition, 1999).

14. Daniels, supra note 12 (1).

15. N. Daniels, "Wide Reflective Equilibrium in Practice" provides the most accessible material on methodology in bioethics, but the claim to have used the method in practice is boldest and most interesting in *From Chance to Choice: Genetics and Justice*, 371; and also 22–23, 308–309.

16. In *Justice and Justification: Reflective Equilibrium in Theory and Practice*, Daniels discusses reflective equilibrium, especially wide reflective equilibrium, in the first part of the book—the "Theory" part—but not in the second. Chapters 1–8 in the first part deal with the theory of reflective equilibrium. In the second part (chapters 9–16)—the "Practice" part—reflective equilibrium is mentioned only in the title of chapter 16, and never developed. In chapter 9, the first of the practice chapters, Daniels points to some general implications of his account and rightly recognizes "the many difficulties that face drawing implications from ideal theory for nonideal settings" (199). As I read Daniels, he is a persuasive spokesperson for the defense and extension of Rawls's theory of justice, but he does little to implement transparently the method of reflective equilibrium or to show its implications for practical ethics.

17. N. Daniels, *From Chance to Choice: Genetics and Justice*, supra note 12, 371.

18. The book *Reflective Equilibrium*, ed. Webren van der Burg and Theo van Willigenburg (Dordrecht: Kluwer Academic Publishers, 1998), is composed of 19 essays on the subject. It supposedly discusses how the idea of reflective equilibrium offers a model for practical moral problems. While there is philosophical discussion of the practical implications of the model, I cannot find actual examples of the use of the method to address practical problems.

19. B. Gert, *Morality: A New Justification of the Moral Rules*. This theory is brought to bear on various problems in bioethics in B. Gert, C. M. Culver, and K. D. Clouser, *Bioethics: A Return to Fundamentals* (New York: Oxford University Press, 1997).

20. A. MacIntyre, *After Virtue*, 2nd edn. (Notre Dame: University of Notre Dame Press, 1984), 17, 175, 187, 190–203. See also A. MacIntyre, "Does Applied Ethics Rest on A Mistake?" *Monist* 67 (1984): 498–513.

21. H. Brody and F. G. Miller, "The Internal Morality of Medicine: Explication and Application to Managed Care," *Journal of Medicine and Philosophy* 23 (1998): 384–410, especially 386.

22. Brody and Miller, supra note 21, 393–397; italics added.

23. Brody and Miller, supra note 21, 397.

24. F. G. Miller & H. Brody, "Professional Integrity and Physician-Assisted Death," *Hastings Center Report* (1995): 8–17, especially 12–16.

25. Brody and Miller, supra note 21, 393–394, 397; italics added.

26. J. Moreno, "Ethics by Committee: The Moral Authority of Consensus," *The Journal of Medicine and Philosophy* 13 (1988), 413.

27. D. Dennett, "Conditions of Personhood," in *The Identities of Persons*, ed. A. O. Rorty (Berkeley: University of California Press, 1976), 175–196; J. Feinberg and B. Baum Levenbook, "Abortion," in *Matters of Life and Death: New Introductory Essays in Moral Philosophy*, 3rd edn., ed. T. Regan (New York: Random House, 1993); M. A. Warren, "Abortion," in *A Companion to Ethics*, Peter Singer, ed. (Cambridge, MA: Blackwell Reference, 1991); 303–314; M. A. Warren, *Moral Status: Obligations to Persons and Other Living Things* (New York: Oxford University Press, 1997); and *Kennedy Institute of Ethics Journal* 9 (December 1999), Special Issue on Persons, ed. Gerhold K. Becker.

28. G. Dworkin, *The Theory and Practice of Autonomy* (New York: Cambridge University Press, 1988). The most interesting book in bioethics on autonomy, in my judgment, is O. O'Neill, *Autonomy and Trust in Bioethics* (Cambridge: Cambridge University Press, 2002); however, this book does not present a theory or conceptual analysis of autonomy.

29. Dworkin, supra note 28, 20.

30. No such work has as yet been put forward in bioethics, but some beginnings are available in ethical theory. See H. G. Frankfurt, "Freedom of the Will and the Concept of a Person," *Journal of Philosophy* 68 (1971): 5–20, as reprinted in *The Importance of What We Care About* (Cambridge: Cambridge University Press, 1988): 11–25; and J. Christman, "Autonomy and Personal History," *Canadian Journal of Philosophy* 21 (1991): 1–24, esp. 10ff. Christman's account is a nuanced version of the theory of nonrepudiated acceptance that uses the language of nonresistance. Although it is not clear that Frankfurt has a theory of autonomy, see his uses of the language of "autonomy" in his *Necessity, Volition, and Love* (Cambridge: Cambridge University Press, 1999), chaps. 9, 11. Frankfurt's early work was on persons and freedom of the will. In his later work, he seems to regard the earlier work as providing an account of autonomy, which is a reasonable estimate even if it involves some creative reconstruction.

31. The articles or essays closest to this ideal are J. L. Bernat, B. Gert, and R. P. Mogielnicki, "Patient Refusal of Hydration and Nutrition: An Alternative to Physician-Assisted Suicide or Voluntary Active Euthanasia," *Archives of Internal Medicine* 153 (December 27, 1993): 2723–2728; D. W. Brock, *Life and Death: Philosophical Essays in Biomedical Ethics* (New York: Cambridge University Press, 1993); T. L. Beauchamp, "The Justification of Physician-Assisted Suicide," *Indiana Law Review* 29 (1996): 1173–1200; and J. McMahan, "Killing, Letting Die, and Withdrawing Aid," *Ethics* 103 (1993): 250–279.

14

THE FAILURE OF THEORIES OF PERSONHOOD

What it is to be a person is a principal topic of metaphysics. Ideally, a metaphysical theory expresses a morally detached interest in how to distinguish persons from nonpersons. However, the metaphysics of persons has often been put to work to defend a preferred moral outcome, placing metaphysics in the service of ethics. Metaphysics is invoked to inquire whether individuals have rights and whether the theory of persons can address practical problems of abortion, reproductive technology, infanticide, refusal of treatment, senile dementia, euthanasia, the definition of death, and experimentation on animals.

The different objectives of theories of persons can be clarified by a distinction between metaphysical and moral concepts of persons.[1] Metaphysical personhood is composed entirely of a set of person-distinguishing psychological properties such as intentionality, self-consciousness, free will, language acquisition, pain reception, and emotion. The metaphysical goal is to identify a set of psychological properties possessed by all and only persons. Moral personhood, by contrast, refers to individuals who possess properties or capacities such as moral agency and moral motivation. These properties or capacities distinguish moral persons from all nonmoral entities. In principle, an entity could satisfy all the properties requisite for metaphysical personhood and lack all the properties requisite for moral personhood.

However, most published theories of persons are not clearly distinguishable into these types or even attentive to the distinction between metaphysical and moral personhood. Proponents of these theories have generally not even approached the subject using these distinctions. Their goal has primarily been to delineate the distinctive properties of personhood—moral or non-moral—that are necessary for and confer moral status on an individual. For three decades, and arguably for several centuries,[2] the dominant trend in the literature on persons has been to delineate nonmoral, principally *cognitive*, properties of individuals in a metaphysical account, from which conclusions can be drawn about moral status. A good example is Michael Tooley's well-known analysis moving from metaphysical premises to moral conclusions (1972, sec. 3):

> What properties must something have in order to be a person, i.e., to have a serious right to life? The claim I wish to defend is this: An organism possesses a serious right to life only if it possesses the concept of a self as a continuing subject of experiences and other mental states, and believes that it is itself a continuing entity.

Tooley (1983, p. 51; cf. p. 35) observes that

> [I]t seems advisable to treat the term "person" as a purely descriptive term, rather than as one whose definition involves moral concepts. For this appears to be the way the term "person" is ordinarily construed.[3]

In this account, "person" has descriptive content ("an entity that possesses either self-consciousness or rationality"), but is not a purely descriptive term; the person-making properties in this metaphysical account endow their possessors with moral rights or other moral protections.

The belief persists in philosophy and beyond that some special cognitive property or properties of persons such as self-consciousness or rationality confers a unique moral status, and perhaps forms the exclusive basis of this status.[4] I believe, by contrast, that no cognitive property or set of such properties confers moral status and that metaphysical personhood is not sufficient for either moral personhood or moral status, though some conditions of metaphysical personhood may be *necessary* conditions of moral personhood.[5] I also maintain that moral personhood is not a necessary condition of moral status. I claim, in this way, that metaphysical personhood does not entail either moral personhood or moral status and that personhood of either type is not the only basis of moral status.

THE CONCEPT OF METAPHYSICAL PERSONHOOD

The common-sense concept of person is, roughly speaking, identical with the concept of human being. Human psychological properties continue to play a pivotal role in philosophical controversies over personhood. However, there is no warrant for the assumption that only properties distinctive of membership in the human species count toward personhood or confer moral status. Even if certain properties that are strongly correlated with membership in the human species qualify humans more readily than the members of other species, these properties are only contingently connected to being human. It just so happens, if it is so at all, that individuals possessing these properties are of a particular natural species. The properties could be possessed by members of nonhuman species or by entities outside the sphere of natural species such as computers, robots, and genetically manipulated species.[6]

Fortunately, a metaphysical account of persons need have no reference to properties possessed only by humans. In some of the theories mentioned previously (e.g., Tooley's), an entity is a person if and only if it possesses certain *cognitive* rather than singularly human properties. Cognitive conditions of metaphysical personhood similar to the following have been promoted by several classical and contemporary writers[7]: (1) self-consciousness (of oneself as existing over time), (2) capacity to act on reasons, (3) capacity to communicate with others by command of a language, (4) capacity to act freely, and (5) rationality.

Presumably these characteristics are put forward to distinguish persons from nonpersons irrespective of species, origin, or type. If so, it is an open question whether a robot, a computer, an ape, or God qualifies for metaphysical personhood. Methodologically, the properties of personhood are presumed to be determinable a priori by consulting our shared concept of person; such a theory does not require empirical discovery. The only empirical question is whether an entity in fact satisfies the conceptual conditions. A classical example of this method is found in John Locke's analysis of a person as a "thinking intelligent being, that has reason and reflection, and can consider itself as itself, the same thinking thing in different times and places" (1975, 2.27.9; see also 2.27.24–26). Locke pointed out that despite the close association between "man" and "person," the two concepts are distinct, a claim he defended by presenting cases to show that the same man need not be the same person.

Sometimes it is said by those who defend criteria resembling (1) through (5) that only one of these criteria must be satisfied for metaphysical personhood—for example, self-consciousness, rationality, or linguistic capacity. Other writers suggest that each condition must be satisfied and that the five conditions are jointly necessary and sufficient. Another view is that some subset of these five conditions is both necessary and sufficient.

PROBLEMS IN THEORIES OF METAPHYSICAL PERSONHOOD

These cognitive theories fail to capture the depth of commitments embedded in using the language of "person," and they sometimes confuse the most important issues by moving from a purely metaphysical claim to a claim about either moral personhood or moral status. By themselves these cognitive properties have no moral implications. Such implications occur only if an analysis assumes or incorporates an independent moral principle, such as "respect for persons." Such a principle, being independent of a metaphysical theory, would have to be defended independently and given suitable content.

Suppose that some being is rational, acts purposively, and is self-conscious. How is moral personhood or any form of moral status established by this fact? Do moral conclusions follow from the presence of these properties? An entity of this description need not be capable of moral agency or able to differentiate right from wrong; it may lack moral motives and all sense of accountability. It may perform no actions that we can judge morally. It might be a computer, a dangerous predator, or an evil demon. No matter how elevated our respect for this entity's cognitive capacities, these capacities will not amount to moral personhood and will not establish any form of moral status. Capacities of language, rationality, self-consciousness, and the like lack an intrinsic connection to moral properties such as moral agency and moral motivation.

A property often cited in the metaphysical hunt, as we saw in Tooley's theory, is self-consciousness—that is, a conception of oneself as persisting through time and having a past and a future. If animals such as birds and bears lack self-awareness and a sense of continuity over time, they lack personhood (see, e.g., Buchanan & Brock, 1989, pp. 197–199; Dworkin, 1988, esp. Chapter 1; Harris, 1985, pp. 9–10). The hypothesis is that although animals exhibit goal-directed behaviors such as building a nest, they do so without any sense of self, which is thought to be essential to personhood or to any condition that confers moral status. However, it is more assumed than demonstrated in these theories that nonhuman animals lack a relevant form of self-consciousness or its functional equivalent. The prima facie evidence of various types and degrees of animal self-awareness is striking and the possibility of self-consciousness cannot be dismissed without careful study. Language-trained apes appear to make self-references, and many animals learn from the past and then use their knowledge to forge plans of action for hunting, stocking reserve foods, and constructing dwellings (see Griffin, 1992). These animals are aware of their bodies and their interests, and they unerringly distinguish those bodies and interests from the bodies and interests of others. In play and social life, they understand assigned functions and decide for themselves what roles to play. A few appear to recognize themselves from reflections in mirrors (cf. DeGrazia 1997, p. 302; Gallup, 1977; Miles, 1993; Patterson & Gordon, 1993).

There may, then, be reason to attribute at least elementary self-consciousness to these animals, and to think of this ability as admitting of degrees in the several criteria that might be used to analyze it.

One possible strategy to avoid this conclusion is to increase the demands built into the concept of self-consciousness. Harry Frankfurt's (1971) account, sometimes presented as a theory of autonomy, could be adapted to this end (see also Dworkin, 1988, Chapters 1–4; Ekstrom, 1993). In this theory, all and only persons have a form of self-consciousness involving distanced self-reflection. Persons reflectively judge and identify with their basic, first-order desires through second-order desires, judgment, and volition. Second-order mental states have first-order mental states as their intentional objects, and considered preferences are formed about first-order desires and beliefs. For example, a long-distance runner may have a first-order desire to run several hours a day, but also may have a higher-order desire to decrease the hours and the level of commitment. Action from the second-order desire is autonomous and is characteristic of the person; action from the first-order desire is not autonomous and is typical of animal behavior. The capacity to rationally accept or repudiate lower-order desires or preferences, which involves a lofty cognitive ability of distanced self-reflection, is the centerpiece of this account.

Several problems haunt this theory. First, there is nothing to prevent a reflective acceptance or repudiation at the second level from being caused by and assured by the strength of a first-order desire. The individual's acceptance of or identification with the first-order desire would then be no more than a causal result of the already formed structure of preferences, not a new structuring of preferences, and so not a particularly attractive criterion of personhood. Second-order desires would not be significantly different from or causally independent of first-order desires, other than being second-order. Second, the conditions of distance and reflective control are so demanding in this theory that either many human actors will be excluded as persons or their actions will be judged nonautonomous. It is doubtful that an identification at the second level is present in most of the actions that we commonly perform. A potential moral price of this demanding theory is that individuals who have not reflected on their desires and preferences at a higher level deserve no respect for actions that derive from their most deep-seated desires and preferences.[8]

As the quality or level of required cognitive activity is reduced in a theory to accommodate these problems, the volume of humans who qualify will increase, but so will the volume of nonhuman animals. Less demanding conditions—understanding and self-control, say—will likely be satisfied to a greater or lesser extent. A threshold line will have to be drawn in a theory that separates an adequate degree of understanding and self-control from an inadequate degree. Again, a high threshold will exclude many humans that we normally regard as autonomous persons; a low threshold will include at least some nonhuman animals. Nonhuman animals are especially likely to qualify in a theory that uses low cognitive criteria by contrast to lofty cognitive criteria.[9]

Virtually all criteria of personhood or autonomy admit of degrees, and most develop over time. Rationality and understanding clearly admit of degrees (though self-consciousness is a more challenging case). A theory that embraces such degrees of autonomy—and perhaps thereby degrees of personhood—must allow for the possibility that some nonhuman animals will be positioned at a higher level of autonomy or personhood than some humans.[10] The fact that humans will generally score higher under these criteria than other species of animals is a contingent fact. A nonhuman animal may overtake a human whenever the human loses a sufficient measure of cognitive abilities. If, for example, the primate in training in a language laboratory exceeds the deteriorating Alzheimer's patient on the relevant scale of cognitive capacities, the primate gains a higher degree of personhood, and may gain a higher moral status. However, metaphysical theories of persons that appeal exclusively to cognitive criteria entail no such conclusions about either moral persons or moral status, two topics to which I now turn.

THE CONCEPT OF MORAL PERSONHOOD

By comparison to metaphysical personhood, moral personhood is relatively uncomplicated. I will not attempt an account of the necessary and sufficient conditions of moral personhood, but it seems safe to assume that a creature is a moral person if (1) it is capable of making moral judgments about the rightness and wrongness of actions and (2) it has motives that can be judged morally. These are two jointly sufficient conditions of personhood. They are moral-capacity criteria and also cognitive criteria, but they are not sufficient conditions of morally correct action or character; an individual could be immoral and still qualify for moral personhood. These criteria will require for their explication some cognitive conditions discussed previously. For example, the capacity to make moral judgments may require rationality. A general theory of moral person-hood, then, would be needed to defend the aforementioned two conditions and to relate them to the cognitive conditions discussed previously.

However, such a general theory is not needed for the two primary theses that I now will defend. The first thesis is that moral personhood, unlike cognitivist theories of metaphysical personhood, is sufficient for moral status. Moral agents are paradigm bearers of moral status. Any entity qualifying for moral personhood is a member of the moral community and qualifies for its benefits, burdens, protections, and punishments. Moral persons understand moral reciprocity and the communal expectation that they will treat others as moral persons. It is central to the institution of morality itself that moral persons deserve respect and are to be judged as moral agents. Moral persons know that we can condemn their motives and actions, blame them for irresponsible actions, and punish them for immoral behavior. The moral protections afforded by this community may be extended to the weak and vulnerable who fail to qualify as moral persons, but moral status for these individuals must rest on some basis other than moral personhood.

The second thesis is that nonhuman animals are not plausible candidates for moral personhood, though the great apes, dolphins, and perhaps other animals with similar properties could turn out to be exceptions.[11] Here I borrow from Charles Darwin (1981, Chapter 3). He denies that animals make moral judgments while affirming that they sometimes display moral emotions and dispositions. For example, he maintains that animals do not make genuine judgments of blame when they punish their peers for misbehavior, but that they do display love, affection, and generosity. Darwin described conscience (the moral sense in humans) as "the most noble of all the attributes" found in the human animal: "I fully subscribe to the judgment of those writers who maintain that of all the differences between man and the lower animals, the moral sense or conscience is by far the most important." Darwin thus regarded nonhuman animals as failing the test of moral personhood.[12]

Humans, too, fail to qualify as moral persons if they lack one or more of the conditions of moral personhood. If moral personhood were the sole basis of moral rights (a view I do not hold), then these humans would lack rights—and precisely for the reasons that nonhuman animals would. Unprotected humans would presumably include fetuses, newborns, psychopaths, severely brain-damaged patients, and various dementia patients. I will now argue that these individuals do possess some rights and merit moral protections, but not because they satisfy the conditions of moral personhood. In this respect, these humans are in the same situation as many nonhumans: Moral status for them is not grounded in moral personhood any more than it is grounded in metaphysical personhood.

MORAL STATUS IN THE ABSENCE OF PERSONHOOD

It is fortunate for animals and humans who lack moral personhood that moral status does not require personhood of any type. The reason is that certain non-cognitive and nonmoral properties are sufficient to confer a measure of moral status.

At least two kinds of properties qualify a creature: properties of having the capacity for pain and suffering and properties of emotional deprivation. As Jeremy Bentham pointed out, the capacity to feel pain and undergo suffering is more relevant to moral status for nonhuman animals than are cognitive properties.[13] The emotional lives of animals, though seldom discussed until very recently, are no less important. Animals experience love, joy, anger, fear, shame, loneliness, and a broad range of emotions that can be radically altered, distorted, or numbed by their circumstances (Griffin, 1976; Masson & McCarthy, 1995; Orlans et al., 1998).

Nonpersons have many interests in avoidance of pain, suffering, and emotional deprivation. In principle, the status of such an individual could be so morally considerable as to outweigh certain moral rights and interests of persons. For example, the interests of animals could override the inherently limited rights of humans to do research, own zoos, run museums, and operate farms.

The injunction to avoid causing suffering, emotional deprivation, and many other forms of harm is as well established as any principle of morality. This injunction is fashioned to protect individuals because harm is bad in itself, not because it is bad for members of a certain species or type of individual, and not because the individual is or is not a moral person. Animals have interests in avoiding harms other than those of pain, suffering, and emotional deprivation. For example, they have interests in not being deprived of freedom of movement and in continued life. The range of their interests is beyond the scope of my arguments. I have merely maintained that we have at least some obligations to animals independent of their status as persons and that noncognitive, nonmoral properties that confer moral status form the basis of these obligations. This conclusion holds equally for humans lacking metaphysical and moral personhood.

WHICH ANIMALS HAVE RIGHTS?

Thus far I have not discussed whether moral status includes rights for animals other than the human animal. In a well-known article, Carl Cohen maintains that a right is a claim that one party may validly exercise against another and that claiming occurs only within a community of moral agents who can make claims against one another and are authorized to do so. These rights "are necessarily human; their possessors are persons" with the ability to make moral judgments and exercise moral claims. Animals cannot have rights, he says, because they lack these abilities (Cohen, 1986, p. 865; 1990), which is to say that they lack moral personhood. Kant seems to hold this view, which is also embraced by many contemporary contractarians. They regard us as having only indirect obligations to animals.

Though widely embraced, this view endangers animals and humans alike. A better account is that both humans and animals can be rights holders regardless of whether they are metaphysical or moral persons. This conclusion follows from my arguments about the diverse bases of moral obligations, but those arguments need to be combined with the widely accepted doctrine in law and morals that rights are correlative to obligations. On this account, obligations always imply corresponding rights if they are bona fide moral obligations, by contrast to merely self-assumed obligations or personal moral ideals, such as "obligations" of charitable giving.[14] "X has a right to do or to have Y" therefore means that the moral system of rules (or the legal system, if appropriate) imposes an obligation on someone to act or to refrain from acting so that X is enabled to do or have Y. The language of rights is always translatable in this way into the language of obligations, and vice versa. For example, if a research investigator has obligations to animal subjects to feed them and abstain from extremely painful procedures during the conduct of research, then animal subjects have a right to be fed and not to have the pain inflicted. More generally, if we have direct rather than merely indirect obligations to animals, then animals have correlative rights. From this perspective, a polarization into two fundamentally different types of theory, premised on a difference about rights and obligations, makes no sense. Correlativity requires that anyone who recognizes obligations logically must recognize that animals have whatever moral rights correspond to those obligations. Since Cohen and most thoughtful persons believe in some range of human obligations to nonhuman animals that derive from some source, it follows that they accept the view that the animals have correlative rights.

Possession of a right is also independent of being in a position to assert the right. A right-holder need not be the claimant in a particular case. For example, small children and the mentally handicapped may not be able to understand or claim their rights. Nonetheless, they possess them, and claims can be made for them by appropriate representatives. Similarly, animals have all the rights correlative to obligations that humans owe them, and they have these rights regardless of whether they or any surrogate is in a position to exercise the rights.

Whatever the precise set of rights of animals and of humans who fall short of moral personhood, and whatever their precise level of moral status, that set of rights will not be the same as the set of rights enjoyed by moral persons. Because bears and beagles lack the accountability and moral agency found in moral persons, their rights are different. A theory of moral personhood should help us understand why some entities have a full moral status, but the theory will not be sufficiently powerful to exclude other entities from a partial moral status. This point is not trivial, because some of the most important moral questions about our uses of both humans and nonhumans—for example, as sources of organs and as subjects of research—turn on the precise moral status of these individuals.

THE PROBLEM OF VAGUENESS IN THE CONCEPT OF PERSONS

Conceptual unclarity is another problem about theories of personhood that deserves attention. Literature on the criteria of persons is mired in an intractable dispute over a wide range of cases, including fetuses, newborns, the irreversibly comatose, God, extraterrestrials, and the great apes. Facts about these beings are not the source of the dispute. The problem is created by the vagueness and the inherently contestable nature of the ordinary language concept of person,[15] with its commitments to a human individual composed of a rather open-textured set of mental traits.

The vagueness of this concept is not likely to be dissipated by general theories of personhood, which will invariably be revisionary of the concept. Theories typically reflect the concept's vagueness and kindle more disagreement than enlightenment.[16] They give us no more than grounds for a claim that there are alternative sets of sufficient conditions of personhood. The possibility of necessary and sufficient conditions of person in a unified theory now seems dim. The concept of person is simply not orderly, precise, or systematic in a way that supports one general philosophical theory to the exclusion of another.

There is a solution to this problem of vagueness in the concept of person: Erase it from normative analysis and replace it with more specific concepts and relevant properties. I favor this option for both metaphysical personhood and moral personhood because it would enable us to go directly to the heart of substantive moral issues instead of using the oblique detour now made through theories of personhood. That is, we could inquire directly about the moral implications of possessing specific nonmoral and moral properties, such as reason and moral motivation, or we could discuss the substantive bases of ascriptions of rights. Questions about whether fetuses can be aborted, whether xenotransplantation is permissible, and whether anencephalics can be used in human experiments would then be recast in terms of whether and, if so, on what moral grounds such actions can be performed.

My suggestion is not that we should abandon philosophical theories of metaphysical persons and moral persons. My interest is exclusively in eliminating the abuse of these theories in normative analysis, not in eliminating the theories themselves.

CONCLUSION

I have said relatively little about specific normative problems or about the practical implications of the conclusions I have reached, but not because these questions are unimportant. I conclude with a comment on how very important they are.

Much has been made of the potential breakdown of the lines that have traditionally distinguished human and nonhuman animals. If nonhumans turn out to possess significantly more advanced capacities than customarily envisioned, their moral status would be upgraded to a more human level. However, this possibility remains speculative and may be less important than the thesis that because many humans *lack* properties of personhood or are less than full persons, they are thereby rendered equal or inferior in moral status to some nonhumans. If this conclusion is defensible, we will need to rethink our traditional view that these unlucky humans cannot be treated in the ways we treat relevantly similar nonhumans. For example, they might be aggressively used as human research subjects and sources of organs.

Perhaps we can find some justification of our traditional practices other than a justification based on status as persons or nonpersons. However, if we cannot find a compelling alternative justification, then either we should not be using animals as we do or we should be using humans as we do not.[17]

References

Beauchamp, Tom L. 1992. "The Moral Status of Animals in Medical Research." *Journal of Law, Medicine, and Ethics* 20: 7–16.

Benn, Stanley. 1976. "Freedom, Autonomy and the Concept of a Person." *Proceedings of the Aristotelian Society* 76: 123–130.

_____. 1988. *A Theory of Freedom.* Cambridge: Cambridge University Press.

Bentham, Jeremy. 1948. *The Principles of Morals and Legislation.* New York: Hafner.

Biernbacher, Dieter. 1996. The Great Apes—Why They Have a Right to Life. *Etica & Animali* 8: 143.

Buchanan, Allen, and Brock, Dan. 1989. *Deciding for Others: The Ethics of Surrogate Decision Making.* Cambridge: Cambridge University Press.

Cohen, Carl. 1986. "The Case for the Use of Animals in Research." *New England Journal of Medicine* 315: 865–870, esp. 865.

_____. 1990. "Animal Experimentation Defended." In *The Importance of Animal Experimentation for Safety and Biomedical Research,* ed. S. Garattini and D. W. van Bekkum, 7–16. Boston: Kluwer Academic.

Darwin, Charles. 1981. *The Descent of Man.* Princeton: Princeton University Press.

DeGrazia, David. 1996. *Taking Animals Seriously: Mental Life and Moral Status.* New York: Cambridge University Press.

_____. 1997. "Great Apes, Dolphins, and the Concept of Personhood." *Southern Journal of Philosophy* 35: 301–320.

Dennett, Daniel. 1976. "Conditions of Personhood." In *The Identities of Persons,* ed. Amelie O. Rorty, 175–196. Berkeley: University of California Press.

Dworkin, Gerald. 1988. *The Theory and Practice of Autonomy.* New York: Cambridge University Press.

Ekstrom, Laura W. 1993. "A Coherence Theory of Autonomy." *Philosophy and Phenomenological Research* 53: 599–616.

Engelhardt, H. Tristram, Jr. 1996. *The Foundations of Bioethics.* 2nd ed. New York: Oxford University Press.

English, Jane 1975. "Abortion and the Concept of a Person." *Canadian Journal of Philosophy* 5: 233–243.

Feinberg, Joel. 1989. "The Rights of Animals and Future Generations." In *Animal Rights and Human Obligations*, 2nd ed., ed. Tom Regan and Peter Singer, 190–196. Englewood Cliffs, NJ: Prentice Hall.

_____and Levenbook, Barbara Baum. 1993. Abortion. In *Matters of Life and Death: New Introductory Essays in Moral Philosophy*, 3rd ed., ed. Tom Regan, 195–234. New York: Random House.

Francione, Gary L. 1995. *Animals, Property, and the Law*. Philadelphia: Temple University Press.

Frankfurt, Harry G. 1971. "Freedom of the Will and the Concept of a Person." *Journal of Philosophy* 68: 5–20.

Frey, Raymond. 1988. "Moral Status, the Value of Lives, and Speciesism." *Between the Species* 4 (3): 191–201.

_____. 1996. "Medicine, Animal Experimentation, and the Moral Problem of Unfortunate Humans." *Social Philosophy and Policy* 13: 181–211.

Gallup, Gordon G. 1977. "Self-Recognition in Primates." *American Psychologist* 32: 329–338.

Gervais, Karen G. 1986. *Redefining Death*. New Haven: Yale University Press.

Goodman, Michael. 1988. *What Is a Person?* Clifton, NJ: Humana Press.

Griffin, Donald R. 1976. *The Question of Animal Awareness: Evolutionary Continuity of Mental Experience* (2nd ed., 1981). New York: Rockefeller University Press.

_____. 1992. *Animal Minds*. Chicago: University of Chicago Press.

Harris, John. 1985. *The Value of Life*. London: Routledge.

Locke, John. 1975. *An Essay Concerning Human Understanding*, ed. Peter Nidditch. Oxford: Clarendon Press.

Lomasky, Loren. 1987. *Persons, Rights, and the Moral Community*. Oxford: Oxford University Press.

Marras, Ausunio. 1993. "Pollock on How to Build a Person." *Dialogue* 32: 595–605.

Masson, Jeffrey M., and McCarthy, Susan. 1995. *When Elephants Weep: The Emotional Lives of Animals*. New York: Delacorte Press.

Miles, H. L. 1993. "Language and the Orang-utan: The Old Person of the Forest." In *The Great Ape Project*, ed. Paola Cavalieri and Peter Singer, 52. New York: St. Martin's Press.

Orlans, F. Barbara, et al. 1998. *The Human Use of Animals: Case Studies in Ethical Choice*. New York: Oxford University Press.

Patterson, Francine, and Gordon, Wendy. 1993. "The Case for the Personhood of Gorillas." In *The Great Ape Project*, ed. Paola Cavalieri and Peter Singer, 58–77. New York: St. Martin's Press.

Pollock, John. 1989. *How to Build a Person*. Cambridge, MA: MIT Press.

Puccetti, Roland. 1969. *Persons*. New York: Harder and Harder.

Rachels, James. 1990. *Created From Animals: The Moral Implications of Darwinism*. New York: Oxford University Press.

_____. 1993. "Why Darwinians Should Support Equal Treatment for Other Great Apes." In *The Great Ape Project*, ed. Paola Cavalieri and Peter Singer, 152–157. New York: St. Martin's Press.

Regan, Tom. 1983. *The Case for Animal Rights*. Berkeley: University of California Press.

Rodd, Rosemary. 1990. *Biology, Ethics, and Animals*. Oxford: Clarendon Press.

Sapontzis, S. F. 1987. *Morals, Reason, and Animals*. Philadelphia: Temple University Press.

Savulescu, J. 1994. "Rational Desires and the Limitation of Life-Sustaining Treatment." *Bioethics* 8: 191–222.

Strawson, Peter. 1959. *Individuals*. London: Methuen.

Tooley, Michael. 1972. "Abortion and Infanticide." *Philosophy and Public Affairs* 2 (Fall): 37–65.

_____. 1983. *Abortion and Infanticide*. Oxford: Clarendon Press.

_____. 1984. "In Defense of Abortion and Infanticide." In *The Problem of Abortion*, 2nd ed., ed. Joel Feinberg, 120–134. Belmont, CA: Wadsworth Publishing Company.

Warren, Mary Anne. 1973. "On the Moral and Legal Status of Abortion." *The Monist* 57: 43–61.

_____. 1991. "Abortion." In *A Companion to Ethics*, ed. Peter Singer, 303–314. Cambridge, MA: Blackwell Reference.

Notes

1. Other philosophers have used this or a similar distinction, but not as I analyze the distinction (cf. Dennett, 1976, esp. 176–178; Feinberg & Levenbook 1993; Sapontzis 1987, 47ff).

2. A respectable case can be made that Aristotle, Boethius, Descartes, Locke, Hume, and Kant either presupposed or argued for this position. However, Kant's apparent inclusion of moral autonomy renders him a borderline case, and other qualifications would need to be made for some of these figures.

3. Tooley's clarification of the distinction between the descriptive and the normative functions of "person" is useful. For a concise and persuasive account of the descriptive (factual) and normative (implying rights and duties) uses of the concept of person and the philosophical importance of the distinction, see Biernbacher (1996, 143). However, neither account captures the notion of *moral personhood*, which is more descriptive than normative. The normative dimension is best understood in terms of the moral status of persons, irrespective of whether that status is attributed on the basis of metaphysical or moral personhood. This point seems generally overlooked in the relevant literature (see, e.g., Gervais, 1986, 181).

4. Throughout the histories of philosophy and law, there has been little resistance to the postulate that animals have no moral or legal standing because they lack the properties that confer moral status. Animals have been given almost no legal standing in British and American systems of law, but questions of their moral status are far from decided (see Beauchamp, 1992; DeGrazia, 1997; Francione, 1995, Chapter 4; Frey, 1988, esp. 196–197; Rachels, 1990; Regan, 1983).

5. I do not deny the possibility of a theory of metaphysical personhood. My objections do not apply to some of the early and influential metaphysical accounts in contemporary philosophy, such as Strawson (1959) and Puccetti (1969). Locke, as cited earlier, is another example.

6. On the relevance and plausibility of robots and physical-mental systems that imitate human traits, see Pollock (1989) and Marras (1993).

7. See Tooley (1972, 1983); also see Engelhardt (1996, Chapters 4, 6); Lomasky (1987); Tooley (1984); and Warren (1973, esp. sec. 2; 1991, esp. 310–313). See, too, the articles and bibliography in Goodman (1988).

8. There are more demanding theories than these second-order reflection theories. Some theories require extremely rigorous standards in order to be autonomous or to be persons. For example, they demand that the autonomous individual be authentic, consistent, independent, in command, resistant to control by authorities, and the original source of values, beliefs, rational desires, and life plans (see Benn, 1976; 1988, 3–6, 155f, 175–183; see also Savulescu, 1994).

9. See Donald R. Griffin, *Animal Minds* (Chicago: University of Chicago Press, 1992).

10. Some measure of personhood is gained or lost over time as critical capacities are gained or lost. These capacities are often gained or lost gradually, feeding the hypothesis of degrees of personhood.

11. For the kinds of capacities and action that appear to constitute an exception, see the study of gorillas in Patterson and Gordon (1993, esp. 70–71).

12. Darwin argues that moral sensitivity is itself the product of evolution. He maintains that some humans display a high level and other humans a low level of moral responsiveness; the highest level of morality is reached when persons extend their sympathies beyond their own group and indeed beyond their own species to all sentient creatures.

13. Bentham (1948, Chapter 17, sec. 1) reasons as follows: "If the being eaten were all, there is very good reason why we should be suffered to eat such of them as we like to eat: we are the better for it, and they are never the worse. They have none of those long-protracted anticipations of future miserys which we have. The death they suffer in our hands commonly is, and always may be, a speedier, and by that means a less painful one, than that which would await them in the inevitable course of nature. . . . But is there any reason why we should be suffered to torment them? Not any that I can see. Are there any why we should not be suffered to torment them? Yes, several. . . ."

Donald Griffin has argued that no good reason exists to place a special weight on the distinction between perceptual awareness in animals and a reflective consciousness. Griffin (1992, esp. 248) proposes multiple levels of mentation shared across species, from basic pain receptors to intentionality (see also DeGrazia, 1996; Rodd, 1990).

14. See Joel Feinberg's (1989) argument that animals can have rights because they have, or at least can have, interests that we are obligated to protect. For example, animals have the right to be treated humanely, which follows from an obligation of justice. Feinberg and others have argued that we have a strong moral obligation not to cause unnecessary suffering in animals, and that correlative to this obligation are rights for animals—even if the fulfillment of that obligation has the consequence of losing benefits for humans.

15. For an early and influential analysis of this problem, see English (1975); see also DeGrazia (1996, esp. 305–315).

16. Some theories appeal to human characteristics, others to beings with moral status, and still others to those with properties such as second-order volition (Frankfurt), moral volition (Kant), and the capacity to experience pain and suffering (Bentham). Each account is tied to some larger philosophical doctrine. Without judging the merits of the latter, it is difficult if not impossible to judge the former.

17. My conclusion here has been influenced by private discussions with Raymond Frey (see Frey, 1996); see also the engaging essay by Rachels (1993).

15

LOOKING BACK AND JUDGING OUR PREDECESSORS

It seems widely believed, as the chairman of the Chemical Manufacturers Association recently opined, that "You cannot judge people or a company based on today's standards or knowledge for actions taken 40 to 60 years ago" ("Ex-owner," 1994). The claim is that people cannot be judged or held responsible for forms of waste disposal, research practices, types of marketing, and the like that were common and rarely challenged a half-century ago. The Advisory Committee on Human Radiation Experiments (ACHRE) has recently shown that this thesis cannot be sustained, at least not without heavy qualification.

The Advisory Committee's framework of distinctions and principles is found in Chapter 4 of its *Final Report*, entitled "Ethics Standards in Retrospect" (ACHRE, 1995). I accept the major components of the moral framework of principles presented by the Advisory Committee, but I will argue that the Advisory Committee does not altogether adhere to the language and commitments of that framework of principles in later chapters of the *Final Report*. My concern is with how the Advisory Committee's principled framework was used and how it could and should have been used to make retrospective judgments about *wrong-doing* and *culpability*. I will here limit my comments to plutonium cases (see ACHRE, 1995, Chapter 5), and I will emphasize the University of California at San Francisco (UCSF) case. However, these conclusions are generalizable to the entire report, especially to the "Findings" in Chapter 17.

Although there are imperfections in the Advisory Committee's use of its own framework in reaching judgments of culpability, these shortcomings are significantly offset by its persuasive and well-documented judgments of wrongdoing. Furthermore, this committee's weaknesses look like strengths when compared to the more serious deficiencies in the *Report of the UCSF Ad Hoc Fact Finding Committee on World War II Human Radiation Experiments* (UCSF, 1995). The latter report, I will argue, effectively has no framework and reaches no significant judgments of either wrongdoing or culpability, although it was positioned to do so.

STANDARDS FOR RETROSPECTIVE JUDGMENT

In its *Final Report,* the Advisory Committee presents a well-developed set of distinctions, principles, explanations, and arguments pertinent to retrospective moral judgments. It delineates "An Ethical Framework" (ACHRE, 1995 [GPO, pp. 197–212; Oxford, pp. 114–124]), which I will call "the framework." Its core, for my purposes, is (1) a distinction between *wrongdoing* and *culpability;* (2) the identification of three kinds of ethical standards relevant to the evaluation of the human radiation experiments (basic principles, government policies, and rules of professional ethics); and (3) an account of culpability and exculpation, including mitigating conditions that are exculpatory. I will first review what the *Final Report* says about these three parts of the framework, and then turn to critical appraisal later.

The Wrongness of Actions and the Culpability of Agents

The distinction between the wrongness of actions and the culpability of agents derives from the need to distinguish whether one is evaluating the moral quality— in particular, the wrongness—of actions, practices, policies, and institutions or evaluating the blameworthiness (culpability) of agents. The Advisory Committee correctly concluded that past actions regarding the conduct of human radiation research can be judged instances of wrongdoing without at the same time judging the agents who performed them to be culpable. From the fact that an action was wrong or that someone was wronged by the action, it does not follow that the agent(s) who performed the actions can be fairly blamed, censured, or punished. This distinction is of the highest significance and is appropriately given a prominent position in the Advisory Committee's Ethical Framework (ACHRE, 1995 [GPO, pp. 208–212; Oxford, pp. 121–124]).

Universal Moral Principles and Contemporaneous Policies and Rules

The Advisory Committee identifies six basic ethical principles as relevant to its work: "One ought not to treat people as mere means to the ends of others"; "One ought not to deceive others"; "One ought not to inflict harm or risk of harm"; "One ought to promote welfare and prevent harm"; "One ought to treat people fairly and with equal respect"; and "One ought to respect the self-determination of others" (ACHRE, 1995 [GPO, p. 198; Oxford, p. 114]). These principles state general obligations. The Advisory Committee held that they are widely accepted and that the validity of the principles is *not time-bound*. A hundred years or a thousand years ago would not alter their moral force (ACHRE, 1995 [GPO, p. 199; Oxford, p. 115]). By contrast, policies of government agencies and rules of professional ethics do not have this universal quality and are often specific as to time and place (ACHRE, 1995 [GPO, pp. 214–221; Oxford, pp. 125–130]).

Culpability and Exculpation

Third, building on the wrongdoing–culpability distinction, the Advisory Committee added an account of culpability and exculpatory conditions (ACHRE, 1995 [GPO, p. 208ff; Oxford, p. 121ff]). The Advisory Committee found that several factors limit our ability to make judgments about the blame-worthiness of agents. These include lack of evidence; the presence of conflicting obligations; factual ignorance; culturally induced moral ignorance, in which "cultural factors … prevent individuals from discerning what they are morally required to do" (ACHRE, 1995 [GPO, p. 209; Oxford, p. 121]); an evolution in the delineation of moral principles; and indeterminacy in an organization's division of labor and designation of responsibility.

Although these conditions are exculpatory—that is, they *mitigate* or *tend to absolve* of alleged fault or blame—satisfaction of the conditions does not always exculpate and only two of the conditions affect judgments of wrongdoing (ACHRE, 1995 [GPO, p. 204; Oxford, p. 118]). The conditions are satisfied by degrees, and exculpation can involve balancing several different considerations (ACHRE, 1995 [GPO, p. 210; Oxford, p. 122]). Presumably at the heart of the Advisory Committee's work is an examination of whether these exculpatory conditions were present in particular cases in order to determine whether the persons involved are excul-pated—that is, are free or relatively free of blame for what they did.

The Advisory Committee understood its first task to be that of evaluating the rightness or wrongness of actions, practices, and policies. It emphasized the impor-tance of discovering whether judgments ascribing blame to individuals or groups can and should be made. It noted that "unless judgments of culpability are made *about particular individuals,* one important means of deterring future wrongs will be precluded" (ACHRE, 1995 [GPO, p. 212; Oxford, p. 123], emphasis added).

THE UCSF CASE

One case considered by the Advisory Committee, and the only one I will consider in detail, originates at UCSF and eventuates in the Ad Hoc Committee report previously mentioned. I will use this case as an example of the Advisory Committee's application of its framework to assess a case and as a means of evaluating the UCSF Ad Hoc Committee's judgments.[1]

Plutonium Injections from 1945 to 1947

The salient facts in this case are as follows. From April 1945 to July 1947, 17 patients were injected with plutonium at three university hospitals—UCSF, the University of Chicago, and the University of Rochester—and 1 patient was injected at Oak Ridge Hospital in Tennessee. Three of the 18 (known as CAL-1, 2, and 3) were injected at UCSF. Eventually allegations surfaced that the injections of plutonium were toxic to the patients and that they never consented to involvement as subjects of the research.

These patient-subjects were part of a secret research protocol initiated by the Manhattan Engineer District, a government program responsible for the production of atomic weapons. The purpose of this scientific research was to determine the excretion rate of plutonium in humans so that the government could establish safety levels and standards for workers who handled this radioactive element. Although performed largely in secret, some of this work was known publicly as early as 1951. It was discussed in the 1970s and 1980s, but did not generate a substantial controversy until 1993, as a result of the work of a persistent investigative reporter in Albuquerque, N.M.

The 1995 Report of the UCSF Ad Hoc Committee

On January 7, 1994, UCSF Chancellor Joseph Martin appointed an Ad Hoc Committee to investigate these allegations by studying the history of UCSF involvement. After a year of investigating documents and debating the issues, this committee filed its report in February 1995. The Ad Hoc Committee confirmed UCSF involvement and confirmed that at least one of the three initial patients had been included in the secret government protocol. The UCSF report notes that the "injections of plutonium were not expected to be, nor were they, therapeutic or of medical benefit to the patients" (UCSF, 1995, p. 27).[2]

The Ad Hoc Committee found that written consent was rare, disclosure narrow, and the permission of patients not typically obtained even for nontherapeutic research during this period. They found that it is not known and could not be known exactly what these research subjects were told or what they understood (UCSF, 1995, pp. 26, 34). They also found that the word *plutonium* was classified at the time; it is therefore certain that it was not used in any disclosures or explanations that might have been made to patient-subjects. The committee noted that in a recorded oral history in 1979, Kenneth Scott, one of the three original UCSF investigators, said that he never told the first subject what had been injected in him. Scott went on to say that the experiments were "incautious" and "morally wrong" (UCSF, 1995, pp. 26–27).[3]

Nonetheless, the Ad Hoc Committee wrote, "At the time of the plutonium experiments, [today's issues about proof of consent] were not discussed. The Committee is hesitant to apply current-day standards to another historical period," although "overall, the Committee believes that practices of consent of the era were inadequate by today's standards, and even by standards existing at the time.... [T]he Committee believes that researchers should have discussed risks with potential subjects" (UCSF, 1995, pp. 32, 34).

The Ad Hoc Committee concluded that this experimentation offered no benefit to subjects but also caused no harm because patients did not develop any medical complications. It also found that the experiments themselves were "consistent with accepted medical research practices at the time" (UCSF, 1995, p. 33). The Ad Hoc Committee concluded that the subjects were *wronged* and the experimentation was "unethical" *if* the patients did not understand or agree to the interventions; in this event, they were wronged because their integrity and dignity were violated. However, the Ad Hoc Committee found that since it could not establish what the patients understood, no basis existed for saying that they actually were wronged (UCSF, 1995, pp. 28–34).

In an appendix to the Ad Hoc Committee's report, a lawyer and committee member, Elizabeth Zitrin, concluded that even if the experiments were consistent with accepted medical practices at the time, "it does not make them ethical. And they were not consistent with the highest standards of the time articulated by the government, the profession, or the public." The chairman of the Ad Hoc Committee, Roy Filly, responded that this comment by the lawyer held investigators to an unrealistically high research standard.[4] I will consider this issue momentarily, but first one further development in this case merits attention.

One day after the Ad Hoc Committee filed its report in February 1995, it received a recently declassified memorandum about this research that had been written on December 30, 1946. The memo was written by the chief of the

Operations Branch, Research Division, at the Oak Ridge Atomic Facility. His subject was the preparations being made "for injection in humans by doctors [Robert] Stone [one of the three original UCSF investigators] and [Earl] Miller." The memo reports that:

> These doctors state that the injections would probably be made *without the knowledge of the patient* and that the physicians assumed full responsibility. Such injections were not divergent from the normal experimental method in the hospital and the patient signed no release (Chapman, 1946, p. 1).

This memorandum and other known facts in the UCSF case indicate, despite an excessively restrained Ad Hoc Committee report (discussed later in this essay), that these patients were seriously wronged, even if they were not physically or mentally harmed (ACHRE, 1995 [GPO, pp. 249–252, 256–258, 264–269; Oxford, pp. 149–152, 154–155, 160–163]). The UCSF committee was unwilling to reach conclusions about wrongdoing, preferring, like the chairman of the Chemical Manufacturers Association, the position that it is too demanding to judge people or institutions for actions taken a half-century ago. Nowhere did the Ad Hoc Committee consider culpability, but its conservative conclusions strongly hint at exculpation on grounds of the limited evidence available to the committee.

No analysis of this case or the other plutonium cases will be adequate if it evades examination of questions of wrongdoing and culpability. The Advisory Committee's framework makes this demand. But how does the Advisory Committee fare in making the judgments its framework calls for, and does it fare better than the Ad Hoc Committee?

THE ADVISORY COMMITTEE'S FRAMEWORK

A section entitled "Applying the Ethical Framework" in the Advisory Committee's *Final Report* evaluates "human radiation experiments conducted between 1944 and 1974" (ACHRE, 1995 [GPO, pp. 212–221; Oxford, pp. 124–130]). I will first examine what, in my judgment, the Advisory Committee could be expected to have decided in light of its own framework and, second, ways in which the Advisory Committee deviated from what could be expected.

The Advisory Committee's framework and discussion of its application indicate that it undertook three assignments:

1. to locate moral wrongdoing that violates either basic moral principles or guidelines in the government policies and professional ethics of the period;

2. to place the violations in the context of mitigating or exculpatory conditions; and
3. to decide which persons and institutions are culpable and which exculpated, as well as which lie on a continuum between the two.

Through a resourceful and historically innovative examination of the actual policies of government agencies and rules of professional ethics of the period, the Advisory Committee unhesitatingly addressed the first assignment:

> [T]hese experiments were unethical.... [T]wo basic moral principles were violated—that one ought not to use people as a mere means to the ends of others and that one ought not to deceive others.... The egregiousness of the disrespectful way in which the subjects of the injection experiments and their families were treated is heightened by the fact that the subjects were hospitalized patients...[leaving] them vulnerable to exploitation (ACHRE, 1995 [GPO, pp. 267–268; Oxford, p. 162]).

This evaluation of wrongdoing contrasts with the vacillation and indecisiveness in the UCSF Ad Hoc Committee report. Although, with the exception of the memo, both committees had basically the same documentary evidence before them, the ways in which that evidence was used for retrospective judgments is striking. This contrast makes for an excellent bioethics case study of different approaches to the evidence for retrospective moral judgment.

The Advisory Committee tackled the second assignment with the same decisiveness and conscientious use of historical documents. In the UCSF case and other radiation cases, it noted that judgments of excusability, culpability, and the like depend, at least to some extent, on whether proper moral standards for research involving human subjects were acknowledged in government agency policies and in the culture of medicine. If relevant standards and duties were entirely undeveloped at the time, this lamentable circumstance becomes exculpatory for persons accused of wrongdoing. Such circumstances would be very different from a situation in which there existed well-developed and officially endorsed policies for human subjects research.

The Advisory Committee determined, however, that exculpation does not come easily, because policies that included vital elements that would today be considered central to the ethics of research involving human subjects existed even in the mid-1940s. For example, the Advisory Committee concluded from the evidence that "it was common to obtain the voluntary consent of healthy subjects who were to participate in biomedical experiments that offered no prospect of medical benefit to them" and that ill subjects were not a relevantly different class of subjects (ACHRE, 1995 [GPO, p. 217; Oxford, p. 127]). The Advisory Committee also found that "even fifty years ago, [the six basic] principles were pervasive features of moral life in the United States" that every medical investigator could be expected to observe (ACHRE, 1995 [GPO, p. 204; Oxford, p. 118]).

In light of these discoveries and conclusions, the Advisory Committee often reacted to proposed exculpatory conditions with the same strength and decisiveness with which it reacted to violations of principles. An example is found in its conclusion that the mitigating condition of culturally induced moral ignorance does not apply to many government officials, because they simply failed to implement or communicate requirements that were already established as their responsibility: "The very fact that these requirements were articulated by the agencies in which they worked is evidence that officials could not have been morally ignorant of them" (ACHRE, 1995 [GPO, p. 215; Oxford, p. 126]).

Throughout its assessments under assignment 2, the Advisory Committee relied on the aforementioned cluster of factors, including factual ignorance and culturally induced moral ignorance, that limit the ability to make judgments of agent culpability. These criteria and the conclusions drawn from them contrast markedly with the work of the UCSF Ad Hoc Committee, which attempted to place a maximal distance between the policies of the 1940s and those of the 1990s, rather than to locate their similarities. The Ad Hoc Committee was willing to find mitigating conditions that either exculpate or suggest exculpation at almost every point in the trail of evidence, whereas the Advisory Committee placed the evidence in a broader and more revealing context.

The mood and strategy shift, however, in the Advisory Committee's handling of the third assignment. There is a sharp deviation from what I hypothesize to be the expected path the Advisory Committee would take. Instead of assessing culpability and exculpation for individuals and institutions, the Advisory Committee focused almost entirely on the wrongness of actions. Despite its statement, previously quoted, that "judgments of culpability [should be] made *about particular individuals,*" no such judgment is reached in the *Final Report,* not about the plutonium cases or any other cases, apparently because the Advisory Committee found the trail of warranting evidence to run out at this point.

This outcome is surprising in light of the Advisory Committee's assessment that many of the individuals involved in these cases had an obligation to the norms governing conduct and yet often failed to take them seriously. For example, the Advisory Committee found that various physicians could and should have seen that using sick patients as they did in the plutonium cases was morally worse than using healthy people, for in so doing one was violating not only the basic ethical principle not to use people as a mere means but also the basic ethical principle to treat people fairly and with equal respect (ACHRE, 1995 [GPO, p. 219; Oxford, pp. 128–129]).

Following these indictments of the *actions* of physicians—and government officials, in corresponding passages—the reader is poised for the next step: a treatment of mitigating conditions that are exculpatory, followed by an assessment of culpability or exculpation. Surprisingly, this analysis never develops, or at least does not develop for the evaluation of specific individuals. Only in the final sentence of Chapter 5 does the Advisory Committee hint at the issue, using a new language of "accountability." It determined that responsible officials at government agencies and medical professionals responsible for the plutonium injections were *"accountable* for the moral wrongs that were done" (ACHRE, 1995 [GPO, p. 269; Oxford, p. 163], emphasis added).

Clearly these professionals were accountable (i.e., responsible and answerable), but were they culpable (blameworthy and censurable)? The term *accountable* may also here be functioning to pronounce blame, but the terms do not have the same meaning, and the subtlety of the point will escape even close readers. The Advisory Committee makes no connection in its *Final Report* between being accountable and being culpable; nor does it present an argument to indicate that in reaching the aforementioned judgment of accountability the Advisory Committee is blaming the individual physicians responsible for the injections or any of the other parties mentioned.

Some of this lost ground is recovered in the Advisory Committee's "Finding 11" in Chapter 17, where it finally restores the language of blame and returns to its earlier style of reaching decisive conclusions:

> The Advisory Committee finds that government officials and investigators are blameworthy for not having had policies and practices in place to protect the rights and interests of human subjects who were used in research from which the subjects could not possibly derive medical benefits (nontherapeutic research in the strict sense). By contrast, to the extent that there was reason to believe that research might provide a direct medical benefit to subjects, government officials and biomedical professionals are less blameworthy for not having had such protections and practices. We also find that, to the extent that research was thought to pose significant risk, government officials and investigators are more blameworthy for not having had such protections and practices in place (ACHRE, 1995 [GPO, pp. 787–788; Oxford, pp. 503–504]).

This passage is particularly important for understanding what the Advisory Committee believed it could and could not conclude in light of the massive body of evidence before it. The Advisory Committee apparently thought that it could blame only individuals and groups of individuals in institutions such as government agencies and the medical establishment. While this blaming is amorphous and anonymous, the Advisory Committee managed to reach a critical general assessment:

> [G]overnment officials and biomedical professionals should have recognized that when research offers *no prospect* of medical benefit, whether subjects are healthy or sick, research should not proceed without the person's consent. It should have been recognized that despite the significant decision-making authority ceded to the physician within the doctor-patient relationship, this authority did not extend to procedures conducted solely to advance science without a prospect of offsetting benefit to the person (ACHRE, 1995 [GPO, p. 788; Oxford, p. 504]).

These forms of blame are improvements over the weaker conclusions in Chapter 5 about the plutonium cases. They also, once again, contrast noticeably with the inconclusiveness in the UCSF Ad Hoc Committee report, which assesses no form of blame, general or particular. Nonetheless, nowhere in the Advisory Committee's *Final Report* is a named agent, other than the federal government and the medical profession, ever found culpable. This is true not only in the Advisory Committee's discussion of the plutonium cases, but also throughout the Advisory Committee's report. This outcome is not what one would have expected after the Advisory Committee's indictments of the intentional actions of wrongdoing mentioned throughout its *Final Report,* and it raises questions of what might have been decided within the Advisory Committee's framework had it not held out for exceptionally high standards of historical and testimonial evidence before assessing individual blame (as is discussed in the Conclusion of this essay).

WHAT FINDINGS SHOULD HAVE BEEN REACHED ABOUT THE VIOLATIONS OF STANDARDS?

I will now consider the judgments the Advisory Committee should have reached, given its framework and objectives. In some cases, it did reach these judgments; in others, it did not. Again the UCSF case will serve as the principal example. In asking whether the UCSF investigators violated moral standards, we could be asking one or both of two questions, as the Advisory Committee notes. A first question is whether these investigators violated well-articulated *rules of professional ethics* or *government policies.* A second question is whether *universal rights* or *principles* were violated. The Advisory Committee offers convincing answers to both questions. However, its answer to the second needs assessment before proceeding to the more important questions of mitigating conditions.

Were Universal Standards Violated?

The Advisory Committee notes that the first *two* of its principles were violated, namely, that persons may not be used as mere means to the ends of others and that persons may not be deceived by others; elsewhere in the *Report* it adds a violation of its fifth principle, "One ought to treat people fairly and with equal respect" (ACHRE, 1995 [GPO, pp. 219, 267; Oxford, pp. 128–129, 162]). The claim that three principles were violated is justified, but the mention of only three principles is puzzling. The evidence assembled in the UCSF case, and in other cases before the Advisory Committee, is sufficient to conclude that *all six* of the principles identified by the Advisory Committee were violated.

The third principle is, "One ought not to inflict harm or risk of harm." Given what was known and not known about plutonium at the time, it is reasonable to infer that the physicians involved placed their patients at risk of harm, though perhaps risk at an uncertain level. Whether this principle was violated was a matter of debate during the Advisory Committee's deliberations, but the available evidence seems to warrant a conclusion that violations of the principle did occur. It is not credible that a physician could inject a patient with plutonium without any awareness that doing so involved risk for the patient. The fourth principle is, "One ought to promote welfare and prevent harm." In the context of the plutonium experiments, it does not appear that a serious attempt was made to prevent harm from occurring and certainly there was no affirmative promotion of welfare. There was an attempt to refine the methods used so as to reduce the likelihood and magnitude of harm, but no more. Finally, the sixth principle is, "One ought to respect the self-determination of others." This principle was violated beyond a reasonable doubt, because the investigators routinely ignored the right to consent to bodily invasions following adequate disclosures.

The Advisory Committee thus *implicitly* recognized that all six of its principles were violated in the plutonium cases, but its failure to reach the *explicit* conclusion that all six principles were violated is not insignificant. The Advisory Committee identified its set of principles in order to provide a comprehensive account of what could be reasonably expected of persons. It aimed for a complete assessment of past practices in order to reduce the risk of errors and abuses in future human experimentation. The Advisory Committee insisted that, in light of these goals, a "complete and accurate diagnosis requires not only stating what wrongs were done, but also explaining who was responsible for the wrongs occurring" (ACHRE, 1995 [GPO, p. 212; Oxford, p. 123]).

Underassessment of the number of principles violated and those responsible for violations outcomes are an unfortunate outcome. Perhaps it is but a minor error in the Advisory Committee's report, but the same type of error afflicts the report of the UCSF Ad Hoc Committee.[5] If the Advisory Committee hoped to affect the thinking of future committee members on committees such as the one at UCSF, it would have been instructive to show that and how all six principles had been violated.

What Findings Should Have Been Reached About Exculpatory Conditions?

Is the ineffectual professional ethics during the period in question a condition that mitigates blame—an exculpatory condition? Yes. Does this condition erase the wrongs done to research subjects? No. Judgments of wrongdoing are not affected by exculpatory conditions. Does the ineffectual professional ethics exculpate the agents involved? No. A weak professional ethics merely mitigates (i.e., tempers or lessens the severity of) blame; it does not clear of blame or exculpate. I will address exculpation in a moment. The immediate question is about exculpatory conditions and how they are related to the void in professional standards: What conditions are exculpatory? Why are they exculpatory? To what degree do they exculpate?

As previously noted, the Advisory Committee identified a set of exculpatory or mitigating conditions: lack of evidence; the presence of conflicting obligations, including obligations to protect national security; factual ignorance; culturally induced moral ignorance; an evolution in the delineation of moral principles; and indeterminacy in an organization's division of labor and designation of responsibility. To these conditions we might add that blame could be mitigated by culturally induced misunderstandings, by a person's good character, and by what in law is called "excusable neglect," which is neglect caused by an unavoidable hindrance or accident. Only three of these conditions need assessment here because of the role they play in the plutonium cases: (1) factual ignorance, (2) culturally induced moral ignorance, and (3) obligations to protect national security.

Factual Ignorance

The Advisory Committee never argues that a significant measure of nonculpable factual ignorance was operative in the UCSF case. The Advisory Committee holds that claims of nonculpable factual ignorance can too easily function as an excuse for wrongful actions and, by inference, as an excuse for failures to make retrospective moral judgments:

[J]ust because an agent's ignorance of morally relevant information leads him or her to commit a morally wrong act, it does not follow that the person is not blameworthy for that act. The agent is blameworthy if a reasonably prudent person in that agent's position should have been aware that some information was required prior to action, and the information could have been obtained without undue effort or cost on his or her part (ACHRE, 1995 [GPO, p. 208; Oxford, p. 121]).

Culturally Induced Moral Ignorance

A claim of culturally induced moral ignorance lacks credible backing in the UCSF case. Even if we grant that there were no strong cultural incentives to abstain from the research and little instruction in medical ethics, it is not too much to expect these physicians to have been aware that their actions required a justification other than the experiment's utility for others. Never in the history of civil medicine has it been permissible to exploit patients by using them to the ends of science in nontherapeutic research that carries risk of harm. In the plutonium cases, the problem is not merely that no *informed* consent was obtained. No consent at all was obtained.

Culturally induced beliefs, such as the belief that consent is not morally required in a hospital setting, are most likely to constitute a valid excuse for wrong actions when alternative views are unavailable or are not taken seriously in the context. But alternative views were available and were considered matters of the utmost significance in sources available to the relevant parties. It was known or easily knowable at the time that (1) a debate had occurred during the mid-1940s about experimentation in Nazi Germany; (2) the American Medical Association's Judicial Council had sided in 1946 with what would soon be the Nuremberg thesis that voluntary consent to participation in research is essential; (3) the Hippocratic tradition required physicians to put the care of patients first, not to deviate radically from accepted therapies, and not to risk harm to patients through nontherapeutic interventions; and (4) there was a long tradition of post-Hippocratic writings in medical ethics that included Thomas Percival, Claude Bernard, and Walter Reed, each of whom recognized nontherapeutic experimentation as valid only if subjects had consented. Thus, requirements such as voluntary consent to experimentation and protection against harmful interventions had long been present in the medical community and even were present in some government policies traceable to the early 1940s (see Lederer & Moreno, 1996).

In light of this history, the UCSF physicians could not plausibly appeal to nonculpable moral blindness, because they and the officials at their institutions, as well as responsible higher officials in medicine, could have been expected to remedy contextual moral ignorance. There was ample opportunity for

remediation of inadequate moral beliefs and therefore culpability for the con-
tinuance of those beliefs. The excuse of *nonculpable ignorance,* then, is not
credible.

Conflicting Obligations—The National Security Exception

The matter of mitigating conditions is more complicated than nonculpable
ignorance, because it might be argued that there was reason to believe that the
research constituted a justifiable *exception* to ordinary physician obligations and
government policies requiring compliance with established standards. In the
UCSF case and others considered by the Advisory Committee, obligations to
protect national security might be viewed as conflicting with and overriding
obligations to protect human subjects. The so-called "national security exception" suggests that in order to survive as a nation and preserve a culture of
freedom, we can justifiably forfeit some measure of individual rights and interests—a classical utilitarian justification that promotes the public interest by
asking for some sacrifice on the part of individual citizens. The Cold War
struggle in the late 1940s could magnify the importance of this proposed exception; perhaps it could even serve as justifying the research done with human
subjects.

The Advisory Committee considers this argument and rightly blunts its force.
The Advisory Committee maintains that appeals to national security would have
unjustifiably caused investigators to lose sight of firm requirements of voluntary
consent. Those requirements could have been satisfied by asking subjects for their
permission after telling them that they would be injected with a radioactive
substance that might be dangerous and would not be beneficial, but would help
protect the health of persons involved in the war effort.

The culpability of agents in the plutonium cases might be mitigated by their
conscientious and understandable interpretation of the need to protect workers in
projects of great national significance, leading them to authorize or to perform the
research. Government officials and possibly the physicians with whom they
contracted could perhaps be found blameless because of the massive confusion
surrounding the Cold War commitments and their general lack of familiarity with
research medicine, but the Advisory Committee rightly rejected the plausibility of
this claim, especially for government employees.

In some respects this defense is even less plausible for physicians. The special
nature of the patient–physician relationship places a more stringent obligation on
physicians to attend to the welfare of the patient, and not merely their patients,
but any patient with whom they are professionally involved. In clinical circumstances, patients defer to their physicians' judgment, and it seems transparent that

these physicians capitalized on this deference and failed to adequately protect the welfare of their patients, a violation of the Advisory Committee's fourth principle.

The Advisory Committee also discredited the thesis that national security was ever formally invoked to justify these research efforts.

[I]n none of the memorandums or transcripts of various agencies did we encounter a *formal* national security exception to conditions under which human subjects may be used. In none of these materials does any official, military or civilian, argue for the position that individual rights may be justifiably overridden owing to the needs of the nation in the Cold War (ACHRE, 1995 [GPO, p. 206; Oxford, p. 120]).

In short, the evidence does not indicate that the agents themselves viewed their actions in this light, and even if they did, there were alternatives to the forms of exploitation of patients that occurred in the plutonium cases.

Culpability or Exculpation?

The final problem is whether judgments of exculpation or judgments of culpability follow from the foregoing analysis. Were the mitigating conditions sufficient to exculpate the agents? To this question, the answer is, emphatically, "No." Weak training in professional ethics, embryonic federal policies, and parallel forms of ignorance, together with other mitigating conditions, temper the reach and level of possible judgments of blame, but they are not sufficient conditions of exculpation. These conditions are only weakly exculpatory. Violation of the six basic universal principles is, by itself, sufficient for a judgment of culpability.

Any intentional act of taking patients who were seriously ill and placing them at risk without their knowledge or consent in nontherapeutic research indicates culpability. The evidence suggests both that the physician-investigators knowingly exploited these patients and that sufficient opportunities existed for physicians to obtain relevant information in order to determine whether their actions were warranted. Even if responsibilities were not clearly assigned to individuals in institutions, and even if the effort involved numerous persons, sufficient guidelines and historical precedents still existed to make judgments of culpability. That federal officials and physicians associated with the plutonium cases were culpable seems to follow from the Advisory Committee's thesis that if the means to overcome cultural biases or relevant forms of ignorance are available to an agent and the agent fails to take advantage of these means, then the agent is culpable.

In reaching such conclusions, the Advisory Committee was right to insist that we can and should assess persons other than the UCSF investigators, including

persons in positions of authority or responsibility for initiating the research and
for overseeing it—government authorities as well as those with oversight responsibilities in medical and research institutions. Those responsible for setting,
implementing, and overseeing standards for the conduct of research are at least
as culpable as those who conducted the research.

CONCLUSIONS

All things considered, the performance of the physicians and government officials
involved in the plutonium cases is inexcusable. However, the fairest conclusion in
these cases may be that the various exculpatory conditions excuse the agents
involved *to some degree*. The moral culpability of agents admits of degrees, and
there are many degrees on the scale, depending on what is known, what is
believed, what is intended, and what is widely recognized and disseminated. For
example, there are degrees of culpable moral ignorance in these cases, and it
would be difficult to pinpoint the degree of culpable ignorance for any particular
agent.

Perhaps it is enough to conclude that whatever the degrees of culpability,
culpability there must be. A milder conclusion is that it is enough to judge persons
or institutions deficient in conduct, which carries a loss of status and reputation,
without attaching the stigma of blame or inflicting punishments such as formal
censure, invalidation of a license, or fines. Which among these possible conclusions did the Advisory Committee reach, and was it correct to take the course it
did?

The Advisory Committee's even-handed Findings 10 and 11 (ACHRE, 1995
[GPO, pp. 785–789; Oxford, pp. 502–504]) provide a clue. Here the Advisory
Committee determines that physicians and government officials were "morally
responsible in cases in which they did not take effective measures to implement"
available government and professional standards. The most favorable interpretation of these findings, in light of the rest of the *Final Report*, is that the Advisory
Committee is *blaming* government officials and associated physicians for moral
failures. Despite its relatively polite language of "accountability" and "responsibility," the Advisory Committee's view strongly suggests that government officials
and physicians in positions of leadership were culpable for serious moral failures.

In the attempt to be even-handed and not to stretch beyond the evidence—a
key consideration in the Advisory Committee's deliberations and findings
(Buchanan, 1996)—the Advisory Committee reached conclusions that do not
extend all the way to the culpability of individual physicians and government
officials. In eschewing questions of individual culpability, the Advisory
Committee risks reproach for indecisiveness, much as I have criticized the

UCSF Ad Hoc Committee, and some reproach is in order. However, in assessing the fairness of such criticism of both the Advisory Committee and the UCSF committee, these committees did have a responsibility not to overstep the evidence, a task that becomes increasingly difficult in assessing the culpability of particular individuals.

It would also be rash to judge the Advisory Committee harshly for not investigating each government official and physician who might be blamed for wrongdoing. The Advisory Committee existed for little more than a year and did not have the means for a broad-scale investigation of individuals. Nonetheless, I believe that sufficient evidence exists and was available to the Advisory Committee for judgments of culpability in the case of a number of individuals involved in the human radiation experiments. In the UCSF case alone, investigator Kenneth Scott himself testified to physician culpability during the aforementioned interview. The evidence also indicates that principal investigator Robert Stone was guilty of the kind of negligence, errors of judgment, and moral failures that are sufficient for culpability.

If we cannot judge particular persons blameworthy in a case as clear as that of the UCSF plutonium injections, it is hard to see how to stop short of either exculpation or paralysis of judgment in a great many cases of serious past moral wrongs. This problem of line drawing cannot be dismissed, as the Advisory Committee recognized, on grounds that it is too difficult for human judgment. We should be cautious but not incapacitated in the work of retrospective moral judgment. Cautiousness in making claims to have sufficient evidence of culpability is a virtue, but suspending judgment in the face of sufficient evidence is simply a failure to make the proper judgment.

The matter is complicated by questions of the proper criteria of sufficient evidence. More than one standard of evidence can be defended, and significant epistemological problems surround the defense of one standard over another. All evidence gathering assumes a theory of what counts as evidence, and two or more theories may support competing standards, making assertions of sufficiency inherently contestable. While this problem is of indisputable relevance to assessments of culpability, it does not provide an adequate reason to doubt the availability of a reasonable standard for making such assessments. In the present case, I do not believe that the standard would vary significantly from those used by the Advisory Committee for assessing wrongdoing.

The bigger problem is the amount of time it would have required to assemble the evidence properly in each particular case, given the lapse of 50 years and the many gaps of information as to what did and did not happen. Time was not available for all cases to be handled appropriately, nor could all the desired evidence have been acquired (Buchanan, 1996). Since it generally is less time consuming to assemble evidence of sufficient quality to assess culpable nonperformance within the professions than to assemble comparable evidence for culpable wrongdoing on the part of each individual, it is easy to understand why the Advisory Committee reached the conclusions it did. But with more careful collection and sifting of the evidence in individual cases, the quality of the evidence may turn out to be as good as the evidence of general institutional culpability in medicine and government.

A judgmental person is a fool, but fear of rendering a foolish judgment some-times induces an unwarranted reserve. Such restraint appears to have unjustifi-ably inhibited decision making by the UCSF Ad Hoc Committee. The Advisory Committee cannot be similarly evaluated, because it was decisive beyond what might reasonably have been anticipated in light of its broad and diverse mission. However, it seems likely that the Advisory Committee's revealing findings are no more than a starting point for judgments of individual culpability that we can expect and should encourage in the ongoing work on the subject of the human radiation experiments.

References

Advisory Committee on Human Radiation Experiments (ACHRE). 1995. *Final Report.* Washington, DC: U.S. Government Printing Office. Subsequently published as *The Human Radiation Experiments.* New York: Oxford University Press, 1996. Pagination for both volumes is provided in the textual citations.
Buchanan, Allen. 1996. "The Controversy over Retrospective Moral Judgment," *Kennedy Institute of Ethics Journal* 6 (1996): 245–250.
Chapman, T. S. 1946. "Memorandum: To Area Engineer, Berkeley Area (30 December 1946)." ACHRE No. DOE-112194-D-3.
Davidson, Keay. 1995. "Questions Linger on 1940s UCSF Plutonium Shots," *The San Francisco Examiner* (23 February 1995): A6.
"Ex-owner of Toxic Site Wins Ruling on Damages." 1994. *New York Times* (18 March 1994): 5B.
Lederer, Susan E., and Moreno, Jonathan D. 1996. "Revising the History of Cold War Research Ethics," *Kennedy Institute of Ethics Journal* 6: 223–237.
UCSF. University of California at San Francisco. 1995. *Report of the UCSF Ad Hoc Fact Finding Committee on World War II Human Radiation Experiments* (February, 1995, unpublished but released to the public.)

Notes

1. In presenting the facts in the UCSF case, some parts of my discussion derive from the Advisory Committee's *Final Report,* but most derive from the Ad Hoc Committee's Report. All the facts were well known to the Advisory Committee, which discusses the UCSF case in Chapter 5.

2. The amount of plutonium injected was approximately 0.1% of the LD50 in rats and 0.35% of the LD50 in dogs.

3. The oral history was conducted by medical historian Sally Hughes.

4. See Elizabeth A. Zitrin and Roy A. Filly, UCSF, "Report of the UCSF Ad Hoc Fact Finding Committee," Letters, Appendices. Filly's response is reported by Keay Davidson (1995).

5. For an example of this error, see the personal statement by UCSF committee member Mack Roach III (UCSF 1995, Appendices).

INDEX

Abandonment of patients, 40, 87
Abuse (of patients and subjects), 74, 116, 133, 136, 271
Access
  to clinical trials, 36
  to drugs, 26
  to health care, 40, 133–37
  to medical records, 74
  to results of research, 26
  See also Allocation of scarce resources; Justice; Research
Accountability, 250, 255, 269, 276
Ad Hoc Committee of UCSF (Plutonium experiments), xxv, 261–78
Addiction, 92, 105, 111
Advance directives, 46, 177, 183
Advisory Committee on Human Radiation Experiments, xii, xxv, 29, 261–76
Agency. *See* Autonomy
AIDS, 26
Allocation of scarce resources, 154, 212, 216. *See also* Access; Justice
Allowing to die. *See* Euthanasia; Killing and letting die; Refusal of treatment
American Medical Association (AMA), 14, 48, 50, 52, 58, 273
Analogy, its place in methods of ethics, 160–64, 171. *See also* Casuistry
Animals (nonhuman), xxiv–xxv, 91, 93–96, 250–56, 259–60. *See also* Moral status
Appelbaum, Paul, 39
Applied ethics, xi, xiv, xxii, 47, 211–226, 243
Aristotle, 95, 216, 259
Arnold, Denis, xi
Arras, John, ix–x, xx

Autonomy
  autonomous actions contrasted with autonomous persons, 79, 89, 93, 96
  autonomous authorization, 63–65, 79–80
  autonomy-limiting principles, 102–06, 129
  balanced with beneficence. *See* Paternalism
  the concept of, 79–80, 89, 239–41
  its connection to informed consent, 63–65, 82, 88, 142–44
  degrees of, 88, 252
  diminished, 24, 37, 70, 80, 137, 142–44
  Dworkin's theory of, x, xxiv, 89, 219, 240–41, 250–51
  Frankfurt's theory of, xviii, 89–92, 95, 99, 240, 251
  intentionality a condition of, 63–66, 71–72, 80, 83–85, 88, 94–95, 270
  metaphysical contrasted to moral, 79, 94–96
  paradigm cases of, 82
  principle of respect for, xvii–xviii, 7, 24, 36–38, 42, 46, 64–65, 74, 79–82, 90–93, 97, 104, 109, 111–12, 166, 215, 220, 240
  theories of, 81–97, 240
  understanding a condition of, 37, 60, 63–65, 68, 83–86, 88, 93, 251–52
  voluntariness a condition of, 86–88, 90
  See also Advance directives; Informed consent; Kantian theory; Liberty; Paternalism; Refusal of treatment; Suicide

Culpability and wrongdoing, xiv, xxvi,
  261–63, 266–69, 274–78. *See also* Blame
  and blameworthiness
Cultural Relativity. *See* Pluralism and
  relativism (moral)
Culturally induced moral ignorance, 263,
  268, 272–74
Culver, Charles, x, 15, 219, 233
Customs, 67, 181, 185

Damages, 66, 68
Daniels, Norman, xi, xxiii–xxiv, 189,
  216–17, 230, 236–37, 240
Darwin, Charles, 96, 253
Davidson, Arnold, xi
Davis, Wayne, ix
Deception, 52–53, 192, 196, 214, 263, 267, 271.
  See also Lying
DeGrazia, David, ix, xi, xxi, 15–16, 49, 175,
  180, 182–85, 188, 250
Dementia, 96, 134, 247, 253
Deontological theory, 27, 220. *See also*
  Kant; Kantian theory
Depression, 80, 107
Descriptive ethics, 180–81, 187, 192, 194,
  197–200
Dignity, xix, xxiv, 9, 22, 95, 100, 135, 265
Dilemmas, xxiii, 12, 140–41, 172, 183, 223,
  229
Disabled persons, 7, 69, 134, 204. *See also*
  Vulnerabilities; Vulnerable persons
  and groups
Discernment (virtue of), 160, 166
Disclosure
  its connection to law and liability,
  66–68, 73
  and informed consent, 50–55, 58, 60–63,
  142–44, 157–58, 219–20
  nondisclosure of pertinent information,
  37, 65, 114–15, 239, 265, 271
  See also Confidentiality; Informed
  consent; Veracity
Discretion, 19, 25, 44, 155
Discrimination, 136, 156, 199, 214. *See also*
  Bias; Disabled persons; Justice;
  Prejudice; Vulnerabilities; Vulnerable
  persons and groups

Distress, 114, 128, 134, 136, 141–42, 235.
  See also Harms; Pain
Distributive justice, 41, 145, 217, 230, 236.
  See also Justice
Donagan, Alan, 6, 43, 190, 230
Double-blind studies, 55. *See also* Clinical
  trials
Dworkin, Gerald, x, xxiv, 89, 219, 240–41,
  250–51

Economically disadvantaged subjects, xi,
  xix–xx, 22, 132–46. *See also* Justice;
  Poverty; Vulnerabilities; Vulnerable
  persons and groups
Egalitarian theories, 41
Emanuel, Ezekiel (Zeke), x
Emergencies (and emergency medicine),
  73, 112
Emotions, 72–73, 86, 94, 96–97, 166,
  253–54
Empirical justification (in the study of
  ethics), xxii, 47, 55–56, 59–60, 146,
  178–81, 183, 186, 191, 194, 200–04, 249
Engelhardt, H. Tristram, ix
Equal consideration, 41, 185
Equity, 144
Ethics of care, 172. *See also* Virtues and
  virtue theory
Ethnicities, 186
Euthanasia, 46, 130, 213, 216, 241, 247.
  See also Killing and letting die;
  Physician-hastened death
Evil, 169–70, 192, 196–98, 216
Exculpatory conditions, xxvi, 262–77
Experimentation
  Advisory Committee on Human Radiation
  Experiments, xii, xxv, 29, 262–76
  on drugs, 55, 72,
  the Jewish Chronic Disease Hospital
  case, 56–57
  Nazi, 20, 25, 56
  non-therapeutic, 37
  involving prisoners, 72, 116–17
  Tuskegee syphilis case, 19–20, 25,
  57, 71
  Walter Reed's Yellow Fever, 53
  See also Clinical trials; Research

Research (*Continued*)

National Commission for the Protection of Human Subjects of Biomedical and Behavioral Research, ix, xiii–xv, 4–11, 18–30, 36, 69–70, 116–17

paternalism in research ethics, 72, 116–17, 136, 142

payment schemes for research subjects, 137–42

President's Commission for the Study of Ethical Problems in Medicine and Biomedical and Behavioral Research on, 58–60, 69–70, 148–49

prisoners as research subjects, 19, 58, 69–72, 116–17, 134–36

rights of research subjects, 13, 57, 134–35, 144, 269ff

scandals that motivated development of research ethics, 19–21, 56–57

utilitarian justifications of, 7, 25–26, 274–75

See also Animals (nonhuman); Autonomy; Double-blind studies; Experimentation; Informed consent; IRBs; Placebo-controlled trials; Therapeutic misconception; Tuskegee Syphilis Study; Vulnerable persons and groups

Respect for autonomy (principle of). *See* Autonomy; Principlism and principles (in bioethics)

Respect for persons (principle of), 4, 7–9, 13, 21, 24–27, 93–94, 214, 240, 250

Retrospective moral judgments, xxv–xxvi, 262–78

Richardson, Henry, x, xii, 182

Rights

of animals, 253–56, 260

autonomy-based, xvii, xix, 37, 65, 79ff, 102, 157, 232

connection to persons and theories of persons, xxv, 247–48, 254–55

correlativity with obligations, 255

to health care, 157

legal and political, 41, 54, 58, 116

prima facie obligations and rights, xvi, 41, 44–47, 103, 113, 115, 168, 242, 250, 275

of research subjects, 13, 57, 134–35, 144, 269ff

See also Autonomy; Balancing moral norms; Specification

Risk. *See* Balancing moral norms; Beneficence; Harms

Robertson, John, ix

Role responsibilities in professions, xxiii, 42, 56, 101, 156, 158, 169–70, 237, 272

Ross, W.D., 6, 23, 44

Rothman, David, 30

Ryan, Kenneth, ix

Sacrifice (personal), 40, 274

Safeguards, 22, 70, 134, 238

Secrecy, 214. *See also* Confidentiality

Seldin, Donald, ix

Self-defense, 126

Self-determination, 24–25, 51, 54, 73, 79, 157, 263. *See also* Autonomy

Self-governance. *See* Autonomy

Singer, Peter, 230

Slavery, 186

Slippery-slope arguments, 184

Smith, David, x

Socrates, 211, 213, 224–26

Specification, x, xvi, 27, 41, 43–47, 155–63, 182–85, 199, 201, 215. *See also* Principlism and principles (in bioethics)

Standing (moral). *See* Moral status

Stereotypes, 135

Strong, Carson, ix–xi, xiv, xviii, xx, 70

Suffering. *See also* Distress; Harms; Nonmaleficence; Pain; Physician-hastened death; Suicide

Suicide, xix, 104, 107–14, 117, 128, 130, 184, 238, 241. *See also* Killing and letting die; Physician-hastened death

Sunstein, Cass, 108

Supererogation, *See* Ideals (moral)

Surrogate decision makers

authority, rules of, 44, 73, 117, 154

guardians as, 73, 81, 104, 115, 255

Taylor, James Stacey, x, xvii

Terminal sedation, 128, 241

Therapeutic misconception, 86